Y0-BSM-647

RESEARCH DEPARTMENT
IRWIN MEMORIAL BLOOD BANK OF THE
SAN FRANCISCO MEDICAL SOCIETY
270 MASONIC AVENUE
SAN FRANCISCO, CALIFORNIA 94118

To Susie,

with love and with appreciation for her excellent assistance.

Herbert A. Perkins

HEPATITIS AND
BLOOD TRANSFUSION

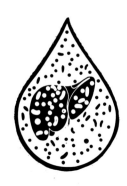

Proceedings of
a Symposium held at the
University of California,
San Francisco,
March 25-26, 1972

HEPATITIS AND BLOOD TRANSFUSION

Edited by

Girish N. Vyas
Herbert A. Perkins
Rudi Schmid

Grune & Stratton   New York and London

Grune & Stratton, Inc.
111 Fifth Avenue
New York, New York 10003

Library of Congress Catalog Card Number 72-6498
International Standard Book Number 0-8089-0779-4
Printed in the United States of America

CONTENTS

CONTENTS

Section V: POST-TRANSFUSION HEPATITIS
Chairman: J. M. Stengle

CONTENTS

Section VI: PROPAGATION OF VIRAL CANDIDATES
Chairman: F. Deinhardt

PARTICIPANTS

I. ORGANIZING COMMITTEE

Julius R. Krevans, M.D., University of California
Edwin Lennette, M.D., Ph.D., California State Department of Public Health
Piero Mustacchi, M.D., University of California
Herbert A. Perkins, M.D., Irwin Memorial Blood Bank, San Francisco
Judith Pool, Ph.D., Stanford University
Rudi Schmid, M.D., Ph.D., University of California
Girish N. Vyas, Ph.D., University of California, *Program Chairman*

II. SPECIAL INVITEES

George Brecher, M.D., Chairman, Department of Clinical Pathology and Laboratory Medicine, University of California, San Francisco, California
John Byrne, M.D., U.S. Department of Health, Education and Welfare, Center for Disease Control, Atlanta, Georgia
Robert J. Byrne, D.V.M., National Institutes of Health, Bethesda, Maryland
Marcel E. Conrad, M.D., Walter Reed Army Medical Center, Washington, D.C.
Dr. M. Duca, World Health Organization, Geneva, Switzerland
June K. Dunnick, Ph.D., National Institutes of Health, Bethesda, Maryland
Tibor J. Greenwalt, M.D., Blood Program, The American National Red Cross, Washington, D. C.
Michael B. Gregg, M.D., U.S. Department of Health, Education and Welfare, Center for Disease Control, Atlanta, Georgia
Bengt Gullbring, M.D., Karolinska Institute, Stockholm, Sweden
Leon Jacobs, M.D., Hepatitis Task Force, National Institutes of Health, Bethesda, Maryland
Elvin A. Kabat, Ph.D., Columbia University, College of Physicians and Surgeons, New York, New York
Robert W. McCollum, M.D., Yale University, New Haven, Connecticut
Henry S. Parker, M.D., National Academy of Engineering, Washington, D. C.
James K. Roche, M.D., National Blood Resource Branch, National Institutes of Health, Bethesda, Maryland
Louis F. Saylor, M.D., California State Department of Public Health, Berkeley, California
Paul J. Schmidt, M.D., Clinical Center, National Institutes of Health, Bethesda, Maryland
David Sensor, M.D., Communicable Disease Center, Atlanta, Georgia
V. M. Viliarejos, M.D., LSU-ICMRT, San Jose, Costa Rica
Patricia E. Taylor, Ph.D., Canadian Communicable Disease Center, Ottawa, Ontario, Canada

III. FACULTY

Richard A. Aach, M.D., Division of Gastroenterology, Washington University School of Medicine, St. Louis, Missouri

Harvey J. Alter, M.D., Blood Bank, Clinical Center, National Institutes of Health, Bethesda, Maryland

Lewellys F. Barker, M.D., Division of Biologic Standards, National Institutes of Health, Bethesda, Maryland

Baruch S. Blumberg, M.D., Ph.D., The Institute for Cancer Research, Fox Chase, Philadelphia, Pennsylvania

Howard E. Bond, Ph.D., Electronucleonics Laboratories, Inc., Bethesda, Maryland

James Boyer, M.D., Yale University School of Medicine, New Haven, Connecticut

Vincent Caggiano, M.D., Sacramento Medical Foundation Blood Bank, Sacramento, California

Thomas Chalmers, M.D., Clinical Center, National Institutes of Health, Bethesda, Maryland

Friedrich Deinhardt, M.D., Department of Microbiology, Presbyterian-St. Luke's Hospital, Chicago, Illinois

John L. Gerin, Ph.D., Rockville Laboratory of the Molecular Anatomy Program, Oak Ridge National Laboratory, Rockville, Maryland

David J. Gocke, M.D., Columbia University, College of Physicians & Surgeons, New York, New York

Martin Goldfield, M.D., New Jersey State Department of Health, Trenton, New Jersey

Irving Gordon, M.D., Department of Microbiology, University of Southern California Medical School, Los Angeles, California

George F. Grady, M.D., Commonwealth of Massachusetts Department of Public Health, Boston, Massachusetts

William T. Hall, Ph.D., Electronucleonics Laboratories, Inc., Bethesda, Maryland

Paul V. Holland, M.D., Blood Bank, Clinical Center, National Institutes of Health, Bethesda, Maryland

F. Blaine Hollinger, M.D., Baylor College of Medicine, Houston, Texas

Graham A. Jamieson, Ph.D., Blood Program, American National Red Cross, Washington, D. C.

Julius R. Krevans, M.D., School of Medicine, University of California, San Francisco, California

Saul Krugman, M.D., Department of Pediatrics, New York University School of Medicine, New York, New York

George Le Bouvier, M.D., Department of Epidemiology and Public Health, Yale University School of Medicine, New Haven, Connecticut

Joshua Lederberg, Ph.D., Stanford University School of Medicine, Stanford, California

Edwin H. Lennette, M.D., Ph.D., The Viral and Rickettsial Disease Laboratory, California State Department of Public Health, Berkeley, California

Robert Q. Marston, M.D., National Institutes of Health, Bethesda, Maryland

James E. Maynard, M.D., Ecological Investigators Program, Center for Disease Control, Phoenix Laboratories, Phoenix, Arizona

Joseph L. Melnick, Ph.D., Baylor College of Medicine, Houston, Texas

Irving Millman, Ph.D., Clinical Research Unit, The Institute for Cancer Research, Fox Chase, Philadelphia, Pennsylvania

James W. Mosley, M.D., University of Southern California School of Medicine, Los Angeles, California

Milton M. Mozen, Ph.D., Cutter Laboratories, Inc., Berkeley, California

Robert K. Ockner, M.D., Gastroenterology Unit, University of California School of Medicine, San Francisco, California

Herbert A. Perkins, M.D., Irwin Memorial Blood Bank, San Francisco, California

Nicholas Petrakis, M.D., University of California School of Medicine, San Francisco, California

Herbert F. Polesky, M.D., Minneapolis War Memorial Blood Bank, Minneapolis, Minnesota

Alfred M. Prince, M.D., The New York Blood Center, New York, New York

PARTICIPANTS

Robert H. Purcell, M.D., National Institutes of Allergy and Infectious Diseases, National Institutes of Health, Bethesda, Maryland

Allan G. Redeker, M.D., University of Southern California School of Medicine, Los Angeles, California

Ronald R. Roberto, M.D., California State Department of Public Health, Berkeley, California

Rudi Schmid, M.D., Ph.D., Professor of Medicine, University of California School of Medicine, San Francisco, California

Nathalie J. Schmidt, Ph.D., California State Department of Public Health, Berkeley, California

N. Raphael Shulman, M.D., Clinical Hematology Branch, National Institute of Arthritis and Metabolic Diseases, National Institutes of Health, Bethesda, Maryland

James Stengle, M.D., National Blood Resource Program, National Heart and Lung Institute, National Institutes of Health, Bethesda, Maryland

Howard F. Taswell, M.D., Mayo Clinic Blood Bank, Rochester, Minnesota

Girish N. Vyas, Ph.D., Department of Clinical Pathology and Laboratory Medicine, University of California School of Medicine, San Francisco, California

John H. Walsh, M.D., Veterans Administration Center, Los Angeles, California

Robert Ward, M.D., University of Southern California School of Medicine, Los Angeles, California

Romeo M. Zarco, M.D., Cordis Laboratories, Miami, Florida

A. J. Zuckerman, M.D., London School of Hygiene and Tropical Medicine, London, England

IV. ADDITIONAL CONTRIBUTORS

S. Adelberg, University of California School of Medicine, San Francisco, California

A. Aronoff, Clinical Research Unit, The Institute for Cancer Research, Fox Chase, Philadelphia, Pennsylvania

Pamela M. Baines, London School of Hygiene and Tropical Medicine, Hepatitis Unit, London, England

K. R. Berquist, Center for Disease Control, Phoenix Laboratories, Phoenix, Arizona

Joanne Bill, New Jersey State Department of Health, Trenton, New Jersey

Henry Black, New Jersey State Department of Health, Trenton, New Jersey

Betsy Brotman, The New York Blood Center, New York, New York

Victor J. Cabasso, Cutter Laboratories, Inc., Berkeley, California

E. Chen, Irwin Memorial Blood Bank and the University of California School of Medicine, San Francisco, California

C. R. Coleman, National Institute of Arthritis and Metabolic Diseases, Clinical Hematology Branch, National Institutes of Health, Bethesda, Maryland

Marcel E. Conrad, Walter Reed Army Institute of Pathology, Washington, D. C.

V. Coyne, Clinical Research Unit, The Institute for Cancer Research, Fox Chase, Philadelphia, Pennsylvania

R. Y. Dodd, The American National Red Cross, Washington, D. C.

C. Ehrich, The New York Blood Center, New York, New York

N. C. D. C. Finlayson, New York Hospital — Cornell Medical Center, New York, New York

H. Gault, Clinical Research Unit, The Institute for Cancer Research, Fox Chase, Philadelphia, Pennsylvania

Joan P. Giles, The Willowbrook State School, Staten Island, New York

T. J. Greenwalt, The American National Red Cross, Washington, D.C.

Edwin J. Hacker, Jr., Department of Medicine, Washington University School of Medicine, St. Louis, Missouri

Robert L. Hirsch, Greater New York Blood Program, New York, New York

S. N. Huang, Clinical Research Unit, The Institute for Cancer Research, Fox Chase, Philadelphia, Pennsylvania

A. B. Ibrahim, University of California School of Medicine, San Francisco, California

I. Ikram, The New York Blood Center and Cornell Medical Center, New York, New York

Ricardo Katz, University of Chile School of Medicine, El Salvador, Chile

C. S. Knepp, National Institute of Arthritis and Metabolic Diseases, Clinical Hematology Branch, National Institutes of Health, Bethesda, Maryland

D. H. Krushak, Center for Disease Control, Phoenix Laboratories, Phoenix, Arizona

R. F. Lange, National Institute of Arthritis and Metabolic Diseases, Clinical Hematology Branch, National Institutes of Health, Bethesda, Maryland

J. J. Levin, The American National Red Cross, Washington, D. C.

A. Lippin, The New York Blood Center, New York, New York

Marilyn Aliene Mason, University of California School of Medicine, San Francisco, California

Louisa Ni, The American National Red Cross, Washington, D.C.

A. O'Connell, Clinical Research Unit, The Institute for Cancer Research, Fox Chase, Philadelphia, Pennsylvania

J. M. Panick, Columbia University, College of Physicians & Surgeons, New York, New York

Charles W. Parker, Washington University School of Medicine, St. Louis, Missouri

S. L. Perkins, Irwin Memorial Blood Bank, San Francisco, California

Wayne Pizzuti, New Jersey State Department of Health, Trenton, New Jersey

Julio Rodriguez, Hospital del Salvador, El Salvador, Chile

Duane D. Schroeder, Cutter Laboratories, Inc., Berkeley, California

Sunthorn Srihongse, New Jersey State Department of Health, Trenton, New Jersey

M. Stryker, The New York Blood Center, New York, New York

W. Szmuness, The New York Blood Center, New York, New York

Elizabeth W. Williams, University of California School of Medicine, San Francisco, California

PREFACE

Viral hepatitis continues to be a major problem in public health and transfusion therapy. Despite significant advances in our understanding of the natural history of the disease, of its laboratory diagnosis, and of some of its major epidemiological characteristics, many questions remain unanswered. The discovery of Australia antigen (termed Au, SH, HA, HAA and, recently HBAg for hepatitis B antigen), its intimate association with hepatitis B virus (HBV) its serologic heterogeneity (the *ad* and *ay* subtypes) and some of its physicochemical characteristics have raised additional questions to which answers must promptly be obtained before its full role in the diagnosis and prevention of hepatitis type B can be evaluated. The extraordinary and rapid accumulation of new data and concepts have made it highly desirable to assess the available information in order to distinguish what is known from what is conjectural or uncertain and to define areas in which further research is urgently needed.

To accomplish these objectives, a local committee was charged with the organization of a structured Symposium to bring together a group of investigators and teachers recognized for their recent contributions to the problems related to hepatitis. The Symposium was organized in connection with a meeting of the contract investigators of the National Blood Resource Branch of the National Heart and Lung Institute, which brought a number of the leading investigators to the University of California Medical Center in San Francisco. The Organizing Committee took pains to invite speakers and discussants for selected topics in order to cover all major clinical, laboratory and epidemiological aspects of viral hepatitis, giving special emphasis to the transfusion-transmitted form of the disease. Acceptance of our invitations and enthusiastic cooperation from all participants encouraged the Center for Continuing Education of the University of California to plan the organizational details of the Symposium on short notice. The result of this teamwork was, we believe, a well-balanced, informative and stimulating Symposium conducted at the University of California in San Francisco on March 25 and 26, 1972.

We feel that the stated objectives of the Symposium have been more than accomplished, for which we are grateful to the distinguished guest faculty that we were privileged to host at the University of California. The value and importance of the Symposium were underlined by the presence of Dr. Robert Q. Marston, Director of the National Institutes of Health, who took the time and trouble to come to San Francisco on his way to Moscow and to open the Symposium with an inaugural address. Dr. A. J. Zuckerman from London, Dr. M. Duca from Geneva, representing the World Health Organization, Dr. Bengt Gullbring from the Karolinska Institute, Stockholm, and Dr. Patricia Taylor from Ottawa extended the scope of participation in the Symposium beyond the geographic boundaries of the United States. The Symposium was presented jointly by the Department of Clinical Pathology and Laboratory Medicine, University of California School of Medicine, and the Center for Continuing Education in the Health Sciences, University of California, San Francisco, with the cooperation of Stanford University, the California State Department of Public Health, the National Institutes of Health, the U.S. Public Health Service, the National Research Council, the Center for Disease Control, the American National Red Cross and the American Association of Blood Banks.

The design of this Symposium not only provided a comprehensive review of the most recent information in the selected topics but focused particularly on problems and controversies, as well as on prospective issues related to viral hepatitis and blood transfusion. The present volume containing the proceedings of the Symposium is intended as a reference source for investigators and teachers in the field of hepatitis who wish to be brought up to date on the "state of the art." In editing the proceedings, changes and alterations were kept to a minimum in order to retain the originality and expression of views of the individual contributors and discussants. In this endeavor the editors were generously assisted by Dr. K. R. Rao, Mary Martin and Virginia Hayes. Prompt publication of this volume was made possible by the fact that most of the speakers fulfilled their promise to submit a completed manuscript at the time of the Symposium and by the many hours of overtime work by Marilyn Archbold, Barbara Mohammad, Judy Garza and Virginia Hayes, who typed the final version. We found that a consolidated bibliography for the entire volume saved considerable space while providing an up-to-date reference source for the entire field. We wish to acknowledge the help and cooperation of Messrs. John de Carville and George Brown, of Grune & Stratton, publishers of the volume. The support of Chancellor Phillip Lee, Dean Seymour Farber, Dean Julius Krevans and Professor George Brecher contributed most valuably to the success of the Symposium. Last but not least, we appreciated the participation of the many physicians, scientists and blood bankers who attended the Symposium as registrants in Continuing Education and made for an unusually interested and enthusiastic audience.

Girish N. Vyas
Herbert A. Perkins
Rudi Schmid

STATEMENT OF NOMENCLATURE*

The generic term *viral hepatitis* embraces at least two clinically similar entities due to infection with immunologically distinct etiologic agents (designated as virus A and virus B in the 1940's, but still not conclusively identified in the laboratory). Although referred to by a variety of names over the years (including epidemic hepatitis, homologous serum jaundice, post-vaccinal jaundice, post-transfusion hepatitis, etc.), common usage has largely settled on infectious hepatitis (IH) for the short-incubation disease associated with virus A and serum hepatitis (IH) for the long-incubation disease associated with virus B. However, the application of this terminology for clinical and reporting purposes has often been imprecise owing to the lack of specific reliable laboratory tests for differential diagnosis.

In the late 1960's epidemiologic dogma concerning the exclusively parenteral transmission of virus B was upset with the first clear demonstration of non-parenteral transmission. At the same time, the specific association of Australia antigen with hepatitis virus B infection was firmly established. This opened up the long-sought serologic approach to clinical diagnosis and epidemiologic study. As research efforts and publications rapidly increased, new terms were introduced. Australia antigen, Au or Au(1) antigen, serum hepatitis antigen (SH antigen), Au/SH antigen, hepatitis antigen (HA) and hepatitis-associated antigen (HAA) apparently all referred to one and the same thing. Related terminology referring to the antibody found to react with this antigen included Au antibody, anti-Au antigen antibody, Au/SH antibody, etc. This welter of terms and symbols has often been confusing to clinicians, epidemiologists and laboratory investigators.

The Committee on Viral Hepatitis (the Division of Medical Sciences, National Academy of Sciences-National Research Council),** after considering the need to bring some order out of the existing chaos, has adopted the following terminology for its own working purposes until such time as specific recommendations are made by an appropriate international body. The generic term *viral hepatitis* is used when referring to both diseases collectively or to unspecified types, and the terms *viral hepatitis type A* and *viral*

*This statement of nomenclature was kindly provided by Dr. R. W. McCollum.

**The Committee on Viral Hepatitis: R. W. McCollum, Chairman, M. B. Gregg, E. A. Kabat, S. Krugman, J. L. Melnick, A. G. Redeker, and P. E. Taylor.

Editorial Note: A detailed statement has recently been published by the Center for Disease Control in the *Morbidity and Mortality Weekly Report* (vol. 21, no. 16, for the week ending April 22, 1972). Despite our editorial attempt to conform to this recommended nomenclature, certain inconsistencies were considered unavoidable in order to accomplish rapid publication of the proceedings of the Symposium.

hepatitis type B are used when referring to infectious hepatitis and serum hepatitis and their synonyms, respectively. In keeping with these terms, the Committee has agreed that the following designations be used:

Hepatitis A virus	HAV
Hepatitis B virus	HBV
Hepatitis B antigen	HB Ag
Hepatitis B antibody	HB Ab or anti HB Ag

If an antigen is found to be associated with hepatitis type A, the designation HA Ag and HA Ab will be used for the antigen and its antibody.

SECTION I

CLINICAL ASPECTS OF VIRAL HEPATITIS

Chairman: R. Schmid

1. INAUGURAL REMARKS

Robert Q. Marston

Director, National Institutes of Health
Bethesda, Maryland

It gives me a great deal of pleasure to participate in this Symposium on Viral Hepatitis and Blood Transfusion and to deliver these opening remarks, not only because of the importance of the subject itself, but also because research in hepatitis illustrates several timely aspects of the process of biomedical science.

Viral hepatitis is one of the most serious infectious diseases affecting the American public today. It is a matter of great concern in public health agencies, clinics, and research laboratories throughout the country. Although hepatitis is a disease which has been recognized for centuries, little progress has been made in determining its etiology.

Volunteer studies in the late 40's and early 50's were stimulated by the enormous increase in hepatitis during the second World War. Two primary types of hepatitis, A and B, were identified and characterized, and a presumed viral etiology for each was ascertained. However, interest and progress in hepatitis research waned after some of the volunteer studies experienced an unacceptably high mortality rate; and the studies were consequently terminated.

But the problem is too serious to be neglected. Moreover, it has been aggravated by the extensive but necessary use of blood transfusions and blood products and by the increased risks attributed to the drug culture.

Transfused blood is estimated to cause more than 30,000 cases of overt hepatitis and 1,500 to 3,000 deaths every year in the U.S. Since there are many subclinical cases of viral hepatitis, the actual incidence has been estimated as high as 150,000 cases annually.

Recent discoveries will reduce the impact of the hepatitis-contaminated blood problem, but will not result in a quick solution of the overall hepatitis problem. The greatest obstacle to development of effective preventive measures is the need to isolate and identify the causative agents, presumably viruses. The whole history of infectious disease research supports the view that once the causative agents can be isolated and grown, developments in diagnosis, treatment and vaccines can be targeted.

Progress in the hepatitis field provides a striking example of the benefits of fundamental research. The discovery of the Hepatitis B antigen is a case history which underscores the importance of research on a broad scientific base and the need for insuring communication between different scientific disciplines.

You are familiar with the story--how a clue was found in a most unexpected way. A medical geneticist, Dr. Baruch S. Blumberg, (who had worked at NIH in the 1960's and continued his investigation as a grantee), headed a scientific team studying blood proteins in primitive peoples of the South Pacific. A previously unidentified protein was detected (at the NIH) in the blood of an Australian Aborigine. The discovery was crucial, and in time realization of its significance emerged through continued work of the original team, and through the work of a growing number of virologists and other investigators.

Successful exploitation of the discovery like the hepatitis antigen requires the commitment of ever increasing numbers of scientists and of research facilities. The work on the problem proceeded in many laboratories over the nation and in six different components of the NIH.

At one point, a large number of frozen and stored blood samples which had been collected in 1952 for a study in the Division of Biologics Standards was tested. The samples were known to be contaminated with hepatitis agents, and in what DBS Director Murray called "serologic archeology", the newly discovered antigen was found in almost three-fourths of the specimens.

In the hepatitis B antigen story, the mutual dependence of targeted and non-targeted research is illustrated.

The importance of an obscure clue was sensed, then verified, and this stimulated a new wave of interest in the scientific community. Hepatitis research burgeoned. Interim research reagents for hepatitis B antigen were made available by the NIH to investigators to evaluate their test systems for detection of the antigen. With the use of high speed ultra-centrifuges, a group of scientists began extracting hepatitis B antigen from positive human sera.

Scientists thus had available carefully characterized reagents which permitted more accurate comparisons of research results.

Special publications were initiated by the NIH to facilitate quick and informal exchange of information between scientists and their colleagues around the world.

The promise of significantly decreasing the incidence of post-transfusion hepatitis by identifying and eliminating blood which is positive for hepatitis B antigen became a reality early last year with the final issuance of Federal standards for the antibody to be used in testing for hepatitis B antigen.

At this time hepatitis B antibody is now commercially available from seven federally licensed manufacturers. The current supply of the product is more than adequate to meet the national needs for testing all blood and plasma donors.

Hepatitis B antigen testing has moved from the experimental laboratory to the blood banks with extraordinary rapidity. The development of more sensitive, practical and reproducible tests is under intensive study; within the next few years, other tests-- some involving new principles--may be introduced.

Progress is being made with primates as animal models of serum hepatitis in order to gain a better understanding of the disease and ways that it may be prevented or treated.

Published reports of transmission of hepatitis A to the marmoset, a subhuman primate, offer hope for progress against this human virus.

Several laboratories have reported success in transmitting the virus hepatitis B to subhuman primates, including chimpanzees and rhesus monkeys. These findings, though not yet published, offer promise for markedly increasing our understanding of the virus of hepatitis B.

The search for a vaccine is also continuing, and some progress in this direction has recently been reported. But there are several preliminary steps which must be taken before we can proceed to vaccine development--proving the viral character of hepatitis

agents, growing them in animals or tissue culture, finding a safe
strain of virus, producing prototype vaccines, and testing them for
potency and safety. Despite all the new discoveries, therefore,
full control of hepatitis is still very much in the future.

I have already mentioned the necessity for close communication
and coordination among a number of scientific disciplines in the
field of hepatitis. We have faced this matter squarely at the
National Institutes of Health, where at least five of our Institutes
and Divisions are engaged in programs related to hepatitis.

The Division of Biologics Standards has the responsibility for
establishing and maintaining standards of quality and safety for all
biologic products, including human blood for transfusion, products
prepared from blood, and the test materials and methods used to
assure that products meet standards.

The National Blood Resource Program of the National Heart and
Lung Institute is responsible for initiating research on improving
blood resources and usage. This includes development of new technology to assure safety.

The National Institute of Allergy and Infectious Diseases is
charged with research on the causative agents of viral hepatitis,
with developing new methods for detecting hepatitis virus, and with
vaccine development.

The National Institute of Arthritis and Metabolic Diseases
has a general responsibility for research in liver diseases, including clinical diagnosis, medical management and the fundamental
processes underlying these diseases.

The Clinical Center, in its use of blood and blood products,
is an intrinsic part of our research effort on hepatitis. Also,
the broad virologic and immunologic capabilities of the National
Cancer Institute are being called on to help solve some of the
basic problems involved as well as to assure that new vaccines
are free of tumor-inducing viruses.

It is essential that these efforts be coordinated, both in the
interest of program efficiency and economy and in order to apply
the results of research findings to human health as quickly and
expeditiously as possible. Last year, therefore, I established an
NIH Task Force on Research on Viral Hepatitis to coordinate our
efforts within the NIH and to mesh this with related work of other
agencies. The Task Force also serves as an information exchange
in this field.

NIH has also recently sponsored formation of a National
Academy of Sciences/National Research Council Committee on Viral

Hepatitis. This Committee is assisting in coordinating hepatitis research activities on a national level to assure optimal use of new information and biological materials and to encourage development of a standardized system of terms.

The problem of viral hepatitis, as the title of your Symposium indicates, is closely linked to the need for an adequate and safe supply of blood and blood components for transfusion. Blood services have not kept pace with the Nation's expanding demands for medical care. The President identified this need as a matter of national concern in his Health Message to the Congress earlier this month. He directed the Department of Health, Education, and Welfare to study this problem and recommend a plan "for developing a safe, fast and efficient nationwide blood collection and distribution system".

The problems inherent in developing such a plan are obviously great. In addition to the medical considerations, there are legal, social, and economic factors that must be kept in mind. We will need to draw on the skills of modern management and technology. Above all, however, we will need the input of the medical and research communities. We are making every effort to consider all aspects of the problem and to keep all our policy options open. I invite your serious attention to this problem of national importance.

I hope too that this Symposium will encourage many of you to participate in the search for solutions to the many unanswered questions about viral hepatitis. You are zeroing in on a field of lively interest indeed, one in which the opportunities are great. I feel sure that this Symposium will serve its announced purpose of providing a constructive framework for·the cross-fertilization of ideas in the hope of furthering our knowledge and understanding of one of the most serious infectious diseases in this country.

2. VIRAL HEPATITIS: NATURAL HISTORY OF THE DISEASE

Saul Krugman and Joan P. Giles

Department of Pediatrics, New York University
School of Medicine, and the Willowbrook State
School, Staten Island, New York

The term "viral hepatitis" includes at least two diseases, one caused by hepatitis A virus (HAV) and the other by hepatitis B virus (HBV). The clinical, pathological, epidemiological and immunological aspects of viral hepatitis, types A and B share many similarities and some differences.

The term viral hepatitis type A is synonymous with "infectious hepatitis", an ancient disease described by Hippocrates and long known under such aliases as "acute catarrhal jaundice", "epidemic jaundice", and epidemic hepatitis. The fulminating form of the disease was called "acute yellow atrophy of the liver".

The term viral hepatitis, type B, is synonymous with "serum hepatitis", a disease with a more recent history since the first known outbreak occurred in 1883 among a group of shipyard workers who were vaccinated against smallpox with glycerinated lymph of human origin [301]. Later, an increased incidence of the disease was observed among patients attending venereal disease clinics, diabetic clinics, and other facilities where multiple injections were given with inadequately sterilized syringes and needles. The most extensive outbreak occurred in 1942 when yellow fever vaccine containing human serum caused 28,585 cases of hepatitis B infection with jaundice among United States military personnel. It was unknown at the time of vaccination that the human serum component of the vaccine was contaminated with virus. During the past three decades the increasing use of blood and blood products played an important role in the wide dissemination of the infection. The various aliases of viral hepatitis, type B, which are recorded in the literature include: "serum hepatitis", "homologous serum

jaundice", "transfusion jaundice", "syringe jaundice" and "post-
vaccinal jaundice".

Current concepts of the natural history of viral hepatitis
stem from human volunteer studies which were conducted in the
1940's [196, 302, 348, 375, 471]. These studies were initiated
because of the failure to propagate the causative agents of human
hepatitis in laboratory animals. Later, the advent of tissue culture techniques in the 1950's provided new methods for the isolation
and identification of various viruses. Intensive efforts by many
investigators failed to provide reproducible methods for the cultivation of the viruses responsible for hepatitis in man.

The human volunteer studies provided indirect evidence for the
existence of at least two viruses, hepatitis A and hepatitis B
[196, 302, 338, 348, 375, 471]. These studies revealed that viral
hepatitis, type A was primarily an enteric infection, characterized
by a relatively short incubation period (15 to 40 days), viremia,
and fecal excretion of virus. The most common mode of transmission
was the fecal-oral route; parenteral transmission was also possible.

In contrast, limited studies at that time indicated that hepatitis B virus caused a parenteral infection characterized by a
long incubation period (50 to 180 days), and unlike hepatitis A
virus, it was not infectious by mouth. It was thought that hepatitis B infection was transmitted by inoculation only, and that
the infection did not spread by contact.

More recent studies in the 1960's provided evidence for the
existence of two types of viral hepatitis with distinctive clinical,
epidemiological and immunological features [261]. One type, MS-1,
resembled viral hepatitis, type A; it was characterized by an incubation period of 30 to 38 days and a high degree of contagion by
contact. The other type, MS-2, resembled viral hepatitis, type B;
it had a longer incubation period (41 to 108 days). Contrary to
the prevailing concept, the MS-2 strain of hepatitis B virus was
infectious by mouth as well as parenterally, and patients with this
disease were moderately contagious. These studies provided support
for the contention that hepatitis B infection could be acquired by
contact as well as the parenteral route [321, 395].

The discovery of Australia antigen by Blumberg et al. [45, 59],
its association with viral hepatitis, type B [162, 259, 384] and
the development of tests for the detection of hepatitis B antigen
and antibody provided a new technology for studies of the natural
history of viral hepatitis. Knowledge of the course of the disease
was derived from prospective observations of patients at the Willowbrook State School where viral hepatitis has been endemic since
1949.

The background of our studies on the natural history of viral hepatitis at Willowbrook was described in detail in previous publications [259,264,484]. Two diseases have been studied intensively: 1) the MS-1 strain of viral hepatitis, type A, and 2) the MS-2 strain of viral hepatitis, type B. The derivation of the terms "MS-1" and "MS-2" is as follows: the letter "M" refers to the first initial of the last name of a patient with viral hepatitis. The letter "S" refers to the patient's serum. "MS-1" represents the serum obtained during the patient's first attack of hepatitis. "MS-2" represents the serum obtained from the same patient 6 months later when he had a second attack of hepatitis. The first attack of hepatitis was typical viral hepatitis, type A; the second attack resembled viral hepatitis, type B. Moreover, MS-1 serum has consistently produced hepatitis A virus infection, and MS-2 serum has consistently produced hepatitis B virus infection.

During the course of these studies on the natural history of viral hepatitis, the following tests were performed: serum bilirubin, thymol turbidity, immunoglobulin M (IgM), and serum glutamic oxaloacetic transaminase (SGOT). Hepatitis B antigen and antibody were detected by immunodiffusion [49], complement fixation [400], radioimmunoprecipitation assays [275], and passive hemagglutination [477].

VIRAL HEPATITIS, TYPE A

Clinical Aspects. The typical course of viral hepatitis, type A is illustrated in the upper part of Figure 1. After an incubation period of approximately 32 days, SGOT levels become abnormal,

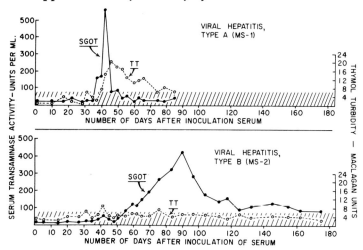

Figure 1. Course of viral hepatitis, type A (MS-1 strain) and viral hepatitis, type B (MS-2 strain). Illustration of serum glutamic oxaloacetic transaminase (SGOT) and thymol turbidity (TT) response. Jaundice, when present, is observed at time of peak SGOT values. From Krugman et al., [261].

usually rising to a peak within 5 to 7 days. This rising phase
of transaminase activity occurs during the preicteric phase of the
disease. It is usually accompanied by fever, anorexia, nausea and
abdominal pain. Jaundice, when present, is detected at the time of
peak transaminase. The period of abnormal SGOT activity is usually
transient, lasting 2 weeks and rarely persisting for more than
3 weeks.

    The thymol turbidity values, which become abnormal after the
SGOT levels rise, are consistently elevated in both anicteric as
well as icteric hepatitis A virus infection. The thymol turbidity
values return to normal levels later than the SGOT. There is a
striking correlation between the IgM levels and the thymol turbidity pattern.

    In general, viral hepatitis, type A, is more apt to be anicteric
and milder in children than in adults. The disease in adults is
characterized by more severe constitutional symptoms and more
prolonged jaundice.

    As indicated in Figure 2, the incubation period of viral hep-
atitis, type A, ranges between 29 and 37 days, average 32 days; it

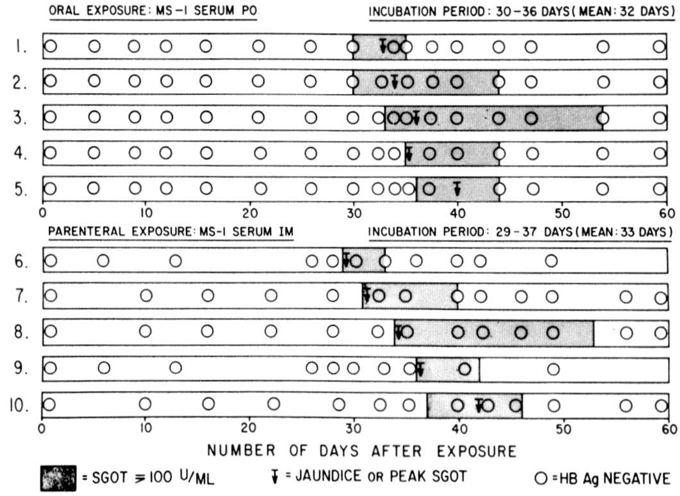

Figure 2. Course of viral hepatitis, type A (MS-1 strain), illustrating incubation period, SGOT activity and absence of hepatitis B
antigen (HBAg) in five patients following an oral exposure (Nos.
1-5), and in five patients following a parenteral exposure (Nos.
6-10). PO signifies by mouth, IM signifies intramuscularly, shaded
area signifies SGOT value >100 units/ml, ↓signifies peak SGOT value
or onset of jaundice, and O signifies HBAg-negative. From Krugman, S., Giles, J.P., [259].

is essentially the same following an oral and parenteral exposure.
Hepatitis B antigen is not present during the course of hepatitis A
infection. Previous reports of the detection of antigen in sera
obtained from patients with viral hepatitis, type A, reflected
errors in diagnosis.

Many physicians labelled a case as "infectious hepatitis" if
there were no history of an inoculation of blood or other potentially
contaminated material. Actually, the true diagnosis was probably
viral hepatitis, type B, which had been acquired as a contact infection.

Epidemiological Aspects. The mode of transmission of hepatitis A infection is chiefly via intestinal-oral pathways, although parenteral transmission is also possible. Experimental
studies have shown that the virus is present in feces of persons
with the active disease regardless of whether the infection was
acquired orally or parenterally [196, 348, 375]. The period of
infectivity of stool and serum during the course of viral hepatitis,
type A, is summarized in Figure 3. Virus was detected in the blood

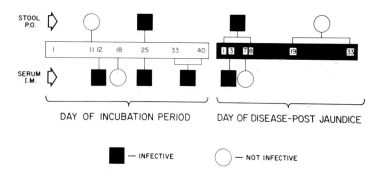

Figure 3. Schematic illustration of the period of infectivity of
serum and stool during the course of viral hepatitis, type A.
Modified from Krugman, S., et al. [266].

during the incubation period, 2 to 3 weeks before onset of jaundice.
Viremia was also detected on the 12th day of the incubation period
and on the 3rd day after onset of jaundice; it was not detected 7
days after onset of jaundice. Virus was detected in the stools
on the 25th day of the incubation period, 2 to 3 weeks before onset of jaundice and within the first 8 days after onset of jaundice;
it was not detected 19 to 33 days after onset of jaundice.

Evidence of hepatitis A viruria was reported by Findlay and
Willcox [153] and by Giles et al. [161]. The infective urine in
both studies was collected on the first day of jaundice.

Immunological Aspects. Studies by Havens [194], by Neefe et al.
[348] and by our group [261] revealed evidence for homologous immunity following hepatitis A virus infection. However, there was
no evidence of heterologous immunity. Hepatitis A virus infection
did not protect against subsequent exposure to hepatitis B virus,
and hepatitis B virus infection did not protect against hepatitis A
virus infection.

VIRAL HEPATITIS, TYPE B

Clinical Aspects. The typical course of viral hepatitis, type
B, is illustrated in the lower half of Figure 1. After an incubation
period of approximately 60 days SGOT values rise gradually reaching
peak levels approximately 30 days later; jaundice, if present,
occurs at this time. The patient may complain of painful joints as
long as 6 weeks before onset of jaundice. Urticaria may be observed
during the early preicteric phase of the disease. Fever, if present,
and anorexia are observed shortly before onset ₤ jaundice. Abdominal pain and tenderness over the liver are also noted at this
time. The SGOT values may be elevated for several months before
subsiding to normal. Thymol turbidity and IgM levels are usually
normal in anicteric hepatitis B infection, but they may be elevated
in icteric infection.

As indicated in Figure 4, the incubation period of hepatitis B
infection is dependent upon the route of infection. A parenteral
exposure was followed by an incubation period of approximately 65
days; it was 98 days following an oral exposure. Studies by Barker
et al. [36] revealed an inverse relationship between dose of hepatitis B virus and incubation period. They noted an average incubation period of 77 days following inoculation of an infectious
undiluted plasma pool; it was 114 days when the plasma was diluted
1000 to 10,000-fold.

The detection of HBAg during the course of viral hepatitis,
type B, is shown in Figure 4. The antigen appears in the blood
approximately 30 to 40 days after a parenteral exposure to MS-2
serum containing hepatitis B virus; it is usually detectable 2
weeks to 2 months before evidence of abnormal SGOT activity. The
occurrence of the antigen in 49 of 50 (98%) cases of viral hepatitis,
type B (MS-2 strain), has confirmed the specificity of the antigen
for hepatitis B virus infection. As indicated in Figure 3, hepatitis B antigen appears about 70 to 80 days after oral exposure
to hepatitis B virus.

The usual sequence of events following a primary infection
with hepatitis B virus is illustrated in Figure 5. The appearance
of complement fixing (CF) hepatitis B antigen (HBAg) preceded

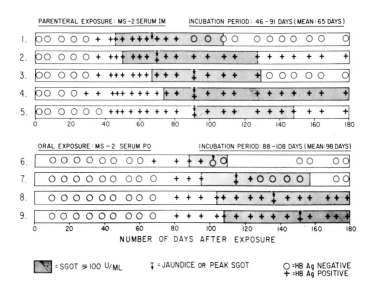

Figure 4. Course of viral hepatitis, type B (MS-2 strain), illustrating incubation period, SGOT activity and appearance of HBAg in five patients following parenteral exposure (Nos. 1-5) and in four patients following an oral exposure (Nos. 6-9). IM signifies intramuscularly, PO signifies by mouth, shaded area signifies SGOT value ≧100 units/ml, ↓signifies peak SGOT value or onset of jaundice, +signifies HBAg-positive and 0 signifies HBAg-negative.

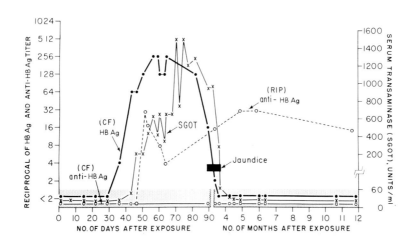

Figure 5. Course of viral hepatitis, type B (MS-2 strain) illustrating 1) early appearance of HBAg on day 36 and its persistence for 3 months; 2) subsequent rise in SGOT value on day 46, returning to normal at 3 1/2 months; 3) absence of detectable complement fixation (CF) antibody (anti-HBAg), 4) appearance of radioimmunoprecipitation antibody (RIP anti-HBAg), and 5) late appearance of jaundice at 3 months. Modified from Krugman, S., Giles, J.P., [259].

evidence of liver involvement as indicated by an elevation of the
SGOT level approximately two weeks later. Jaundice was not detectable until day 90 shortly before CF HBAg titers decreased to
non-detectable levels. Antibody to HBAg (anti-HBAg) was detectable by the sensitive radioimmunoprecipitation (RIP) assay; it
appeared 2 weeks to 2 months after initial detection of antigen.
Antibody was not detectable by the less sensitive CF test.

The duration of HBAg in the blood is variable; it is usually
transient, disappearing about one week to 2 months after onset of
jaundice. Occasionally, however, a chronic carrier state may persist for many years. This carrier state may or may not be associated with chronic active hepatitis.

The variation in response to a parenteral exposure to hepatitis B virus is illustrated in Figure 6. The most common course
is shown by patients Nos. 1 and 2; antigen is detectable by day 30,
followed by abnormal SGOT levels several weeks later, and finally
by the appearance of antibody. Jaundice may or may not be present.

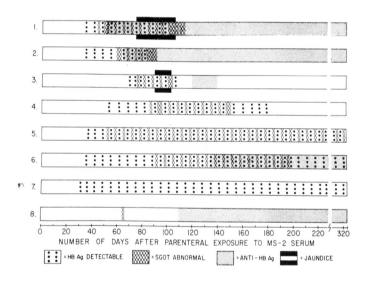

Figure 6. Viral Hepatitis, type B: variation of response fol-
lowing a parenteral exposure to hepatitis B virus (MS-2 strain).
Black dots signify presence of HBAg cross-hatched areas signify
SGOT values >100 units/ml, stippled areas signify antibody to
HBAg and black bars signify jaundice.

Detectable levels of antibody may be transient (patient No. 3) or
non-detectable (patients Nos. 4, 5 and 7). A chronic antigen
carrier state may occur (patients 5 and 6), and in very rare instances, the only manifestation of infection may be the appearance
and persistence of antigen (patient No. 7). In other very rare
instances hepatitis B infection may be characterized by no detectable antigen, a transient appearance of abnormal SGOT values and
subsequent appearance of antibody (patient No. 8).

Epidemiological Aspects. The period of infectivity of patients
with viral hepatitis, type B is dependent upon the presence or absence of a chronic carrier state. Detection of HBAg in the blood
or any secretion is indicative of the presence of hepatitis B virus.
Consequently, all secretions which are contaminated with blood or
serum must be considered infectious if antigen is detectable. As
indicated in Figures 2 and 4, HBAg is detectable during the incubation period and for a variable period of time thereafter.

Immunological Aspects. Evidence of homologous immunity was
observed following infection with hepatitis B virus, MS-2 strain
[259]. As indicated in Figure 7, exposure to MS-2 serum on

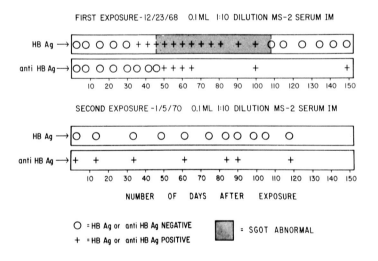

Figure 7. Evidence for homologous immunity one year after first
hepatitis B virus infection. First exposure to a parenteral inoculation of MS-2 serum was characterized by appearance of HBAg on
day 36 and abnormal SGOT levels on day 46. Second exposure to the
same dose of MS-2 serum one year later was not followed by the
appearance of HBAg or abnormal SGOT values. From Krugman, S.,
Giles, J.P., Tr. Assoc. Amer. Phys. 83:133, 1970.

12/23/68 was followed by the appearance of HBAg on day 36, abnormal SGOT values on day 46 and anti-HBAg on day 50. Re-exposure to the same dose of MS-2 serum one year later did not cause hepatitis. Consequently, homologous immunity to viral hepatitis, type B, was observed under the conditions of this study.

We have observed evidence of reinfection which was characterized by transient HBAg of one week's duration, occurring 32 days and 137 days after accidental inoculation of MS-2 serum; the SGOT value was abnormal from day 137 to day 144 post-inoculation.

Antibody to HBAg has not been consistently detected following hepatitis B infection in adults, in spite of the availability of the sensitive RIP and passive hemagglutination tests. Serial samples of blood obtained from 11 adults with viral hepatitis, type B, revealed evidence of detectable antibody in 6. Consequently, the presence of antibody is indicative of past infection and probable immunity. On the other hand, the absence of antibody does not necessarily indicate susceptibility.

Conclusion. Studies on the natural history of viral hepatitis have been conducted by many investigators during the past 30 years. Prospective observations of patients with viral hepatitis, types A and B, have clarified the clinical, epidemiological and immunological aspects of the disease. The discovery of Australia or hepatitis B antigen and its association with hepatitis B virus was followed by the development of tests to detect hepatitis B antigen and antibody. This new technology has accelerated the accumulation of knowledge of the natural history of viral hepatitis.

Acknowledgments. The authors' investigations were done under the sponsorship of the Commission on Viral Infections and was supported in part by the U.S. Army Medical Research and Development Command, under research contract DA-49-193-MD-2331. We are grateful to Dr. Jack Hammond, Director, Willowbrook State School and Mrs. Harriet Friedman and Mrs. Olive Lattimer for their assistance and cooperation.

3. Discussion
VIRAL HEPATITIS: NATURAL HISTORY OF THE DISEASE

A. J. Zuckerman

London School of Tropical Medicine, London, England

Drs. Krugman and Giles have, as usual, presented a masterly account of the natural history of viral hepatitis. The lack of suitable laboratory methods for the study of type A hepatitis has obviously hampered progress, but the discovery of Australia antigen has provided, at long last, a specific marker of infection with the virus of type B hepatitis. The origin of type B virus remains a mystery. It has been suggested that virus B may represent the emergence of a new strain derived from virus A which had undergone some alterations during prolonged survival in the host with viremia and alimentary disease. The transition from A to B, it is further presumed, must have resulted in some loss of infectivity by the oral route. The flaw in this hypothesis is that there is little evidence that survival and excretion of virus A may be prolonged, although Capps et al., [81] demonstrated by transmission studies to volunteers the presence of virus in the feces of one infant with chronic hepatitis 5 months after the onset of illness and in another infant 15 months after onset. It is conceivable that both these infants might have been carrying Australia antigen, since chronic hepatitis after type A infection appears to be uncommon. However, the problem of whether Australia antigen is present in feces is as yet unresolved.

Another aspect which is worth enlarging upon relates to persistence and chronic carriage of Australia antigen. Giles et al. [162] examined serial samples of serum after experimental infection with MS-1 and MS-2. Australia antigen was detected in all the volunteers after infection with MS-2 and in approximately half the patients the antigen persisted in the serum for 200 days and subsequently for at least 3 years after infection. Krugman and Giles [259] later

reported that Australia antigen has been detected in 38 of 104
(36.5%) children, who have been followed up for periods of 4 months
to 13 years. It was concluded that if the antigen is detectable
for more than 4 months, it is likely to persist indefinitely. Nielsen et al. [359] estimated that the susceptibility to persistent
carriage of Australia antigen in the general population after acute
hepatitis is in the order of 3 to 4%, although it must be pointed
out that 128 of their 235 patients were narcotic drug addicts.
Barker and Murray [34] tested for Australia antigen sera collected
from over 100 volunteer prisoners, who participated in hepatitis
studies conducted in 1951-1954 on inactivation of the agent of
serum hepatitis in blood and blood products. Twelve of the volunteers became persistent carriers of Australia antigen. Ten of
these 12 prisoners were examined 1 to 3 years after the inoculations
and all 10 were considered to have either probable or definite
evidence of residual liver dysfunction at that time. It was noted
that persistent carriage of Australia antigen may well be associated
with chronic liver disease.

Drug abuse has been suggested as one of the factors responsible
for the apparently higher incidence of serum hepatitis among males,
particularly since males between the ages of 15 and 29 years have
been identified as a high risk population for abusing parenteral
drugs. Other factors, however, are clearly involved. Szmuness et
al. [454] detected Australia antigen in 35.1% of residents with
Down's syndrome in an institution and 17.2% of a matched sample of
residents with other forms of mental retardation. It was suggested
that early age of exposure, compared to later exposure, increased
the risk of becoming a chronic antigen carrier. It also appeared
that the duration of the carrier state was longer in patients with
Down's syndrome. On the other hand, resistance to the carrier state
seemed to increase both in patients with Down's syndrome and other
forms of mental retardation with chronological age above puberty.
The observed higher incidence of Australia antigen in males was
explained by the age factor, with more males in this study admitted
at an early age than females. Goodman et al. [175], on the other
hand, obtained evidence which clearly indicated sex as the independent primary variable factor responsible for a higher prevalence
of Australia antigen in males than in females in an institution for
the mentally retarded. A survey of 1,077 mentally retarded resident
patients revealed that there is a much lower prevalence of Australia
antigen among karyotypically normal females than in males, whereas
among young patients with Down's syndrome there is a high incidence
of Australia antigen in the females as well as males. It was also
shown that early age of admission to the institution increases the
risk of becoming a carrier of Australia antigen, but less so in
females with a normal karyotype than in other groups.

Washburn et al. [486] studied the sex differences in suscepti-

bility to a number of infections both by a search of the literature
and of the John Hopkins Hospital case records covering the period
1930 to 1963. Special attention was paid to bacterial meningitis
at all ages and bacterial septicemia in children under 15 years
of age. A significant preponderance of males was found and it was
most marked in infancy. The sex difference in susceptibility to
these infections was postulated to be consistent with a genetic
hypothesis concerning a gene locus on the X chromosome of human
beings, which is involved in the synthesis of immunoglobulins.
Small differences in amounts or rates of synthesis of immunoglobulins might be responsible for a slightly greater susceptibility to
infection among some members of one sex. Rhodes et al. [407] investigated 28 women with an additional X chromosome (XXX) and an equal
number of normal men and women matched for age. The mean serum
levels of IgM were found to be highest in the XXX group, intermediate in normal women and lowest in men. IgG levels were also significantly higher in the XXX females than in either normal men or
women. These results and the fact that there is an X-linked basis
for the most common form of congenital agammaglobulinemia support
the suggestion of Washburn et al. [486] that a gene locus on the X
chromosome has at least some regulatory effect on antibody production in man.

The reasons for the high prevalence of Australia antigen in
apparently healthy carriers are not yet known. It has been suggested that the establishment of a complete or at least partial
immunological tolerance to this antigen is the most likely explanation.

It would seem that Australia antigen is not transmitted across
the placental barrier. Smithwick and Go [438] tested for Australia
antigen samples of cord blood collected from 2,225 newly-born infants at a hospital in Brooklyn, New York. Serum specimens from
a random sample of 271 mothers were also examined and in 103 instances paired maternal and cord sera were available. The antigen
was not found in any of the cord blood samples yet the antigen was
detected in 6 out of 271 (2.2%) of the maternal sera. The antigen
was detected in 4 out of 103 (3.9%) of the samples of the mothers
in the group of paired maternal-cord bloods but in none of the 103
cord bloods. Thus, no evidence was obtained for the transplacental
transmission of Australia antigen.

The mode of transmission of Australia antigen to the infants
remains speculative. Three possibilities are suggested: transplacental transmission of the antigen in utero, oral contamination
from the mother's blood during passage in the birth canal or postpartum oral transmission from the mother to the infant as a result
of close contact. Transmission via breast milk is excluded in most
cases since in many of the instances reported, the mothers had not

nursed their infants and, furthermore, Australia antigen has not
been demonstrated to date in breast milk.

Turner et al. [467] concluded that infection of the newborn
can readily occur during parturition and that there is no need to
invoke transplacental transmission. It has been suggested that
familial clustering of Australia antigen is related to genetic
factors. However, the explanation for persistent carriage of the
antigen may lie in mother-to-child transmission and that this
represents the "vertical" transmission of the serum hepatitis virus.
Indeed, Ohbayashi [365] reported two families in Japan in whom
there was a high incidence of familial cirrhosis and positive tests
for Australia antigen. In the two families there were 10 surviving
male and female sibs and all were Australia antigen positive; of
the 13 children of the female sibs, 12 were Australia antigen
positive but all 4 children of the male sibs were antigen negative.

Persistent carriage of Australia antigen is common in patients
with a defective immune response e.g. lymphocytic leukemia, chronic
renal failure (uremia) and lepromatous leprosy. Chronic carriage
of Australia antigen is also usual in patients in whom the immunological mechanisms are impaired therapeutically or suppressed.

The high prevalence of apparent healthy cárriage of Australia
antigen in many tropical countries may similarly be related to
changes in the immunological response [497]. It has been shown
that a background of repeated parasitic infection induces a number
of immunological changes and the immunosuppressive action of malaria is widely recognized. There is also considerable evidence
of an early immune depression in plasmodial infection in mice [415].
An altered immune reactivity in malaria may also affect the outcome
of chronic infection with a virus by. allowing the virus to become
frankly oncogenic and possibly by interfering with the immune reaction to neoplastic cells. Salaman et al. [415] and Wedderburn
[487] demonstrated an increased incidence of malignant lymphoma
caused by murine oncogenic viruses in mice infected with Plasmodium
berghei yoelli. Zuckerman [497] put forward the hypothesis that a
similar relationship might exist between chronic infection with the
serum hepatitis virus and the subsequent development of hepatoma
in the tropics. It is also of interest that an association of Burkitt's tumour and holoendemic malaria has also been suggested by
Kafuko et al. [239]. This subject has recently been reviewed
briefly [21].

4. EPIDEMIOLOGIC IMPLICATIONS OF CHANGING TRENDS IN TYPE A AND TYPE B HEPATITIS

James W. Mosley

University of Southern California School of Medicine,

Los Angeles, California

Total cases of viral hepatitis in a given population at a given time represent the net effect of two etiologic agents capable of transmission by a large number of mechanisms, some of which are common to both. Therefore, to understand the overall pattern in that population at that particular time, we must have as much etiologic and epidemiologic information as possible concerning the individual cases. To remind us of this fact, I recently suggested [330] we apply to both type A and B hepatitis the term prosodemic. Winslow's observations of typhoid fever led him in 1901 [490] to introduce that word to designate infections that maintain themselves by utilizing multiple mechanisms of spread. Winslow's emphasis with respect to typhoid fever must also be our emphasis with respect to type A and type B hepatitis. Extent and mode of propagation in any community at any time produce a composite, with both of the etiologic entities and most of the epidemiologic entities fluctuating according to the action of many independent as well as interdependent factors.

Type A or type B hepatitis transmitted by a particular mechanism often produces a pattern sufficiently distinctive to permit differentiation between the two agents, as well as identification of that mode of spread. Characteristics of importance include the distribution of cases by time of occurrence, by their location in the community, by age, and by sex. These characteristics, in fact, are to the epidemiologist what symptoms and signs are to the clinician. In the absence of a specific laboratory test for diagnosis, the epidemiologist can utilize these characteristics to determine the nature of the problem in the community, just as the practitioner can often diagnose disease on the basis of clinical concurrences.

This approach, however, has limitations for the epidemiologist, just as it does for the clinician.

The epidemiologist investigating viral hepatitis in the community can usually be definite about etiologic agent and epidemiologic mechanism only when cases are sufficient in number to permit statistical validation. Neither the epidemiologist nor the clinician has been able to differentiate reliably between type A and type B hepatitis in most instances of sporadic disease. It is for this reason that the terms "infectious" and "serum" hepatitis became largely meaningless. The latter was more reliable, being applied almost exclusively to transfusion-associated cases and obvious cases of addiction-associated hepatitis. The former ("infectious" hepatitis) was sometimes applied on the basis of adequate evidence, such as household exposure within 6 weeks of onset, but more often was merely presumptive, at least among adults, when no history suggestive of a likely source was elicited.

Just as the advent of a specific diagnostic test often extends for the clinician his concept of disease beyond the "classical" syndrome, the description [49] and documentation [162, 333, 364, 384] of a specific laboratory test for type B hepatitis has enlarged our information about the distribution of its infectious agent. Fortunately, the test for hepatitis B antigen (HBAg) is positive even by relatively insensitive techniques after onset of jaundice in a substantial proportion of cases, and is positive in virtually all patients observed prospectively throughout the incubation period [162]. Fortuitously, the technique of diagnosis now available to us is one far more easily and rapidly applicable than would have been true, at least for some time, if the initially discovered technique were one for isolating the virus in tissue culture or in an experimental animal. Because of this test, we now know that many cases previously called "infectious" hepatitis on a purely presumptive basis are, in fact, "serum" hepatitis or type B disease. As a result, the epidemiologist has been confronted with the assimilation into his concepts of many cases outside the spectrum he previously recognized.

Even more recently, the epidemiologist has been given an additional tool. Reactions of partial identity [176, 242, 283, 290] between HBAg's from selected patients led to recognition that the 22 nm particle carries a number of antigenic determinants, two of which appear to be mutually exclusive. As Dr. Le Bouvier will discuss in detail later in this Symposium, we now recognize two subtypes of the type B virus. The "d" and "y" determinants are characteristics of the viral strain, and the transmission of either gives rise to the homologous subtype in secondary or epidemiologically-related cases [335]. Consequently, for some groups of cases having the same subtype, we suggest and may be able to document new epidemiologic relationships, just as for individual cases the hepatitis B antigen itself permitted us to recognize new epidemiologic relationships.

Having offered these considerations as a background, I would like to begin our review by considering the overall behavior of viral hepatitis in the United States, and the implications of recent changes in pattern. The general trend since viral hepatitis became nationally reportable in 1952 is well known through the periodic summaries in the Center for Disease Control's Morbidity and Mortality Weekly Report, and in its Hepatitis Surveillance Report. I would merely remind you from the background trend in Figure 1 that there have been three periods of epidemiologic up-

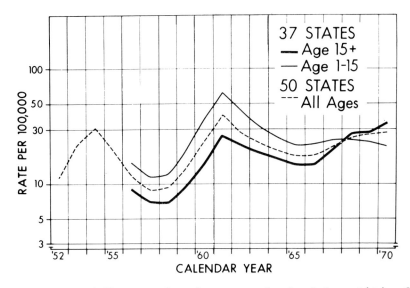

Figure 1. Age-specific trends of reported viral hepatitis from 1956 through 1970 in 37 States reporting consistent data. The overall trend from 1952 through 1970 in all 50 States is shown by the broken line.

swing during that interval: the first reaching a peak in calendar year 1954; the second, in 1961; and the latest, not yet demonstrating a definite peak. So far as predominant pattern is concerned, however, we really have had two periods: that from 1952-53, and after national reporting began, until 1965-66; and that since 1966-67 to the present [332]. A variety of epidemiologic characteristics differ between these two intervals--the recent upswing has been less rapid, the regularity of seasonable variation has been lost, the highest incidence has shifted from non-metropolitan to metropolitan areas, the equal sex distribution has shifted to male predominance, and the age distribution shows heaviest involvement of young adults.

I believe that we can epitomize the change by looking at age-specific secular trends. Unfortunately, this is difficult for the

United States as a whole because of the incompleteness with which
states have compiled and published data concerning age distribution
of cases. Nevertheless, 37 States provided data for the age groups
one to fifteen and fifteen and over since calendar year 1956. These
37 States had an average of 79.7 percent of the population of the
country during this period, and reported an average of 79.2 percent
of all cases. They appear, therefore, to be adequately representative. (Omitted are New Hampshire, Vermont, Indiana, Wisconsin,
Minnesota, Iowa, Nebraska, Texas, Colorado, Arizona, Nevada, Alaska,
and Hawaii).

Figure 1 shows secular trends in the two groups. Children
experienced an epidemic for which the cycle extended from the 1957
low to a 1961 high, and then back to another low in 1965. Since
1965, however, there has been only a very minor wave, so that the
anticipated resurgence in this age group has not occurred.

Persons 15 years of age and over also participated in the
epidemic cycle extending from 1958 through 1965. The semilogarithmic
scale of the graph makes it obvious also that they participated
to an extent approximately equal to that of children during this
time. In fact, the correlation coefficient for children and adults
during this ten-year period is +.94, one of several indications that
the same etiologic and epidemiologic form of viral hepatitis involved them as involved children, albeit adults participated at a
lower level. We have many indications that through the 1950's until
mid-1960's the predominant etiologic form was type A disease for
children and adults, and that contact-associated spread was the
predominant epidemiologic entity [283]. Now, for reasons about
which we can speculate but not necessarily draw any firm conclusions,
contact-associated type A disease has become relatively quiescent.

The second major point to be made from Figure 1 is that since
calendar year 1966 the incidence in adults has been entirely responsible for the epidemic increase, reaching for the first time in
1968 a level above that in children and by 1970 an all time high
for this age group.

Within the group of persons 15 years of age and over, more
detailed analysis is obviously desirable. Even for the period
since 1966, however, consistent data are available only from 41 of
the 52 reporting areas of the United States. These 41 areas, which
had 68.6 percent of the U.S. population, contributed only 63.4 percent of cases in calendar years 1965 and 1966, and 59.7 percent in
calendar years 1969 and 1970. This disproportion is largely due
to the necessary omission of New York City, Florida, Texas, and
California, the metropolitan areas of which have contributed heavily to the national total. Data were deficient or also incompatible
from New Hampshire, Wisconsin, Iowa, Virginia, Alabama, Arizona and
Nevada.

Table 1 shows average annual cases in the 41 areas during calendar years 1965-1966, and during calendar years 1969-70. The

Table 1. Average Annual Reported Morbidity by Age*. "Infectious" and "Serum" Hepatitis reported by 41 areas of the United States** during 1965 and 1966 compared with 1969 and 1970.

Age Group	Average Annual Number of Cases		
	CY 1965 and 1966	CY 1969 and 1970	Percent Change
1-14	8,473	9,102	+ 7
15-24	5,032	15,059	+ 199
25-39	4,037	5,808	+ 44
40 +	2,950	4,055	+ 37

*Source: Annual Supplements to Morbidity and Mortality Weekly Report.
**Omits New Hampshire, New York City, Wisconsin, Iowa, Virginia, Florida, Alabama, Texas, Arizona, Nevada, and California

virtually unchanged tally for children one through fourteen would be expected from the data already shown in Figure 1. For adults, we find, as we would expect from previous reports as well as the general experience of physicians seeing cases of hepatitis, that the major increase among adults is in the youngest group--i.e., those 15 through 24 years of age. There were, however, lesser but still definite increases among persons 25 through 39, and those 40 and over.

Because Table 1 underrepresents the heavily metropolitanized areas of the United States, Table 2 presents data for Los Angeles

Table 2. Average Annual Reported Morbidity by Age*. "Infectious" and "Serum" Hepatitis reported by Los Angeles County during 1965 and 1966 compared with 1969 and 1970.

Age Group	Average Number of Cases		
	CY 1965 and 1966	CY 1969 and 1970	Percent Change
1-14	606	610	+ 1
15-24	634	2,031	+ 221
25-39	577	1,023	+ 77
40 +	324	462	+ 43

*Source: Compilations provided by the Los Angeles County Health Department.

County from compilations of its Health Department. The percent increase in age group 15 through 24 was not much greater than in

the 41 areas included in Table 1, nor was the increase of 43 percent in those 40 and over much larger than the 37 percent increase
in the comparable group shown previously. There was, however, a
greater increase in those 25 through 39 years of age--a 77 percent
increase compared to 44 percent.

The increase in viral hepatitis among young adults since 1966
has coincided with a great increase in percutaneous drug abuse in
the same age group. As a result, we and other groups throughout
the country have found a high frequency of acknowledged self-injection among patients with acute viral hepatitis. Table 3 presents
data for 509 consecutive admissions in 1971 at John Wesley County

Table 3. Patients with Acute Viral Hepatitis Admitting Percutaneous
Drug Abuse within 6 Months of Onset.
John Wesley County Hospital - May - October, 1971

| Age Group | Number of Patients* | Admitted Self-Injection | |
		Number	Percent
15-24	315	147	46.7
25-39	166	60	36.1
40+	24	2	8.3

*Omits 1 patient under 15, and 3 for whom abuse was unknown.

Hospital. Among those 15 through 24 years of age, self-injection
was admitted by 46.7 percent; among those 25 through 39, 36.1 percent, and even 2 of 24 patients 40 years of age or over. This
acknowledgment was obtained on admission, or with only moderately
persistent inquiry at the time an epidemiologic history was taken
several days after admission to the hospital. The percentages
would be higher if suspected instances or acknowledgments subsequent to discharge (at the time of visit to follow-up clinic) were
included.

If I seem to belabor what is accepted by most clinicians as an
obvious fact, it is because some epidemiologists have suggested
that the increase in the 15 through 24 year age group is in part
coincidental with the increase in drug abuse. They point to the
declining incidence of type A hepatitis in childhood, which they
perhaps rightfully relate to improved conditions of living, and
suggest that experience with type A disease has been merely delayed to young adulthood.

With regard to etiology, we cannot at this time document type
A infections, but we do have the means now for documenting type B
hepatitis. Table 4 shows for 207 patients at John Wesley Hospital
admitting drug abuse, the proportion that were HBAg-positive by
counterimmunoelectropheresis (CIEP). Even this relatively

Table 4. Frequency of HBAg Positivity by CIEP; Patients with Acute
Viral Hepatitis Admitting Percutaneous Drug Abuse.
John Wesley County Hospital - May - October, 1971

		HBAg-positive	
Age Group	Number Admitting Self-Injection	Number	Percent
15-24	145*	73	50.3
25-39	60	32	53.3
40+	2	2	-
TOTAL	207	107	51.7

*Omits 2 patients not tested.

insensitive technique (compared with radioimmunoassay) demonstrated
a 51.7 percent positivity overall. Furthermore, the frequency was
no less for the age group 15 through 24, than for those 25 through
39. It seems quite safe to conclude, therefore, that type B
hepatitis could be responsible for no less than half of the cases
among young adults. It may be responsible for much higher proportion, but documentation of that will have to await application
of radioimmunoassay for HBAg, as well as similarly sensitive tests
for antibody response.

The communality of the agent responsible for most cases of
viral hepatitis among drug abusers is further indicated by subtyping. Table 5 shows that a sample (stratified for year of

Table 5. HBAg Subtype Among Patients Admitting Percutaneous Drug
Abuse - John Wesley County Hospital, Stratified Sample, 1969-1971.

Age Group	Total Subtyped	d		y	
		No.	Percent	No.	Percent
15-24	105	14	13.3	91	86.7
25-39	43	6	14.0	37	86.0
40+	3	-	-	3	-
TOTAL	151	20	13.2	131	86.8

admission, age, and sex) of addiction-associated cases at John
Wesley County Hospital were very predominantly of the y subtype
in all age groups. Although Table 5 does not present the data,
there was no significant change in frequency of the y subtype during the three-year period.

Any epidemic in any one part of a community causes concern
about extensions to other parts. In the present situation in
which type B hepatitis is epidemic among young adults practicing
self-injection of drugs, that is a particularly pertinent question.
The prolonged period of viremia in the incubation period, as well

as the production of a chronic carrier state in 2 to 5 percent of
persons with acute HBAg-positive disease, creates the potential
for additional cases in other segments of the population. We must
address ourselves, therefore, to the extent to which the potential
for "spillover" is being realized.

To explore the changes in epidemiologic pattern among the many
groups of potential risk is far beyond the scope allotted to my
presentation today. In view of the interest of this group, therefore, I shall confine my attention to its possible effects upon the
amount of transfusion-associated hepatitis.

The percutaneous drug abuser has supplanted the alcoholic as
the bête noire of the blood banker, and with good reason. There
have been, without question, instances in which blood banks have
improperly relied heavily upon the drug-using population to supply
conveniently their needs at bargain prices [98]. In some metropolitan areas, there has been or still is, a "buyer's market" for
blood and plasma if the blood banker is willing to pay and not be
overly careful in screening. As mentioned, a few blood banks have
deliberately exploited this situation, and the remainder, even the
most careful, have had the integrity of their operation threatened
by this situation. We must ask, therefore, whether there has been
an increase in transfusion-associated hepatitis.

The only practical means for monitoring the behavior of most
diseases is morbidity reporting by physicians to health departments.
Viral hepatitis became reportable in 1952, but not until 1966 did
"serum" hepatitis become separately reportable from "infectious"
hepatitis. We do, however, have data for the period of greatest
interest to us.

As I mentioned previously, "serum" hepatitis to most clinicians
has meant those cases of viral hepatitis in which a percutaneous exposure was strongly suspected as the route of infection. The practical consequence of this usage has been its application almost exclusively to cases of transfusion-associated hepatitis and to the
more obvious cases of addiction-associated hepatitis. That this is
true is demonstrable from data supplied through the Hepatitis Surveillance Program of the Center for Disease Control. Their recent
summary [201] of experience for epidemiologic year 1963-64 through
1967-68 indicates (Table 6) that among children less than 10 years
of age, and adults 40 years of age and over, cases reported as
"serum" hepatitis had a history of prior transfusion within 6 months
in the vast majority of instances. Conversely, as shown in Table 7,
physicians preponderately reported as "serum" hepatitis those cases
in all age groups occurring within 6 months of transfusion. It
seems plausible, therefore, that the trend in serum hepatitis noti-
fications from 1966 through 1970 could serve as at least a rough
index of trend in transfusion-associated disease.

Table 6. Frequency of Transfusion within 6 Months among Cases
Reported as "Serum" Hepatitis - Hepatitis Surveillance Program,
CDC* EY 1963-64 through EY 1967-68.

Age Group	Number Reported as "Serum" Hepatitis	Transfused within 6 Months	
		Number	Percent
<10	38	32	84.2
10-39	3,833	762	19.9
40+	1,520	1,335	87.8

*Source: Hepatitis Surveillance Report No. 31, Jan. 1, 1970.

Table 7. "Etiologic" Classification Applied to Persons Transfused within 6 Months of Onset - Hepatitis Surveillance Program,
CDC* EY 1963-64 through EY 1967-68.

Age Group	Reported as "Serum" Hepatitis		Reported as "Infectious" Hepatitis	
	Number	Percent	Number	Percent
<10	32	72.7	12	27.3
10-39	762	72.1	295	27.9
40+	1,335	83.0	273	17.0

*Source: Hepatitis Surveillance Report No. 31, Jan. 1, 1970.

Table 8. Reporting of Cases as "Serum" Hepatitis by Selected Age
Groups - Trends in the United States* 1966-1967.

Calendar Year	Areas** Reporting One or More Cases	Number of Cases** by Age Group		
		15-24	<10	40+
1966	27	187	4	225
1967	33	332	17	272
1968	36	749	17	316
1969	43	1,602	14	441
1970	46	3,273	22	603

*Source: Annual Supplements of Morbidity and Mortality, Weekly
Report.
**Excludes New York City (but not Upstate New York), Florida,
Texas, and California, which used age groupings incompatible with
the national data.

Table 8 presents data for 48 reporting areas notifying cases
according to the age groupings used for compiling the national
data. The four reporting areas--New York City, Florida, Texas,
and California--that used alternate groupings unfortunately had
large numbers of cases notified. Nonetheless, for the remaining

48 reporting areas, the number of cases in children (<10) remained
approximately the same, but a steady increase occurred among persons 40 years of age and over. We note, however, that the number
of areas reporting even one case increased steadily during this
time, a result of the gradual implementation of separate reporting
of serum hepatitis by health departments, and the acceptance of
the new term for morbidity reporting by physicians. One is left,
therefore, with some uncertainty concerning the meaning of the data.

Table 9 presents similar data for Los Angeles County, where
reporting practices probably have been more homogeneous during
this interval. Cases here also show fluctuations corresponding
to those in the age group 15 through 24. These data, therefore,

Table 9. Reporting of Cases as "Serum" Hepatitis by Selected
Age Groups - Trends in Los Angeles County* 1966 - 1970.

Calendar Year	Number of Cases by Age Groups		
	15-24	<10	40+
1966	64	-	63
1967	242	1	81
1968	793	-	110
1969	530	1	94
1970	439	1	98

*Source: Los Angeles County Health Department

E951   Therapeutic misadventure in infusion or transfusion

This title includes :

Anaphylactic shock
Sepsis
Serum :
  arthritis
  hepatitis   originating from infusion or transfusion
  jaundice   administered for purposes of
  sickness   treatment and not attributable
Other complications,   to the pre-existent condition
    not late effects
Homologous serum jaundice
Post-transfusion hepatitis

Figure 2. Rubric E951 of the Sixth and Seventh Revisions of the
International Lists of Diseases and Causes of Deaths. This classification, in use from 1949 through 1967, includes many complications in addition to viral hepatitis.

THERAPEUTIC MISADVENTURE AND LATE COMPLICATIONS
OF THERAPEUTIC PROCEDURES (E950–E959)

Numbers E950–E959 are not to be used for primary death classification if the condition for which the treatment was given is known.

Figure 3.   Coding instructions from the Sixth Revision of the International Lists of Diseases and Causes of Death. By this rule the individual transfused (e.g.) for leukemia,has his subsequent death from fulminant hepatitis nonetheless attributed to leukemia as the "primary" cause.

are also compatible with an increase in transfusion-associated cases occurring concomitantly with the increase in addiction-associated cases.

An additional and supplemental source of information about trends of transfusion-associated hepatitis should be mortality data. Unfortunately, the rubric for "Therapeutic misadventure in infusion and transfusion" (Figure 2) is a "grab-bag" of unrelated entities. Furthermore, any small value the rubric could have is negated by coding instructions (Figure 3) which relegate wherever possible the death to the condition for which the transfusion was given. The meaninglessness of this rubric may be seen from Table 10, which shows that there have been no more than 173 deaths so coded in any

Table 10. Deaths Coded under Rubric E 951 - "Therapeutic Misadventure in Infusion and Transfusion" - Seventh Revision of "ICD" 1958-1967.

Year	Number of Deaths
1958	103
1959	90
1960	101
1961	99
1962	105
1963	113
1964	142
1965	136
1966	149
1967	173

year, and many of these, of course, are likely to be due to
complications other than viral hepatitis.

We must turn, therefore, from comprehensive data for the
United States as a whole to the special studies carried out before
and since addiction-associated hepatitis became epidemic. In 11
studies (summarized in reference [336]) carried out in the period
from 1946 to 1965, the attack rate per 100 persons transfused
varied from 0.6 to 7.2 and the attack rate per 1000 units from
2.4 to 15.3. The overall rates, for whatever meaning such numbers
have, were 1.7 per 100 persons and 4.1 per 1000 units transfused.
Motivation for data collection in the earlier period was in some
instances to demonstrate high or low rates, as has been pointed
out in another context by Chalmers and co-workers [89]; the extent
to which the high and low centers offset each other is obviously
unknown.

For the period coincident with the increase in addiction-
associated hepatitis, we are fortunate to have prospective estimates
of transfusion-associated hepatitis from 14 centers throughout
the country. These data were a byproduct of the investigation by
Grady and co-workers of globulin prophylaxis [178]. In the
National Transfusion Hepatitis Study, the range for symptomatic
disease per 100 persons transfused was from 0.0 (at one center
with 145 transfused patients) to 8.6, with an overall average of
2.8 percent, somewhat higher than the earlier period. The average
rate per 1000 units was 3.6, somewhat lower than the earlier period.

These morbidity trends as well as the data from the special
studies are obviously unsatisfactory, but suggest that any
increase has not been proportionate to the increase in addiction-
associated hepatitis. In part, this is probably due to recognition of the potential hazard, and the vigorous efforts that
have been made to screen out drug abusers prior to the era of
HBAg testing. There may be, however, other factors.

Table 11 indicates the frequency with which persons admitting or denying self-injection also admitted donations of
blood or plasma within the 6 months prior to the onset of
hepatitis. The frequency of blood donations among drug users was
less than that among those denying use, but service as a plasmapheresis donor was slightly more frequent. The differences,
however, are not significant. Table 12 explores this aspect
further by examining the frequency of blood and plasma donations
by frequency of drug use. Although numbers of donors are small,
both blood and plasma were more frequent among those occasionally
or rarely using drugs than among those using them frequently or
daily. This is perhaps understandable in two terms: 1) The
frequent user is less able to conceal his habit from the technician taking his blood. 2) Five dollars for a unit of blood

Table 11. Blood and Plasmapheresis Donations among Patients
Admitting or Denying Drug Abuse - John Wesley County Hospital
May - October 1971.

Drug Abuse Admitted	Total Patients*	Blood Donations Number of Patients	Percent	Plasmapheresis Donations Number of Patients	Percent
Ever Using	239	6	2.5	4	1.7
Denied	267	14	5.2	2	0.7

*Omits 3 patients for whom drug abuse unknown.

Table 12. Blood and Plasmapheresis Donations by Frequency of
Percutaneous Drug Abuse - John Wesley County Hospital
May - October 1971

Frequency of Drug Abuse	Total Number*	Blood Donations Number of Patients	Plasmapheresis Donations Number of Patients
Daily	48	-	1
Frequently	21	1	-
Occasionally	71	3	1
Rarely	51	2	2

*Omits 34 patients with incomplete information concerning
frequency of drug abuse.

could be a significant supplement to support the habit of a "wino",
and may be of some help to the occasional user; it is probably
insignificant to the person with an expensive habit.

Finally, the predominance of the $\underline{y}$ subtype among drug abusers
should be reflected in its frequency among paid blood donors if
the latter include very many of the former. The data (Table 13)
presently available to us do not suggest that there is any significant difference between volunteer and paid donors, a finding
consistent with the previously discussed indices.

Table 13. HBAg Subtypes - HBAg-positive Blood Donors in Los
Angeles County.

Group	Number Studied	Subtype $\underline{y}$ Number	Percent
Volunteer Donors (Red Cross)	74	10	14
Paid Donors	14	2	14

The indications that we have, therefore, are somewhat re-
assuring that addiction-associated hepatitis is not causing so
much transfusion-associated hepatitis as we feared. I must emphasize, however, that the data are generally inadequate for anything other than a gross impression, and that gross impressions do
not serve our purpose very well.

This meeting is particularly concerned with the possible
effectiveness of various measures to reduce or eliminate the
problem of transfusion-associated hepatitis. Let me emphasize
that the only reasonably reliable estimate of a numerator or a
denominator, from which to estimate rates is the annual survey of
numbers of units transfused. We do not know the number of patients
transfused, the number of cases of overt transfusion-associated
hepatitis, nor the number of deaths from transfusion-associated
hepatitis. It is difficult to see how we are going to determine
effectiveness of preventive measures unless we have better ideas
of what is happening.

A mechanism for effective surveillance of transfusion-associated hepatitis exists in some state health departments, and
through the Hepatitis Surveillance Program of the Center for Disease Control. In particular, the State of New Jersey has done
an outstanding job over the last decade of follow-up of reported
cases, inspection and licensing of blood banks, and establishment
of a carrier registry. I would point out, however, that CDC
received surveillance forms for only 30 percent of all reported
cases in EY 1963-64, and this percentage steadily declined to
22 by EY 1967-68. For transfusion-associated hepatitis, therefore, we have a long way to go to establish truly effective
surveillance. It is time we started.

Acknowledgments. The epidemiologic studies at John Wesley
County Hospital were supported by Grant No. AI 10586-01 of the
National Institute of Allergy and Infectious Disease, and
carried out in collaboration with Miss Virginia Edwards, Dr.
Gerasimos Karvountzis, Dr. Irwing Schweitzer, Mrs. Candice
Norquist, Dr. John Weiner, and Dr. Allan G. Redeker.

EPIDEMIOLOGY OF VIRAL HEPATITIS

R. R. Roberto

California State Department of Public Health,

Berkeley, California

I would like to present some data from California to amplify some of the points made by Dr. Mosley, while showing how experience in California may sometimes differ from national trends.

The secular trend by calendar year of the reported incidence per 100,000 population of infectious hepatitis (hepatitis A) and serum hepatitis (hepatitis B) over the period from 1950 to 1971 is given in Figure 1. The data for 1971 are provisional. Viral hepatitis was not distinguished from other types of hepatitis as a single notifiable disease until 1950. In 1955, a further distinction for reporting purposes was made between hepatitis A and

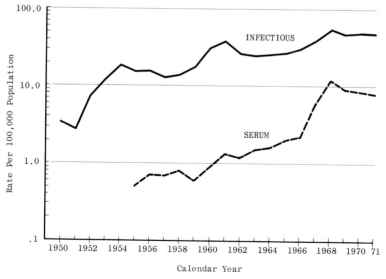

Figure 1. Infectious and Serum Hepatitis, California, 1950-1971

hepatitis B. The cases reported as hepatitis B gave a history of
percutaneous exposure within the six months preceding onset of
symptoms, i.e., transfusion of blood or blood products, self-
injection of drugs or tatooing. All other cases were classified
as hepatitis A. While such a classification into hepatitis A and
B is somewhat arbitrary, it is not totally "meaningless" as
Dr. Mosley has suggested for it does give some notion of the trend
in percutaneous exposure experience. Hepatitis A has shown a
seven year cyclic pattern with three peak years in 1954, 1961 and
1968. Each succeeding peak year has shown an increase in the
incidence rate. The peaks in 1954 and 1961 coincide with the
national pattern; however, unlike the national experience, California continued on the so-called seven year cycle by peaking again
in 1968. Since 1968, the incidence of hepatitis A has not declined abruptly as after the peak years of 1954 and 1961, but has
continued on an essentially plateau course.

The incidence of hepatitis B remained essentially the same
at less than three per 100,000 population until 1967 when a
marked upturn occurred culminating in the peak year of 1968, when
the incidence reached 11.5 per 100,000 population. Since then,
there has been a moderate decline to an incidence of 8.0 per
100,000 population in 1971. Prior to 1967 the majority of reported hepatitis B cases were associated with blood transfusion.
Subsequently the great majority of cases have been associated
with self-injection of drugs. While hepatitis A incidence between the years 1961 and 1968 increased 45 percent, the change
in hepatitis B incidence was 524 percent. The abrupt increase in
hepatitis B incidence seen in 1967 has been associated with marked
changes in life style observed in the youth of California which
coincided with the onset of what might be termed the "Haight-
Ashbury Era".

Coincident with the increasing overall incidence of viral
hepatitis in California there has been a marked change in age-
specific incidence patterns. In Figure 2 we see the age-
specific incidence rates for the peak years of 1954, 1961 and 1968.
The pattern in 1954 shows an age-specific incidence that represents
the classic age distribution of hepatitis A with highest rates
under 14 years of age, and a progressive decline with increasing
age. In 1961 we see a change in age-specific rates from that
noted in 1954. While there was a moderate increase in the under
15 year age group, a much greater increase occurred in those over
15 years of age. In 1968, this change was even more pronounced
with peak age incidence occurring in the 15 to 29 year age group,
with some spillover to older age groups while rates in the under
15 year age group remained essentially unchanged from those in
1954 and 1961. Figure 3 shows that the change in the over 15 year
age group was progressive since first noted in 1961 with peak

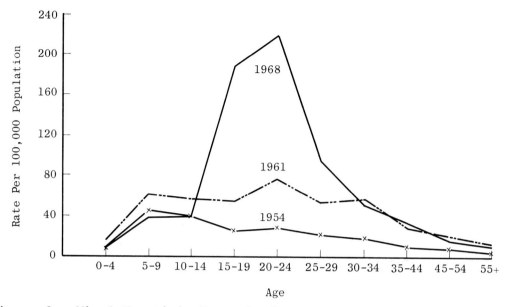

Figure 2.   Viral Hepatitis Rates by Age. California, 1954,1961,1968

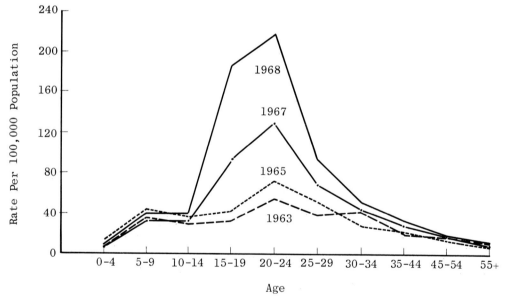

Figure 3.   Viral Hepatitis Rates by Age. California, 1963,1965,1967, and 1968.

age-specific incidence consistently occurring in the 20-24 year age group. From the classic hepatitis A age distribution pattern seen in 1954 there occurred a greater than six-fold increase in age-specific incidence in the 20-24 year age group while the incidence in those under 15 years of age remained unchanged. Although not shown, the age-specific pattern subsequent to 1968 has not changed. The reasons for these marked changes in age-specific incidence since 1954 are not fully understood; however, there are indications that

Table 1. Determinants of HBAg in Various Groups

| Group | Number with HBAg | Number with antigenic determinant | | Percent |
		d+	y+	y+
Healthy Carriers Tonga, 1964 and 1967	62	45	17	27
Hepatitis patients, sporadic - Calif. 1969-1972	27	10	17	63
Hepatitis patients, S.F. Gen. Hosp. 1969-1970	77	5	72	93
Heroin Users Bakersfield, Calif. 1971	30	1	29	97

in large part it is a consequence of the increased use and abuse of drugs and changes in life-style which have led to a deterioration of standards of personal hygiene and sanitary practices in certain segments of our young adult population.

I now would like to comment on what Dr. Mosley said about hepatitis B antigen determinants in patients seen in the Los Angeles area. Table 1 shows data on hepatitis B antigen de- terminants in several groups studied by the California State Department of Public Health Viral and Rickettsial Disease Labora- tory. The tests were performed by Dr. Nathalie Schmidt. Focusing on the bottom two groups, it is seen that of 77 patients with acute viral hepatitis examined at the San Francisco General Hospital in the period 1969-1970 in whom hepatitis B antigen was detected, 72 (93%) were positive for the y sub-determinant. Virtually all of these patients were young adults who gave a history of illicit intravenous drug use. The second group represents 30 young adults positive for hepatitis B antigen among 380 users of intravenous heroin who were seen at a clinic during a large outbreak of narcot- ics-associated induced malaria in 1971. Twenty-nine (97%) were positive for the y sub-determinant. Thus the hepatitis B sub- determinant pattern noted in our laboratory among intravenous drug users is in accord with Dr. Mosley's experience. At this time we do not have information on subdeterminants in hepatitis B antigen positive blood donors, but we are beginning work in this area.

Finally, I would like to comment on post-transfusion hep- atitis in California. A priori, it would be expected that with the increasing incidence of hepatitis A and B there should have been an associated rise in transfusion-associated hepatitis. This has not been the case. In Figure 4 we see the number of reported cases of hepatitis B associated with self-injection of

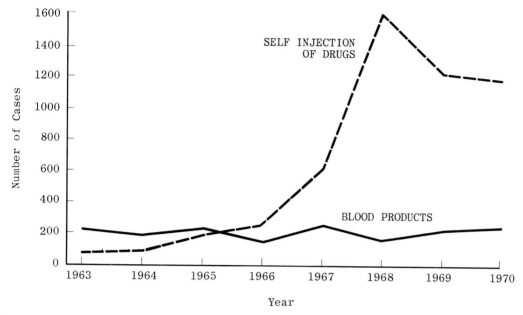

Figure 4. Serum hepatitis cases associated with blood products or self injection of drugs. California, 1963-1970

drugs and the cases associated with transfusion of blood and blood products, both for the years 1963 through 1970. Instead of the expected rise in cases of post-transfusion hepatitis during this period of increasing hepatitis B incidence, it can be seen that the annual number of cases of reported post-transfusion hepatitis has remained essentially constant, averaging slightly over 200 cases per year. Undoubtedly, reporting of post-transfusion hepatitis is incomplete, but this is the case with all forms of viral hepatitis. During the past decade no significant changes in hepatitis reporting procedures have been made which can account for a possible decrease in the reporting of post-transfusion hepatitis. In fact, greater attention has been focused on post-transfusion hepatitis in the lay and medical press, so that if anything, better reporting might be expected.

As Dr. Mosley has suggested, it may be that intravenous drug users do not usually present themselves to blood banks and that if they do, blood banks are fairly efficient in screening out this kind of prospective donor. Whatever the case, continued use of hepatitis B antigen subdeterminant typing gives indication of being a useful marker in the epidemiologic study of transfusion-associated hepatitis.

6. THE CLINICAL AND HISTOLOGIC SPECTRUM OF ACUTE VIRAL HEPATITIS

James L. Boyer

Yale University School of Medicine

New Haven, Connecticut

Viral hepatitis produces a wide spectrum of disease that varies in clinical symptomatology and pathologic effects. Although a systemic infection, the liver is the major target organ.

In previous chapters, the natural history and epidemiology of hepatitis infections have been discussed. As emphasized, the infectious hepatitis, or hepatitis A virus, is an important cause of illness in the military and institutionalized populations and may occur in epidemic form within the community. However, death from liver failure is a rare event, and evidence from long term population surveys indicates that this form of hepatitis does not progress to cirrhosis [69, 344, 349, 494]. Hepatitis A, which is not associated with the Australia antigen, is therefore essentially a benign and self-limited disease.

The serum hepatitis, or hepatitis B virus, is closely related, if not identical to the Australia antigen or hepatitis-associated antigen (HAA), and is an important cause of hepatitis in patients in this country, even though many have no history of parenteral exposure. Although hepatitis B also usually produces self-limited infections, it may result in hepatic failure, chronic active hepatitis or cirrhosis. Therefore, infection with hepatitis B is a much more serious problem.

Although we do not clearly understand the factors that determine the variable clinical response to hepatitis infection, recent evidence indicates that the interaction of virus and host produces a spectrum of clinical disease that is associated with two distinct pathological lesions in the liver.

HISTOLOGIC VARIANTS OF ACUTE VIRAL HEPATITIS

The two histologic lesions which are observed in acute viral hepatitis have recently been described in detail in studies published from the Yale Liver Study Unit [72].

Classic Viral Hepatitis (CH): The most common histologic lesion observed in the liver in liver biopsies from patients with hepatitis is called classic viral hepatitis. The histologic lesion consists of spotty necrosis, a diffuse lobular inflammatory reaction characterized by reticuloendothelial cell hyperplasia, and a portal inflammatory infiltrate which is composed predominantly of round cells. Rosettes, mitotic figures, and thickened parenchymal cell plates are often present, signifying regeneration. The most characteristic feature is the pattern of parenchymal cell necrosis and collapse (Fig. 1). Focal groups of necrotic hepatocytes are scattered diffusely throughout the hepatic lobule but

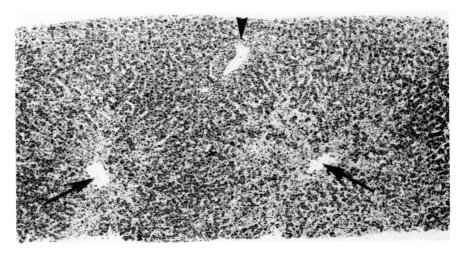

Figure 1. Classic (CH) lesion on 25th day of severe acute viral hepatitis (X128). Note the zones of parenchymal necrosis (light areas) that involve approximately 1/3 of each lobule but do not bridge adjacent portal triads (arrow head) or central veins (arrows). (Reproduced with permission of the New England Journal of Medicine, [72]).

are usually more extensive around central veins or portal triads. This histologic lesion varies greatly in severity, from a few isolated foci of necrotic parenchymal cells with little or no inflammation to lesions where over 50% of the parenchymal tissue is involved in acidophilic necrosis and collapse.

Subacute Hepatic Necrosis (SHN): In the second histologic subtype, called Subacute Hepatic Necrosis (Figure 2), a distinctive

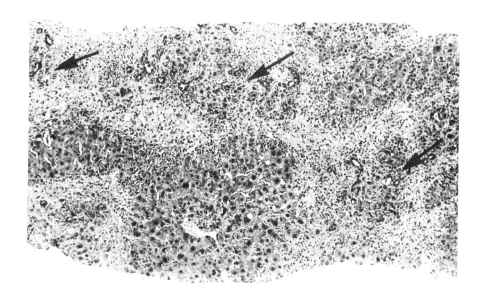

Figure 2. Subacute Hepatic Necrosis-SHN (post-transfusion) on the ninth day of disease (X164). Note the extensive zones of necrosis and collapse (light areas) bridging adjacent portal triads (arrows). Death and autopsy-documented cirrhosis at four months. SHN is best demonstrated in specimen 15-20 mm in length, fixed in Carnoy's solution and stained with Masson's trichrome stain. (Reprinted with permission of the New England Journal of Medicine, 283:1063, 1970.)

pattern of parenchymal cell necrosis is seen which is characterized by zones of collapse that "bridge" between portal triads and/or central veins. Other histologic features of classic viral hepatitis are also observed. When necrosis is extensive, the "bridges" involve entire lobules and may give the appearance of submassive hepatic collapse. Bridging necrosis, which is the hallmark of this lesion, may therefore vary in extent from slender zones, one or two cells in diameter, to complete destruction and collapse of adjacent hepatic lobules.

The clinical significance of these two histologic variants is based on the results of long-term follow-up studies on 170 patients with biopsy documented acute viral hepatitis at the Yale Liver Study Unit. The period of follow-up averaged more than 4 years and revealed striking differences in the clinical sequelae of patients with the two different lesions. As seen in Table 1, none of the 118 patients that had biopsy documented classic viral hepatitis died, or had evidence of chronic progressive liver disease at a later date. Repeat liver biopsies in a sample of 17 patients in this group revealed essentially normal liver histology and there has been no clinical evidence of the development

Table 1.   Sequelae of Classic Hepatitis and Subacute Hepatic
Necrosis.

	Classic Hepatitis (118 patients)	Subacute Hepatic Necrosis (52 patients)
Lost to follow up	10%	4%
Died	0%	19%
Chronic Active "aggressive" hepatitis	0%	13%
Clinical Recovery (with cirrhosis)	90% (0/17 - 0%)	64% (11/21 - 52%)

of chronic liver disease in any of the other patients. Furthermore, with only two exceptions, the classic lesion of hepatitis
was not observed to progress to SHN.   Therefore a benign prognosis
can be predicted when this lesion is found.

    In contrast, recognition of SHN in liver biopsies identified
an important subgroup of patients that were at risk to develop
chronic liver disease, or die of progressive hepatic failure, a
conclusion recently supported in a preliminary report from the
Mayo Clinic [26].   For example, in our own study (Table 1), 19%
of the patients with SHN died of hepatic failure within 4 months
of the onset of hepatitis, while 13% developed a clinical syndrome
that was indistinguishable from chronic active or chronic aggressive hepatitis.   Although the remaining patients eventually
underwent clinical recovery, a third of the 52 patients with SHN
were subsequently found to have histologic evidence of posthepatic
cirrhosis providing further evidence for a causal relationship
between acute viral hepatitis and some cases of chronic liver
disease.

    These studies also emphasized that a liver biopsy was
essential to distinguish between these two groups of patients
since neither CH nor SHN could be differentiated on clinical
grounds unless ascites, edema, or hepatic coma were present,
findings which occurred infrequently and only in patients with
SHN.   Nevertheless, there were certain clinical features which
were more characteristic of patients with SHN (Table 2).

    With an understanding of the histologic variants produced
by viral hepatitis, we can now turn to a review of the clinical
spectrum of disease observed with this infection, recognizing
that a liver biopsy will enable the most accurate determination
of prognosis during the acute phase of the disease.

Table 2. Clinical Characteristics of Patients with Classic
Hepatitis and Subacute Hepatic Necrosis.

	Classic Hepatitis	Subacute Hepatic Necrosis
Age	usually <40	usually >40
Preicteric Phase	" < 2 weeks	" > 2 weeks
Onset	" acute	" insideous
Physical findings		
Ascites	0	~25%
Edema	0	~25%
Coma	0	~25%
Liver Function		
Bilirubin	usually <15 mg%	usually >15 mg%
Pro-time	" >60%	" <60%
Albumin	" >3 g%	" <3 g%

CLINICAL VARIANTS OF VIRAL HEPATITIS (TABLE 3)

Ordinary Acute Viral Hepatitis: The typical case of viral
hepatitis is familiar to every physician and may result from
infection with either hepatitis A or B virus. The classic lesion
is usually present morphologically, and the clinical course is
predictable and self-limited. This form of hepatitis may best be
determined clinically by noting the duration of the preicteric
and icteric phases, and the pattern of jaundice. Symptoms begin
either acutely with a flu-like illness, or insidiously with
anorexia, fatigue and malaise. At this time, in hepatitis B

Table 3. Viral Hepatitis.

Clinical Spectrum	Histologic Spectrum
Benign Disease*	
Ordinary Viral Hepatitis	
Anicteric Hepatitis	
Cholestatic Hepatitis	Classic Hepatitis
Relapsing Hepatitis	
Chronic Persisting Hepatitis ("transaminitis")	
Severe Disease	
Anicteric Hepatitis	
Chronic Active "Aggressive" Hepatitis	SHN
Fulminant Hepatitis	

*Although the majority of patients with the benign forms of
hepatitis have a classic histologic lesion, occasional patients
with subacute necrosis remit spontaneously and behave in a similar fashion to patients with classic hepatitis.

infections, Australia antigen is usually present in the serum [431]. This preicteric phase lasts from several days to one or two weeks, and is then followed abruptly by the appearance of jaundice which is conveniently dated from onset of dark urine. Typically the serum bilirubin rises and reaches a peak within 7-14 days, falling progressively thereafter. Prior to the decline in serum bilirubin, appetite returns, the serum transaminase starts to decline, and detection of the Australia antigen becomes progressively less frequent. Within 4-8 weeks, jaundice and other liver function abnormalities have resolved, and the patient is fully recovered. The characteristic duration of the preicteric and icteric phases of the typical patient with acute viral hepatitis serves as a yard stick against which other patients with hepatitis may be compared.

Anicteric Hepatitis: The most common variants of viral hepatitis are anicteric infections. Many occur in children, are usually caused by the hepatitis A virus which often produces a form of childhood diarrhea, and are recognized only if liver function tests are obtained. In adults, anicteric infection may produce a flu-like illness or persistent malaise. Although anicteric infections are usually associated with classic hepatitis lesions, subacute hepatic necrosis may occur and progress to chronic hepatitis and cirrhosis [248].

The incidence of anicteric infection is not known but as many as 150,000 cases are attributed to transfusions each year, a figure 4-5 times the rate of reported icteric cases [343]. Indeed the incidence of anicteric infections in the population at large is probably at least as high as the Australia antigen carrier rate since a focal hepatitis is usually found when liver biopsies from patients carrying the hepatitis-associated antigen are examined by light microscopy. Thus asymptomatic anicteric forms of hepatitis may be an extremely common phenomenon, particularly in tropical countries where poor hygiene and crowding coexist and where Blumberg and associates indicate that the incidence of Australia antigenemia may be as high as 20% [59].

Cholestatic hepatitis: This form of hepatitis differs from ordinary viral hepatitis because the bile secretory function of the liver is more severely impaired, as reflected histologically, by severe intrahepatic cholestasis. Dubin and associates suggest that a special strain of virus may produce this form of hepatitis [130] but supporting evidence is lacking. Serum bilirubin often reaches levels between 15 and 30 mg%, and the duration of jaundice is prolonged beyond the normal 2-8 week period. Symptoms of cholestasis predominate, and include pruritis, steatorrhea, and vitamin-K responsive hypoprothrombinemia. Despite the severity of jaundice and a prolonged clinical course which may extend over several months, once this form is distinguished histologically from that of SHN, prognosis is assured for eventual recovery.

Relapsing Hepatitis: Five to 20% of patients relapse while in the process of remission or after having recovered from a typical case of viral hepatitis. Recrudesence of biochemical liver function abnormalities may or may not be associated with a recurrence of clinical symptoms. On occasion, there is a complete recapitulation of the original illness. These relapses or recrudesences generally follow within a few months of the initial illness and raise concern about the development of chronic hepatitis, a problem that is resolved by liver biopsy showing features of classic hepatitis. Relapsing hepatitis may occur in patients who prematurely resume physical activity, or use alcohol or drugs while convalescing. This form of hepatitis is particularly prevalent in drug users. The cause of relapsing hepatitis is not known, but the presence of Australia antigen in some suggests that the original viral infection has not been eliminated.

Chronic Persisting Hepatitis: Certain patients, predominantly drug addicts and others with altered immune states, develop an anicteric hepatitis which fails to resolve; others do not remit completely following a typical case of viral hepatitis. This form of hepatitis, which in the absence of clinical symptoms is also called "transaminitis", must by definition persist for at least 4-6 months. It represents an important variant of hepatitis which must be distinguished from more severe chronic forms of hepatitis by liver biopsy (see Dr. Redeker's chapter).

Severe Forms of Hepatitis: Fulminant viral hepatitis (Subacute or submassive necrosis): In the rare patient with hepatitis A(<0.1%) and uncommonly but with greater frequency in hepatitis B (1-10% of jaundiced patients) a fulminant clinical course develops which usually is associated with overwhelming hepatocellular necrosis. A rapidly deteriorating clinical course is heralded by nausea and vomiting and gives way to bleeding, hypoglycemia and coma. Death from hepatocellular failure often occurs within a few days to several weeks after the onset of symptoms. Eighty to ninety percent of patients die after progressing to coma. The cause of this devastating form of hepatitis is not known.

Chronic Active or Aggressive Hepatitis: As mentioned previously (Table 1), certain patients with viral hepatitis, all of whom are believed to have hepatitis B infection and SHN, appear to progress into a clinical syndrome that is indistinguishable from chronic active hepatitis. Further evidence for this relationship is based on the high incidence of Australia antigenemia in both prolonged forms of viral hepatitis and chronic active

Table 4. Australia Antigen in Acute and Chronic Hepatitis.

	Au+/Pts	Percent
Acute Viral Hepatitis		
(<4 mos·)	58/92	62%
Prolonged Viral Hepatitis		
(5 mos - 12 years)	18/43	42%
Chronic Active Hepatitis		
Unknown Etiology	12/54	22%
(? - 12 years)		

hepatitis of unknown etiology (Table 4). Eventually most of these patients develop postnecrotic cirrhosis or die of progressive hepatocellular failure. This form of hepatitis will be discussed in detail in the subsequent chapter.

PATHOGENESIS

At present, the determinants of the host response which result in the variable clinical manifestations to infection with the hepatitis agents are not known with certainty. However, available evidence suggests that a number of interrelated factors may be involved.

The type of infection is clearly important. Only a minority of patients presumed to have hepatitis A infection develop histologic evidence of SHN and in our experience none of these died or progressed to cirrhosis. Rather, as seen in Table 5, death and cirrhosis developed only in patients with hepatitis B infections or sporadic cases where the epidemiology was unknown. Since Prince et al., indicate that the incidence of Australia antigenemia is equally high (50-60%) in both hepatitis B and sporadic cases with unknown epidemiology [390], our findings would suggest that only hepatitis B progresses to chronic or fatal disease, a conclusion which is compatible with long-term follow-up

Table 5. Relation of Virus Type to Mortality and Cirrhosis in 170 Patients with Biopsy Documented Viral Hepatitis.

	Number	Deaths	Cirrhosis
Infectious Hepatitis			
(Hepatitis A)	55	0	0
Serum Hepatitis	51	4	9
(Hepatitis B)			
Unknown	64	6	10

studies of patients with epidemic hepatitis A infection where no significant sequelae have been found [69, 344, 349, 494].

Genetic and acquired factors which alter the immune response to infection may also play an important role as suggested by the difference in the carrier state of Australia antigen in different populations of the world [49, 59], and the tendency of Australia antigen to persist without overt symptoms of hepatitis in patients with uremia, Down's syndrome, lymphoma, leukemia, and lepromatous leprosy, all disorders with depressed cellular and humoral immune responses [49, 59, 298]. It is therefore interesting to speculate that the immune response to Australia antigen might play a major role in the pathogenesis of the clinical and histologic types of hepatitis.

As suggested by electron microscopic studies of Almeida and Waterson [9], the state of the antigen and the antibody response may correlate with the clinical manifestations of the hepatitis infection. For example, antigen but no antibody was observed in serum from a patient who was a chronic carrier. Since no immune complexes were presumably formed, significant tissue damage did not occur. However, in a patient with histologic evidence of chronic active hepatitis, large aggregates composed of antigen-antibody complexes were found and antigen existed in excess. In contrast, in a patient with fulminant hepatitis, antigen was found only in complexes with antibody and antibody existed in excess. In these examples, the clinical form of hepatitis infection appeared to correlate with the magnitude of the antibody response and the type of antigen-antibody complex, suggesting that hepatitis may be an immune complex disease similar to serum sickness. Thus in the ordinary case of acute viral hepatitis, an appropriately quantitative and timed antibody response would clear antigen from the serum producing a moderate degree of tissue damage. Anticomplementary activity would be expected to occur, as demonstrated by Shulman and Barker [432], but antibody would not be detected as it would complex immediately with antigen and be removed from the serum.

Although this concept of the pathogenesis of hepatitis is speculative at the present time, as we learn more about the identity of the infectious agents producing hepatitis, and the nature of the antigens and the immune response that is elicited, it will be important to interpret this information in light of the variable clinical symptoms and histologic damage produced by hepatitis infections.

7. Discussion
THE CLINICAL AND HISTOLOGIC SPECTRUM OF ACUTE VIRAL HEPATITIS

Robert K. Ockner

University of California, School of Medicine,

San Francisco, California

I would like to make a brief comment on a matter of some practical importance in the approach to patients with hepatitis. In his classification of acute viral hepatitis, Dr. Boyer [71, 72] emphasized the importance of histopathology in arriving at a diagnosis and prognosis, and he suggested that the differentiation of benign forms of acute viral hepatitis from subacute hepatic necrosis may not be possible on clinical grounds alone. Conversely, however, it is clear that the caseload of disease processes that fall into the broad category of "hepatitis" is such that it may not be feasible or indeed necessary to biopsy all such patients [331, 416]. Therefore, it is reasonable to ask the question, "Who should be biopsied?"

The approach that I would like to suggest is based on a recognition of two important facts regarding these diseases. First, it is well known that benign acute viral hepatitis may run a course of several months before ultimately resolving [228]. Second, in regard to those patients who ultimately turn out to have subacute hepatic necrosis or active chronic hepatitis, as long as the patient is not deteriorating there is no evidence that a slight delay in arriving at a histologic diagnosis (as the basis for institution of corticosteroid therapy) adversely affects the long term prognosis [72, 163, 324, 403]. With these considerations in mind, the following general guidelines are proposed for arriving at the decision to biopsy a patient with hepatitis.

As seen in Table 1, the first indication, that is, concern as to the accuracy of diagnosis, is obvious and may well be the

Table 1.   Indications for Liver Biopsy in Acute Viral Hepatitis.

Evidence suggesting alternative diagnosis (e.g., ethanol, drug, etc.)
Evidence suggesting more ominous variants
a)   prolonged course (>4-6 months)
b)   severe or progressive course
Evidence of pre-existing chronic liver disease
Cholestasis (selected cases)
Investigational purposes

most frequent indication for biopsy in this situation. Second,
any clinical evidence suggesting that the patient may have one of
the more ominous variants of viral hepatitis would also be reason
for biopsy in order to provide the basis for appropriate therapy.
Such evidence would include a more prolonged course than is
generally consistent with acute viral hepatitis or a course that
is more severe or appears to be progressive. Third, evidence of
pre-existing chronic liver disease might suggest that what appears
clinically to be acute viral hepatitis may in fact be an exacer-
bation of previously inapparent active chronic hepatitis; it would
be important to recognize this because of the implications for
prognosis and therapeutic approach. Fourth, many patients with
cholestasis and a clinical picture suggestive of acute viral hepatitis are exhibiting the cholestatic variant of viral hepatitis
as described by Dr. Boyer. A number of them, however, may
actually have diseases of the extrahepatic biliary tract. Accordingly, and depending on the clinical circumstances, a biopsy
may be helpful in some patients, but in others it may be more
expedient to proceed directly to radiographic examination of the
biliary tree, for example, by means of percutaneous transhepatic
cholangiography. Lastly, it is quite obvious that in the investigation of this disease it has been necessary to obtain
biopsies from a number of patients whose clinical course might
otherwise not have "required" it. Without the information so
obtained, however, we would not have data of the kind presented
by Dr. Boyer and others which have been so important to the
development of our understanding and management of this complex
group of diseases.

8. CHRONIC VIRAL HEPATITIS

Allan G. Redeker

University of Southern California, School of Medicine

Los Angeles, California

Infection with one of the hepatitis viruses is usually followed by complete resolution of the hepatic lesion. Less than 15% of adults with acute icteric hepatitis develop some form of chronic hepatitis. The frequency of this complication is prob- ably higher in children [259] and possibly invariable when the acute infection occurs in neonates [423]. Information derived during the past few years utilizing the detection of the type B antigen (HBAg) has clarified a number of questions regarding the nature of chronic viral hepatitis, while at the same time raising others.

The potential consequences of acute viral hepatitis (AVH) are depicted in Figure 1. The concept is derived largely from

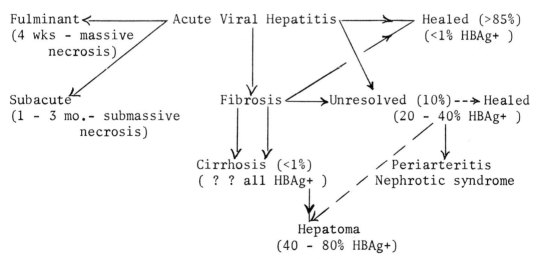

Figure 1. Courses of Acute Viral Hepatitis.

the experience of the Hepatitis Unit at the John Wesley Hospital, Los Angeles, Calif. and our long term follow-up study of hepatitis patients began over 10 years ago. Fatal hepatitis has occurred at the rate of 1% among 3,000 patients with acute icteric viral hepatitis admitted to this unit during the period 1969-1971. Approximately 20% of our patients with fulminant hepatitis and deep coma have survived. However, very severe forms of initial acute hepatitis do not appear to provide an unusual background for the development of chronic hepatitis. We have observed 24 such patients with acute hepatitis and deep hepatic coma who survived and were followed for from 2-5 years. In 23 there was no evidence for any continuing hepatic lesion. One patient developed the features of unresolved (chronic persistent) hepatitis.

Forms of Chronic Viral Hepatitis. Certainly, most patients with AVH have complete resolution of the lesion. The values for serum bilirubin, SGOT and SGPT have usually become normal within three months of the onset of the acute illness. As a rule, the older the patient, the longer the acute icteric phase. Some patients have a very long acute icteric disease, and yet complete healing occurs. We prefer the term "protracted hepatitis" for this course.

There appear to be two major forms of chronic viral hepatitis and since their prognosis and management are so distinctly different, it is important for the clinician to distinguish between them. We prefer the following terminology for these forms:

1. Unresolved viral hepatitis;
2. Chronic active viral hepatitis.

Unresolved Viral Hepatitis (UVH). This lesion has been variously termed unresolved viral hepatitis [405], chronic persistent hepatitis [126], and transaminitis. It is demonstrably the most common sequela of acute hepatitis. Typically, the patients seem to have recovered clinically, but features of a mild inflammatory lesion in the liver persist. Serum transaminase values are persistently or recurrently elevated, providing the biochemical basis for the recognition of the disorder (Figure 2). Persistent or recurrent jaundice does not occur. The serum proteins are essentially normal, with some patients demonstrating a slight hypergammaglobulinemia. Bromsulphalein (BSP) retention is usually abnormal, but is variable and occasionally normal, even when the SGOT and SGPT are elevated. The liver is often palpable and the spleen is occasionally palpable.

The histologic picture is fairly characteristic although variable in terms of the degree of expression. The most uniform histologic feature in a monotonous, cobblestone arrangement of the

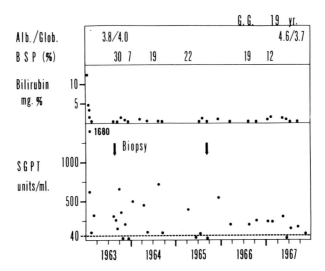

Figure 2. Hepatic tests in a typical case of unresolved viral hepatitis. SGPT values are erratic, periodically being normal.

parenchymal cells, which are swollen and pale, obscuring the sinusoidal pattern. There are occasional foci of hepatocytolysis. The Kupffer cells are not prominent. The portal areas may be some-what widened and infiltrated by lymphocytes. When the lesion is most minimally expressed, there is only the cobblestone pattern of the hepatocytes (Figure 3).

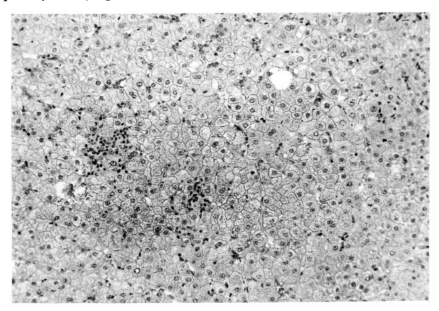

Figure 3. Photograph of the microscopic appearance of the liver with unresolved viral hepatitis. A central vein is at the upper right. The hepatocytes are swollen and the cord pattern is dis-torted. Two areas of focal hepatocytolysis (lower left) are shown with lymphocytic infiltration (H and E x 120).

UVH may follow either icteric or anicteric hepatitis. There is, as yet, no strong evidence favoring development from one compared to the other. In our long term hepatitis follow-up clinic, we have observed the lesion to persist for at least 12 years. None of our patients has developed cirrhosis, in fact, there has invariably been a tendency for all features, biochemical and histological, to become less prominent with time. Thus we feel that the long term prognosis, from the standpoint of hepatic manifestations, is good. On the other hand, we have never observed UVH, when present for at least one year, to subsequently totally resolve. It has been our clinical practice not to apply the term UVH until the lesion has been present for one year, feeling that protracted hepatitis will have come into complete resolution by that time and the histological features of chronic active viral hepatitis (CAVH) will be evident by that time.

From the hepatic standpoint, UVH, as defined above, would appear to be an inconsequential lesion. On the other hand, UVH does appear to have a close association with the virus carrier state. Table 1 details the results of follow-up studies of three

Table 1. Relationship of unresolved viral hepatitis to persistence of HBAg in patients with long term follow-up.

Acute Viral Hepatitis: Follow-up Studies		
Group I 134 Acute hepatitis, HBAg positive (6-18 month follow-up)		
	Number	HBAg +
Healed*	121	1 (0.8%)
Unresolved hepatitis	13 (9.7%)	5 (38.4%)
TOTAL	134	6 (4.4%)
Group II 106 Acute hepatitis, HBAg negative (6-18 month follow-up)		
	Number	HBAg +
Healed*	93	0
Unresolved hepatitis	13 (12.2%)	0
TOTAL	106	0
Group III 706 Acute hepatitis, acute phase, HBAg unknown (1-9 year follow-up)		
	Number	HBAg +
Healed*	620	5 (0.8%)
Unresolved hepatitis	85 (12%)	18 (21.0%)
TOTAL	705	23 ((3.2%)

*Biochemically healed
HBAg determined by AGD and CEP with tenfold concentration of serum

groups of hepatitis patients, showing the frequency of UVH and of persistence of HBAg. These studies, involving adult subjects (over

age 15 years) show that UVH follows icteric hepatitis in 10-12% of
patients, and that the frequency of this lesion is essentially the
same for initial HBAg positive and negative types of hepatitis.
The chronic carrier state for HBAg developed in 4.4% of initial
HBAg positive patients (Group I). Importantly, it is evident (Groups
I and III) that there is a close association between UVH and
persistence of HBAg, with less than 1% of biochemically healed
patients demonstrating persistent HBAg. Since this relationship
is so close, it seems fair to question whether UVH following HBAg
negative hepatitis also marks the carrier state for a different
viral agent. We have observed no beneficial effect on UVH from
rest or corticosteroid therapy.

     Chronic Active Viral Hepatitis (CAVH). From follow-up studies
of patients with acute viral hepatitis, it appears that less than
1% subsequently develop cirrhosis. The ultimate lesion is a liver
reduced in size and presenting a macronodular cirrhosis. Characteristically, there are periods in the course of this lesion when
features of inflammation and necrosis are prominent both histologically and biochemically, hence the inclusion of this type of
chronic viral hepatitis under the larger term "chronic active hepatitis". The terms chronic aggressive hepatitis and chronic active
liver disease have also been used. At the present, we prefer the
broad term chronic active hepatitis, subtype chronic active viral
hepatitis (when the HBAg is present). The other subtypes would
then be: chronic active lupoid hepatitis (when LE cells are present); chronic active toxic hepatitis (oxyphenisatin, or other,
toxicity); chronic active cryptogenic hepatitis (LE cells, anti-
nuclear antibodies and HBAg not present). As a rule, one cannot
distinguish between these forms of CAH from the histologic features. It is somewhat arbitrary and possibly too restrictive to
confine the designation CAVH to only HBAg positive patients, since
some proportion of the "cryptogenic" groups may also be of viral
origin. It has been our clinical experience, however, that most,
by far, of the instances wherein we have observed acute hepatitis
progressing to cirrhosis have been HBAg positive. It has also been
our experience that CAH patients exhibiting the LE phenomenon and
the HBAg positive patients are mutually exclusive. In a group of
73 patients with CAH, we found 22 to have LE cells demonstrable
and 20 to be HBAg positive. There was no overlap between these
two groups. The remaining 31 patients had no "markers" evident,
although 11 did have smooth muscle antibody at high titre. This
lack of association between LE positive and HBAg positive CAH
patients has been confirmed by at least two other reports [75,491].

     There is considerable confusion and some disagreement as to
when the designation CAH should be applied in relation to the histologic features. Obviously, CAVH begins with a morphologically acute
hepatitis and there is then progression at a variable rate to

cirrhosis, with stages in between demonstrating fibrosis in addition to ongoing necrosis and inflammation. Boyer and Klatskin have pointed out that a very early histologic feature of hepatitis progressing to cirrhosis is intra- and interlobular necrosis and collapse of parenchyma (bridging portal areas or central veins or both), and that this lesion is evident during the initial acute hepatitis [72]. However, although this lesion may be the earliest histologic feature of CAVH, their data also shows that an equal number of such patients will go on to complete healing as will progress to cirrhosis. An additional smaller number of such patients develop only unresolved hepatitis (Fig. 1). Thus, the prognosis for CAVH, if the term is applied at this early stage, is not necessarily ominous. However, as necrosis and regeneration continue, the portal and periportal areas become fibrotic and heavily infiltrated by lymphocytes and sometimes plasma cells, and there is increasing commitment to a chronic and aggressive course. Ultimately, nodular regeneration is evident (cirrhosis). It is not uncommon for the clinician to first encounter the patient at this later stage, and he must then presume prior chronic hepatitis of unknown duration. In this regard, it has been our experience that instances of HBAg positive acute hepatitis which have progressed to cirrhosis have usually shown the histologic evidence of cirrhosis within 12 to 18 months after the acute hepatitis. Therefore, it seems that within one year after the onset of acute viral hepatitis the long term lesion, UVH or CAVH, will be histologically apparent in most instances. Certainly there are exceptions to this. The course of patients with CAVH is highly variable, some patients having long periods of biochemical and histologic quiescence while others exhibit periodic or even chronic biochemical and histologic "activity". The titres of HBAg in these patients are quite variable, often low, and periodically HBAg may even be undetectable by CEP and AGD. This is in contrast to unresolved hepatitis, wherein HBAg titres are relatively high at all times.

Chronic Hepatitis in Newborn Infants. Schweitzer et al. have found that over 40% of infants born of mothers who have acute HBAg positive hepatitis at the time of delivery acquire HBAg [423]. The serum transaminase values are elevated and liver biopsy tissue reveals the features of unresolved viral hepatitis [139]. Follow-up studies up to two years have shown uniform persistence of HBAg and anicteric hepatitis. It appears that infection with HBAg in neonates invariably leads to a form of chronic viral hepatitis.

Other Disorders Associated with Chronic Viral Hepatitis. Both polyarteritis nodosa and a membranous glomerulonephritis have been reported in persistently HBAg-positive patients [101,170]. The chronic hepatic lesion in these instances appears to be UVH rather than CAVH. Additionally, numerous reports have appeared indicating an association between chronic HBAg and primary liver cell carcinoma. Many of these patients appear to have CAVH with cirrhosis [463,469].

9. Discussion
CHRONIC VIRAL HEPATITIS

Harvey J. Alter

Clinical Center, National Institutes of Health,

Bethesda, Maryland

The long-term follow-up studies of Dr. Redeker shed considerable light on the confusing and sometimes controversial relationship between the hepatitis antigen and chronic liver disease.

Although this relationship has been implied by the concurrence of HBAg and chronic liver disease [Lancet, 2:117, 1969 and 470] and has been suggested by persistent hepatic abnormalities in carriers of HBAg [359,435], the strongest evidence for this relationship is the histologically proven progression from acute to chronic disease as presented by Dr. Redeker today, and also recently shown by Nielsen, et al. [359]

Of the factors which would predispose to the progression of acute hepatitis to chronic liver disease, two seem to stand out: (1) that the initial hepatitis be HBAg positive and (2) that the disease be mild or anicteric. Dr. Redeker has demonstrated the close association between unresolved viral hepatitis and persistence of HBAg and has also shown that although only 1% of patients went on to develop chronic active hepatitis with cirrhosis, the majority of these had HBAg. Drs. Boyer and Klatskin have also shown that the progression to subacute hepatic necrosis and post-necrotic cirrhosis is almost always related to infection with hepatitis virus B [72].

In regard to the importance of anicteric disease, the data of Dr. Redeker show that unresolved viral hepatitis followed icteric and anicteric hepatitis in about equal proportions. It must be remembered, however, that this is a hospital-based series and that the vast majority of patients with anicteric hepatitis may not be sufficiently symptomatic to seek hospital care. What is significant, then, from Dr. Redeker's data is that anicteric disease can progress to chronic liver disease; the true frequency with which this occurs as compared with overt hepatitis cannot be estimated. Looked at from the other side of the coin, however, the vast majority of people who present with post-necrotic cirrhosis or who present as chronic carriers of HBAg have no previous history of overt hepatitis, suggesting earlier asymptomatic disease.

The seriousness of anicteric hepatitis and its evolution into subacute hepatic necrosis and post-necrotic cirrhosis has been well documented by Dr. Klatskin [248]. Chung [97], Prince [389] and others [281,414] have also stressed the frequency of anicteric onset in cases progressing to post-necrotic cirrhosis. Sherlock [428] described 17 patients with HBAg positive, chronic liver disease. Ten had no history of acute viral hepatitis. Vogel [472] demonstrated HBAg in 40% of patients with hepatoma superimposed on post-necrotic cirrhosis; none had a history of previous hepatitis. Lastly, Barker and Murray's [34] volunteer studies are extremely important in that they demonstrate that all those who became persistent carriers of HBAg had mild anicteric or totally inapparent disease and that all had received highly dilute or modified HBAg positive plasma.

The fact that anicteric hepatitis may have more serious long-term implications than acute clinical disease necessitates caution in the use of any agent which will attenuate, but not prevent, infection with the hepatitis B virus. I raise these points because of the current clamor for prophylactic and therapeutic use of high titer anti-HBAg. I do this not to discourage the proposed control trials, but to raise the spectre that attenuation of HBAg positive disease, while decreasing acute morbidity and mortality in some patients, in the long run, may be increasing chronic liver disease, chronic morbidity and long-term fatality. I also raise the spectre that widespread use of anti-HBAg, if it results in an effective lowering of viral dose and a reduction in severity of disease, may favor persistent antigenemia and thus increase the reservoir of HBAg carriers with all the epidemiologic hazards implicit in this.

I would thus urge, first, that the wave of enthusiasm for anti-HBAg not result in its widespread usage prior to the controlled trials and, second, that these controlled trials be extended in time so that data will be obtained regarding progression to chronic hepatitis and to the persistent carrier state.

10. AUSTRALIA ANTIGEN: THE HISTORY OF ITS DISCOVERY WITH COMMENTS ON GENETIC AND FAMILY ASPECTS

Baruch S. Blumberg

The Institute for Cancer Research, Fox Chase,

Philadelphia, Pennsylvania

The chairman of this Symposium has assigned me the task of reviewing 1) the early history of the discovery of Australia antigen and its relation to hepatitis, and 2) family and genetic studies related to Australia antigen. The historical portion will be adapted from an earlier publication on this subject [62].

The Discovery of Australia Antigen and Its Relation to Viral Hepatitis. It is now clear that Australia antigen, Au(1), is intimately associated with viral hepatitis, and there is considerable evidence to support the hypothesis that Au(1) is, or is on, a virus that can cause hepatitis in some individuals. If this is so, then the virus has been discovered in an unconventional manner, and the approach used has resulted in the accumulation of considerable data on the effects of host and environment on infection with the postulated "Au(1) virus".

There were three steps in the discovery: (a) the development of the concept of using sera from multiply transfused patients as a source of antibody; (b) the discovery of Australia antigen; and (c) the discovery of the association of Australia antigen with hepatitis. The last was followed by studies to test the hypothesis that Australia antigen is a hepatitis virus.

The investigation began as a consequence of our interest in inherited polymorphisms of blood. As part of this investigation we had, in 1961 [6,48] started a systematic investigation of the sera of patients who had received a large number of transfusions. We hypothesized that individuals receiving multiple transfusions would receive some serum constituents different from those in their

own blood and would respond by producing antibodies. It was appreciated that both inherited and acquired antigens might occur in
human serum and cause antibody formation in blood recipients. Using a double-diffusion agar gel technique to detect both antibodies
and antigens, a complex system of inherited antigenic specificities
on the low density (beta) lipoproteins (the Ag system) analogous
to the red blood cell groups was described [50]. Shortly after the
discovery of the lipoprotein antibody, we found precipitating antibodies against another antigen present in the same sera [44]. These
antibodies occurred in high frequency in patients with hemophilia
and in others who had received large numbers of transfusions [49].
The antigen was first found in the serum of an Australian aborigine,
and it was referred to as Australia antigen--abbreviated Au(1).
This non-committal designation, which did not restrict observations
to a specific disease or population, has been useful in the development of experiments and hypotheses.*

We soon learned that Australia antigen was very stable when
stored frozen; sera stored for more than 10 years were still reactive. We were then able to test several thousand sera stored in
the blood collection of The Institute for Cancer Research. From
these, we discovered that Au(1) was very rare in Americans (0.1%),
but quite common in apparently normal people living in tropical and
Asian countries [49, 56, 59, 63].

The entry into this project was through our interest in inherited polymorphisms. In our first paper on Australia antigen [49],
a family clustering of Au(1) was found, and in two subsequent
studies (in Cebu [56] and Bougainville [51]) we were able to show
that family clustering was present and that the segregation of
Au(1) in families followed a pattern of simple autosomal recessive
inheritance. The genetic findings have now been confirmed by
Ceppellini and his colleagues in Turin [87]. (The genetic and
family data will be discussed in detail below.)

We also found that there was an increased frequency of Australia antigen in some forms of leukemia [49]. Later, it was found

---

*We have continued to use this designation rather than, e.g.,
hepatitis-associated antigen HBAg, or any of the several other
names that have been proposed. It is known that Australia antigen
is associated with a variety of other diseases, and is found in
apparently normal people. By analogy, the name "E. B. virus" has
been retained for the agent now known to be associated with infectious mononucleosis, Burkitt's lymphoma, nasopharnygeal tumors, and
possibly other diseases; the use of the terms "infectious mononucleosis virus" or "Burkitt's lymphoma virus" has not been substituted.

that Au(1) was found (mostly) in leukemia patients who had received transfusions, and that the frequency of the antigen in patients with lymphocytic leukemia was significantly higher than in transfused patients with other diseases, confirming the early finding of an association between leukemia and Australia antigen [450]. Returning to 1964, when the relationship to leukemia was first found, we tested the hypothesis that individuals with Australia antigen (those more susceptible to persistent or chronic "infection" with Australia antigen) are more susceptible to leukemia than are individuals in the general population. A corollary is that patients with a high risk of contracting leukemia should have a high frequency of persistent Australia antigen. With this in mind, patients with Down's syndrome (mongolism) who are known to have an increased risk (20-100-fold) of developing leukemia were studied. Australia antigen was found to be much more common in Down's syndrome patients living in large institutions (30%) than in other mentally retarded controls from the same institutions (3%) [45, 46, 52-54, 451], or in the general population (0.1%). In addition to supporting the hypothesis, this observation also provided us with access to patients with Australia antigen who could be observed in our Clinical Research Unit.

The initial observations showed that Au(1) was persistent in the Down's syndrome patients. Those who were positive were persistently positive, and Au(1) did not develop in those who were initially negative. In 1965, we had tested one of our Down's syndrome patients, J.B., and found that he did not have Au(1). In May, 1966, he was retested and found to have Australia antigen in low titer. He was admitted to the Clinical Research Unit for study and while under observation developed anicteric hepatitis with an elevated serum glutamic pyruvic transaminase (SGPT) and a liver biopsy consistent with this diagnosis. This finding was so striking that we immediately set about testing the hypothesis that Australia antigen was associated with viral hepatitis. Two kinds of studies were done. We compared SGPT levels in age- and sex-matched Down's syndrome patients with and without Australia antigen and found that the SGPT levels were significantly higher in the Australia antigen group [451]. In addition to this, there was liver biopsy evidence of inflammatory disease. Subsequent studies have revealed small but significant differences in other "liver chemistries". At the same time we began collecting blood specimens from patients with acute viral hepatitis. Our first observations on the association of Australia antigen with hepatitis were completed in 1966 and were published early in 1967 [52]. In the meanwhile, Dr. Okochi [367] in Japan was studying antilipoprotein antisera (Ag system, see above), and found an unusual precipitin in the serum of a transfused patient. He had heard of our studies on Australia antigen during a visit by one of us to Japan for a field trip and sent the antiserum to Philadelphia for

comparison. His antiserum proved to be identical to anti-Au(1).
He initially found an association with liver disease and subsequently confirmed the association with hepatitis. Beginning in
1966 we distributed standard anti-Au(1) antiserum and antigen to
many laboratories, and by late 1968 the association between Au(1)
and hepatitis had been confirmed in Europe, Japan, and the United
States (for review, see Blumberg et al. [61]).

After our finding that Au(1) was associated with hepatitis,
we set about testing the hypothesis that Australia antigen is
(or is located on) a virus that can cause hepatitis in some individuals infected with it. The results of these investigations
have been described in several publications, and many have been
confirmed in other laboratories. Our results will be summarized
here:

Australia antigen is associated with acute "viral" hepatitis,
both "serum" and "infectious" and with various forms of chronic
hepatitis. Isolated Australia antigen has an appearance compatible
with that of a virus particle of about 200 Å in diameter [39]. The
preparations may contain sausage-shaped figures and larger (400 Å)
particles. Millman and his colleagues [114, 318] have prepared
fluorescent anti-Au(1) antiserum. With this they have shown that
the liver cells of patients with Australia antigen in their peripheral blood and/or hepatitis have, in general, fluorescent granules
in their nuclei. This has been confirmed by studies of liver cells
of leukemia patients with Australia antigen [364]. Huang and his
colleagues [224] have recently identified particles in the nuclei
of liver cells of patients with chronic hepatitis and with Australia antigen in their serum. These particles have the electron
microscope appearance of Australia antigen and bind specific ferritin-labeled anti-Au(1). Patients who are transfused with blood
containing Australia antigen will often develop hepatitis accompanied by Australia antigen in the blood. Isolated and partially
purified Australia antigen has been transmitted to nonhuman
primates (infant African green monkeys) and passaged two times.
The amount of antigen present in the final monkey is greater than
would have been expected by simple dilution [296].

Liver cells from patients with Australia antigen which contain material which reacts with fluorescent anti-Au(1) have been
grown in tissue cultures. After 6 passages of the cells, the
tissue culture cells or supernatant were found to contain Australia antigen in their nuclei and the tissue culture fluid contained Australia antigen (detected by radioimmunoassay) [112].
There have been many epidemiologic studies in which the distribution
of the Australia antigen in populations, in disease groups, and in
institutions is consistent with the distribution of an infectious
agent.

It has been reported that Australia antigen isolated from blood contains about 5 per cent of RNA [237]. This is an extremely small amount if the Australia antigen is a complete virus. It is still not certain if this is a portion of the particle or a contaminant, although the presence of the RNA has been confirmed by other methods [316].

If the RNA finding continues to be supported by additional studies, and if it is assumed that RNA is distributed about equally in each of the particles, then it can be estimated that sufficient nucleic acid is present in each particle to code for only one average size protein. The molecular weight of Au(1) is about 3×10^6, and 5 per cent of this is 150,000. If it is assumed that the RNA is single stranded, then there would be about 450 nucleotides which could code for 150 amino acids. If the RNA is double stranded, then it could code for one-half the number of amino acids. An average protein contains about 100 amino acids. Hence the Australia antigen could code for about one regular protein or a few smaller ones, and the remaining material would have to come from the host. This is unusual for a typical virus.

It is also possible that the RNA is not uniformly distributed throughout all the particles, and that only a few particles have a full complement of RNA. If this were so, then it could be possible to separate the particles containing RNA from the empty ones using gradient density centrifugation. This has not happened in the studies which have been completed.

Irrespective of any theoretical considerations, it is of practical importance to regard Australia antigen as if it were a virus since isolated Australia antigen appears to be highly infectious and persons working with it may contract hepatitis if precautions are not taken.

FAMILY STUDIES ON AUSTRALIA ANTIGEN

The family studies related to Australia antigen will be presented under the following categories.

1. Clustering of Au(1) in families.
2. Segregation analysis of Au(1) in families.
3. Geographic distribution of Au(1).
4. Sex distribution.
5. Age distribution.
6. Maternal effect.
7. Mother child studies.
8. Australia affinity group of diseases.

    9.   The nature of Australia antigen as an "infectious" and
"inherited" agent.
    10.   Relation of Au(1) to other polymorphisms.

    Most of the data presented will be from our investigations
designed to study these points. A comprehensive review of the
investigations on Australia antigen up to the middle of 1970 has
been published recently [61].

    As already mentioned above, our investigations of Australia
antigen began as a consequence of our interest in genetic polymorphisms. Therefore, the very first studies on distribution
included family material [49]. The studies on normal populations
were done on sera collected during field trips designed for other
purposes and stored in the blood collection of the Institute for
Cancer Research. In some cases, family sera were available, and
the results were analyzed to determine if there were a family
aggregation of Australia antigen. Batsheve Bonne, an Israeli
anthropologist, had examined 125 sera obtained from Samaritans
living near Tel Aviv, Israel (Figure 1). This represented nearly
all the members of this highly inbred community. Of these, two
siblings who were the offsprings of a consanguineous marriage
(both of whose parents were double cousins) were the only individuals with detectable antigen. Studies were also completed on

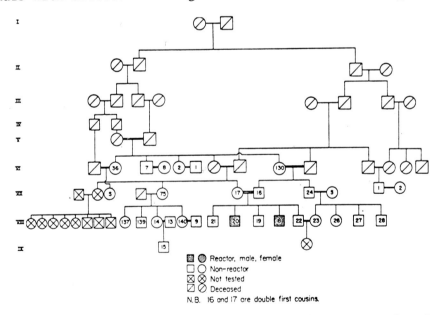

Figure 1. Portion of a pedigree from a Samaritan community in
Israel showing the presence of Australia antigen in two sibs and
the close interrelationship of their parents. This was the initial
observation which formed the basis for the autosomal recessive
inheritance hypothesis.

a Micronesian (Rongelap Atoll) population which included family
material. In this population, there was one father and a son
affected. Of the 47 patients with thalassemia studied, only two
were positive, and they were siblings. Their parents and one aunt
were not reactors. On the basis of these observations, the hypothesis was made that Australia antigen was inherited as a simple
autosomal recessive trait. Our next step was to test this hypothesis in an appropriate family study.

   In order to determine if family clustering did occur and to
perform the segregation analysis, it was necessary to identify an
area where Australia antigen was relatively common, where family
pedigrees could be reliably obtained and where family members would
volunteer to provide blood specimens. A fortunate coincidence
occurred at about this time. We had received about 1,000 blood
specimens from leprosy patients and controls collected on Cebu
Island in the Visayan Islands in the central Philippines. These
were to be tested as part of an extensive genetic study on leprosy
conducted by Drs. Binford, Lechat, Cohen, Guinto and others under
the auspices of the Leonard Wood Memorial (American Leprosy
Foundation). We found that approximately 6% of these specimens
had Au(1). Through the generous cooperation of the Memorial we
went to Cebu to collect blood specimens from the families.

   In testing the inheritance of a blood trait it is useful to
know whether the supposed phenotype is constant during the lifetime of the individual or, if not, the nature of the inconsistency.
If the trait varies considerably, it would be difficult to use
specimens collected at one time in evaluating a genetic hypothesis.
If, in general, the trait is consistent over a significant length
of time, it can be assumed that the conclusions made from a single
observation may be extrapolated to other (although, perhaps not
all) periods of a lifetime. In order to test persistence of the
trait, it would be necessary to ascertain individuals with the
trait and test them periodically over a course of several months
and years. Serial samples of this nature were available from the
population of Rongelap Atoll in the central Pacific.

   Samples from more than 300 different Micronesians from Rongelap Atoll, Marshall Islands were collected during the period from
1958 to 1965. Subsequently, material up to and including the
year 1968 was collected. Serial samples (blood collected over
an interval of two or more years) were available from more than
250 individuals. Of these, about 237 were consistently negative,
i.e., if negative at one point they were negative when subsequently tested. The results of serial studies on the individuals
in whom Australia antigen was found is shown in Figure 2. From
this it was concluded that, in general, an individual's Australia
antigen phenotype is consistent over a fairly long range of his
lifetime.

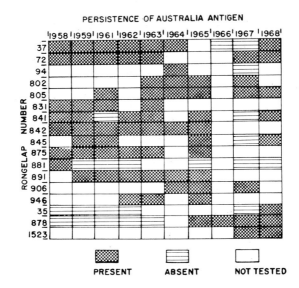

Figure 2. Persistence of Australia antigen in blood samples
collected serially from apparently normal individuals from
Rongelap, Marshall Islands. The subject numbers are given on the
left. Reactions of serum samples collected in the years shown
on the top are given in the body of the figure.

In order to determine if family clustering occurred, a formal
study was undertaken in Cebu. Sixty-four of the sera collected
contained Australia antigen. Blood specimens were collected from
13 families identified through individuals with Au(1) and 40
families through "negatives" (for the purposes of this study a
family was defined as two or more individuals from the same
nuclear family). There were 78 members of the families ascertained
through the positive reactors, of whom 24 were positive, and 153
members of the families ascertained through nonreactors, of whom
two were positive. In each case the index cases were subtracted
from the total number. The frequency of positive reactors in the
families found through reactors is significantly higher than the
frequency of reactors in the family members found through nonreactors and this difference is highly significant ($p = 3.32 \times 10^{-4}$)
(Table 1).

We were now in a position to test the genetic hypothesis
generated in our first observations. The hypothesis states that
individuals homozygous for a gene tentatively designated Au^1
(i.e., Au^1/Au^1) have detectable Australia antigen using the
Ouchterlony double diffusion method (phenotype Au(1)). Individuals
homozygous for the alternate gene (Au/Au) and heterozygotes (Au^1/
Au) do not have detectable Australia antigen (phenotype Au(0))
[56].

Table 1. Australia Antigen in the Families of Persons from Cebu.
Identified through Australia Antigen-Positive and Australia Antigen-
Negative Index Cases [56]. The probability for this distribution
is P = 3.32 X 10^{-4} by Fisher's exact method.

Families Studied	With Positive Index Case	With Negative Index Case
Number of families	13	40
Index cases included:		
Family members	78	153
Positive Australia antigen	24	2
Index cases subtracted:		
Family members	65	113
Positive Australia antigen	11	2
Per cent positive	16.92	1.76

The segregation analysis was performed using the method of
Smith. Since we did not have complete ascertainment of all the
families in the population those portions of the analysis dependent
on such data were not used. In addition to the Cebu families,
several families from other locations were used in the analysis.
The results of the segregation analysis are shown in Table 2. From
this it can be seen that for each of the mating types the expected
number of recessive children (i.e., those with phenotype Au(1)) is
very close to that observed. The criticisms of this study are
given in the reference [56]. Despite these, our general conclusion
was that the simple genetic hypothesis was not rejected by this
study.

The next step then was to test this hypothesis again in
another population [51]. J. Freidlander had collected blood from
1,797 different individuals residing in 18 villages on the island
of Bougainville as part of an intensive genetic and anthropological
study. These sera were tested for Au(1) by the immunodiffusion
method.

In order to determine if there was family clustering the
following procedures were used:

The frequency of Au(1) in the 18 villages varied from 2.9 to
23.9%. IBM cards were prepared for each of the sera, given sequential numbers, and sorted in the IBM 1620 with a random numbers
program. The cards were then examined in turn until the card of
an individual who was scored as Au(1) was found. The next card
of an individual of the same sex and within five years of the
same age, but who was scored as Au(0), was selected as a control.
The cards of the immediate family (mother, father, daughter, son,
brother, sister, grandmother, grandfather, grandson, granddaughter)

Table 2. Segregation of Australia antigen (Au(1)) in families with at least one Au(1) (positive) child. Comparisons by the method of Smith for the Cebu families and the Cebu families plus the additional families (for details of ascertainment, see original paper[56]). In each case the observed number (R_1, R_2) is very close to the expected (E_1, E_2), and the difference between them is always less than the variance (V_1, V_2). The meanings of the other symbols are given in the reference [56].

Number of children in family	Number of families	Observed number of recessive children	Expected number of recessive children	Variance
Cebu families: mating type, positive x negative				
c	m_c		$m_c a_c$	$m_c b_c$
2	1	1	1.333	0.222
3	2	3	3.428	0.980
4	1	3	2.133	0.782
Total	4	$R_1=7$	$E_1=6.894$	$V_1=1.984$
Cebu families: mating type, negative x negative				
c	M_c		$M_c A_c$	$M_c B_c$
3	2	2	2.594	0.526
4	2	3	2.926	0.840
5	1	1	1.639	0.592
6	2	3	3.650	1.552
8	1	4	2.223	1.172
Total	8	$R_2=13$	$E_2=13.032$	$V_2=4.682$
All families: mating type, positive x negative				
c	m_c		$m_c a_c$	$m_c b_c$
1	1	1	1.000	0.000
2	1	1	1.333	0.222
3	3	6	5.142	1.470
4	1	3	2.133	0.782
5	1	1	2.581	1.082
Total	7	$R_1=12$	$E_1=12.189$	$V_1=3.556$
All families: mating type, negative x negative				
c	M_c		$M_c A_c$	$M_c B_c$
1	8	8	8.000	0.000
2	3	4	3.429	0.366
3	3	3	3.891	0.789
4	3	5	4.389	1.260
5	2	3	3.278	1.184
6	3	5	5.475	2.328
7	1	1	2.020	0.970
8	1	4	2.223	1.172
Total	24	$R_2=33$	$E_2=32.705$	$V_2=8.069$

of the individual scored Au(1) were then examined and the frequency of Au(1) was determined. The same was done for the family of the control (Au(0)) individual. Twenty-four pairs were studied in this manner.

The significance of the results was tested with the Sign test. If the frequency of Australia antigen was higher in the family of the Au(1) individual than in that of the control (Au(0)), it was scored as positive; if the reverse were true, as negative. If there were no clustering in the families of individuals with Australia antigen, then an equal number of positives and negatives would be expected; but this was not seen (Table 3). Twenty-one of the twenty-four pairs studied were positive, two were negative, and one was the same; and this is highly unlikely to be due to chance ($p \ll 0.001$). This difference was not due to the differences in Au(1) frequencies in the villages from which the case and controls were selected. From this we concluded that there was family clustering of the trait in this population.

Two methods of segregation analysis were used to test the genetic hypothesis. First, the Smith method used in the Cebu study; the results of this are shown in Table 4. Again, there was a very close fit of the observed to the expected number of recessive children, a finding consistent with the hypothesis. The second method of analysis was that of Li and Mantel. In this the total number of children, T, who are the issue of Au(0) by Au(0) matings, the number of recessives, R, (Au(1)) among these, and the number of children, J, who are the only recessive offspring in the family, are determined. The proportion p' equal to (R minus J) over (T minus J) is 0.250 for an ideal recessive trait. Li and Mantel give the rationale for this calculation and show that it compares favorably with other methods of segregation analysis. The results of these calculations are shown in Table 5 in which they are compared to the calculations for the Cebu data. For the Cebu data the value of p' is 0.2461, a close fit, and for Bougainville, 0.2527, also a close fit. Again, this segregation analysis was consistent with the autosomal recessive hypothesis.

The next test of the genetic hypothesis was provided by Ceppellini and his colleagues [87] in Turin. They found a striking age effect (similar to but more profound than we found in Cebu) with a considerably decreased frequency of Australia antigen in the older age group. A prevalence correction was made; with this the fit of observed to expected was very close. A summary of these findings is given in Table 6 in which the analysis by the Smith method is shown. The analysis by the Li and Mantel method is shown in Table 5.

Table 3. Clustering of Au(1) in families as shown by the Sign test. (Bougainville study [51])

1	2	3	4	5	6	7	8	9	10
Au(1)		Au(0)			Au(1)		Au(0)		
Family members	Au(1), %	Family members	Au(1), %	Sign	Family members	Au(1), %	Family members	Au(1), %	Sign
14	14.7	7	14.7	±	8	37.5	18	16.6	+
3	66.6	11	0	+	33	9.1	24	8.3	+
13	15.4	14	0	+	12	25.0	14	14.7	+
9	22.2	8	0	+	10	10.0	19	31.6	-
12	50.0	10	10.0	+	17	29.4	29	0	+
17	41.1	22	13.5	+	21	9.5	3	0	+
10	20.0	11	0	+	21	9.5	13	0	+
5	40.0	8	37.5	+	33	21.2	13	0	+
21	10.5	8	0	+	27	25.8	16	12.5	+
14	50.0	8	0	+	9	44.4	15	0	+
11	27.2	34	20.6	+	9	11.1	13	0	+
15	6.7	10	30.0	-	17	11.7	13	0	+

The number of family members and the per cent with Au(1) in the family of Au(1) individuals are given in columns 1, 2, 6 and 7. The same data for individuals who are Au(0) are given in columns 3, 4, 8 and 9. When the percentage of Au(1) was greater in the families of the Au(1) individuals than it was in the families of the Au(0) individuals, the doublet was scored as positive: if the opposite was the case, as negative. There were 21 positives and 2 negatives; it is highly unlikely that this is due to change (p << 0.001).

Table 4. Bougainville families. Segregation of Au(1) in families with at least one Au(1) child. The symbols are the same as those used in Table 2 [51].

Number of children in family	Number of families	Recessives Observed	Expected	Variance
		Mating type:	Au(1) x Au(0)	
c	m_c		$m_c a_c$	$m_c b_c$
1	6	6	6.000	0
2	5	5	6.665	1.110
3	4	8	6.856	1.960
4	6	17	12.798	4.692
5	3	6	7.743	3.246
Totals	24	42	40.062	11.008

$\chi^2 = 0.341 \qquad 0.7 > p > 0.5$

		Mating type:	Au(0) x Au(0)	
c	M_c		$M_c A_c$	$M_c B_c$
1	4	4	4.000	0
2	13	15	14.859	1.586
3	13	16	16.861	3.419
4	4	8	5.852	1.680
5	5	9	8.195	2.960
6	1	2	1.825	0.776
8	1	2	2.223	1.172
Totals	41	56	53.815	11.593

$\chi^2 = 0.412 \qquad 0.7 > p > 0.5$

Table 5. Segregation analysis of the family material from Cebu, Bougainville, and Sardinia using the method of Li and Mantel. Here Au(0) parents are assumed to have a genotype Au^1/Au and persons with persistent Au(1) to have the genotype Au^1/Au^1. Theoretical p' value for Au(0) x Au(0) matings is 0.2500 and for Au(1) x Au(0) is 0.5000.

Location	Type of Mating	t	j	r	p'
Cebu	Au(0) X Au(0)	85	20	36	0.2461
Bougainville	Au(0) X Au(0)	124	33	56	0.2527
Sardinia	Au(0) X Au(0)	168	21	49	0.1904
Total	Au(0) X Au(0)	377	74	141	0.2211
Cebu	Au(1) X Au(0)	14	2	7	0.4166
Bougainville	Au(1) X Au(0)	47	6	32	0.5098
Sardinia	Au(1) X Au(0)	30	3	14	0.4074
Total	Au(1) X Au(0)	101	11	53	0.4666

t = Total number of children born to these matings.
j = Number of single recessive (Au(1)) children in a family.
r = Total number of recessive children born to these matings.

$$p' = \frac{r-j}{t-j}$$

Table 6. Sardinian data from Ceppelini et al. [87]. Summary of the tests for the goodness of fit of the autosomal recessive hypothesis. The uncorrected results (a) and the results corrected for incomplete penetrance (b) are both given.

	Tests	Matings	$\chi^2 a$	$\chi^2 b$
1.	No. of recessive children	- x -	0.527	2.960
2.	No. of recessive children	- x +	0.048	0.340
3.	No. of segregating families	- x -	67.565	0.595
4.	No. of segregating families	- x +	8.647	2.029
	Total	(4 d.f.)	76.787	5.924
			P < 0.01	0.3 > P > 0.2

a: not corrected for incomplete penetrance q = 0.183
b: corrected for incomplete penetrance   q = 0.323

Taken altogether, it could be said that these three independent studies, two from the Philadelphia laboratory and the third from an independent laboratory, did not reject the autosomal recessive hypothesis generated by the 1965 study. It was clear from the earliest investigations that factors other than genetic, including sex, age, geographic location and presumably other environmental agents affected the presence or absence of the antigen. Subsequently, a maternal effect has been found. These features of the distribution of the trait will now be described.

Sex. The sex distribution of Australia antigen in several normal populations and in disease groups are shown in Table 7. From this it will be seen that the frequency of Australia antigen is (in all cases but one) greater in males than in females. The difference appears to be primarily due to increased frequency of positive males in the younger age groups, and this decreases with increasing age. Similar results have been reported by other investigators.

It is interesting that a similar sex predilection is seen in many of the diseases associated with Australia antigen. For example, males are affected more commonly than females in lymphocytic leukemia, lepromatous leprosy, Hodgkin's disease, and hepatoma.

Age. In nearly all of the published studies the frequency of Australia antigen is higher in the younger age groups than in the older ones. There have only been a small number of studies in which large numbers of samples were available from very young people. A typical study is shown in Table 8 [57]. The frequency is low in very young children, increases to what appears to be a maximum at about the ages 15-19 and decreases after that.

Table 7. Sex Ratio of Australia Antigen in Patients with Various Diseases (a) and Normal, Non-hospitalized Populations (b). (Immunodiffusion Method).

Disease	Male N	Male Au(1)	Male % Au(1)	Female N	Female Au(1)	Female % Au(1)	Ratio	P
Acute viral hepatitis	112	40	35.7	94	18	19.1	1.87	.013
Chronic hepatitis	12	3	25	19	0	C	*	.095
Down's syndrome	212	67	31.6	92	17	18.5	1.71	.027
Other mentally retarded	145	5	3.4	43	1	2.3	1.48	.900
Leukemia	173	22	12.7	124	11	8.9	1.43	.394
Lepromatous leprosy (Cebu)	396	45	11.4	188	10	5.3	2.14	.029
Lepromatous leprosy (India)	451	32	7.1	101	2	2.0	3.58	.088
Tuberculoid leprosy (Cebu)	343	19	5.5	262	7	2.7	2.07	.128
Tuberculoid leprosy (India)	281	8	2.8	103	0	C	*	.184
Chronic dialysis (renal disease)	5	5	100	4	3	75	1.33	.906

$\chi^2 = 42.3270$ P = .0025

Population	Male N	Male Au(1)	Male % Au(1)	Female N	Female Au(1)	Female % Au(1)	Ratio	P
Marshall Island	243	19	7.8	226	14	6.2	1.26	.612
Cebu, Philippines	678	47	6.9	609	17	2.8	2.48	.001
Cashinahua	45	10	22	44	6	14	1.63	.436
Manila	138	6	4.3	59	3	5.1	.855	.884
Polynesia	597	8	1.3	550	3	.54	2.46	.282
New Hebrides	597	61	10.2	394	19	4.8	2.12	.003
New Caledonia	518	13	2.5	444	7	1.6	1.59	.433
India (South)	116	5	4.3	135	0	0	*	.047
British Solomon Islands	127	7	5.5	160	4	2.5	2.20	.312
New Guinea	532	16	3.0	287	5	1.7	1.73	.389
Micronesia	330	13	3.9	292	6	2.1	1.92	.259
Surinam	310	7	2.3	315	5	1.6	1.45	.729
Bougainville	931	112	12.0	906	97	10.7	1.12	.412

$\chi^2 = 47.6840$ P = .0058

*Au(1) only detected in males.

B. S. BLUMBERG

Table 8. Frequency of Australia antigen by sex and age in individuals from Cebu, the Philippines [57].

	Male			Female			Total		
	No. tested	No. pos.	% pos.	No. tested	No. pos.	% pos.	No. tested	No. pos.	% pos.
0- 5	61	3	4.9 }9.6	43	2	4.7 }8.1	104	5	4.8 }9.0
6- 9	33	6	18.2	19	3	15.8	52	9	17.3
10-19	89	11	12.4	122	1	0.8	211	12	5.7
20-29	209	15	7.2	172	7	4.1	381	22	5.8
30-49	172	9	5.2	175	3	1.7	347	12	3.5
50 over	114	3	2.6	78	1	1.3	192	4	2.1
Total	678	47	6.9	609	17	2.8	1287	64	5.0

Maternal Effect. Australia antigen is much more common in the
offspring of matings in which the mother is positive and the father
is negative than in matings in which the father is positive and the
mother negative [41]. Data are available from four different
locations (Table 9). The studies in Cebu, Bougainville and Turin
have already been referred to. Family material was also available
from two locations (Lau, Balgu) on the Island of Malaita in the
British Solomon Islands. These sera were collected by Dr. Damon
and his colleagues of Harvard University and these studies will be
described in detail elsewhere.

In every population the Au(1) mother had a larger number of
Au(1) children than did the Au(1) fathers and this difference was
significant in several of the populations taken separately and all
the populations considered together. It is difficult at present
to comprehend the significance of this maternal effect. The
higher prevalence could be due to the greater exposure which
children have to their mothers in early life than to their fathers.
It could also be explained by other mechanisms of maternal effect
such as cytoplasmic inheritance.

Other data are available on the question of transplacental
transmission and the relation of Australia antigen and hepatitis in
mothers to Australia antigen and hepatitis in children. This
question has been reviewed by Sutnick [453]. From this it appears
that mothers with acute hepatitis often transmit Australia antigen
to their children, who develop persistent antigen. Mothers with
persistent antigen but who are asymptomatic carriers are less
likely to transmit the antigen to their children. The antigen is
only rarely found in the cord blood and when it does appear in the
children it shows itself later in infancy. In an effort to determine if there is any biological effect of Australia antigen on
mothers, Kukowski and her colleagues [270] completed a systematic

Table 9.   Number of children with Australia antigen (Au(1)) and
without Australia antigen (Au(0)) in matings in which at least one
parent is Au(1).   The matings in which the father is Au(1) and
mother Au(0) are shown in the second column, and the matings in
which the mother is Au(1) and father Au(0) in the next column.   In
every population the Au(1) mother had a larger number of Au(1)
children.   This difference is significant at the .05 level in two
of the populations (Cebu, Bougainville) in the total group and in
the total group minus Bougainville [47].

Location	n	Father Positive Children Au(1)	Children Au(0)	n	Mother Positive Children Au(1)	Children Au(0)	P
Cebu et al.	7	5	15	2	6	1	$.8696 \times 10^{-2}$
Bougainville	28	8	61	36	52	34	$.1662 \times 10^{-9}$
Turin	7	9	17	2	5	2	$.09429$
Lau, Malaita	6	5	12	9	16	13	$.0821$
Baguio, Malaita	2	1	2	11	14	18	$.6096$
Total	50	28	107	59	93	68	$.5513 \times 10^{-10}$
Sub-Total	22	20	46	23	41	34	$.2903 \times 10^{-2}$

study of the sera of 852 pregnant women and 699 of their newborn
offspring seen at a hospital in New Delhi, India over the course
of about a year.   Seven of the mothers had Australia antigen in
their blood; none of the cord bloods contained the antigen.

Using the Mann-Whitney statistic, it was found that the
mothers with Australia antigen had a significantly longer ges-
tation time and were significantly younger than the mothers who
did not have Australia antigen.   There were no other significant
differences found in respect of mother's gravida or the babies'
head circumference or weight.   From this, it would appear that the
presence of Australia antigen could effect biological factors
related to the delivery of children, but the small numbers involved
in the study argue for more extensive information before conclusions
are made.

AUSTRALIA AFFINITY GROUP OF DISEASES.

     There are a group of diseases which are associated with
Australia antigen, but the relationship does not appear to be
etiologic.   In this group of diseases Australia antigen occurs more
frequently than in what would appear to be appropriate controls
[54].   Included among these are the lymphocytic leukemias, Down's
syndrome, Hodgkin's disease, lepromatous leprosy (but not tuber-
culoid leprosy), and (probably) hepatoma.   The genetic hypothesis
has been used to explain some of these relationships.   The

hypothesis states that the Au^1 gene in double dose renders an individual susceptible to persistent infection to the Australia antigen agent as well as a variety of other agents. That is, the agents responsible for hepatitis and those responsible for some of these other diseases are similar in that they are both related to the Au^1 gene. Using the example of lymphocytic leukemia, individuals who have the Au^1 gene in double dose, when exposed to Australia antigen would develop a persistent infection which may or may not be associated with disease. If the same individuals were appropriately exposed to the postulated agent which causes leukemia then they would also develop a persistent infection. In the case of Australia antigen many of the people with persistent infection do not have apparent disease. In the case of the purported leukemia agent persistent infection could be manifested as clinical leukemia. Individuals with other genotypes (Au^1/Au, Au/Au) would develop transient infections when exposed. This could be associated with acute hepatitis in the case of Au(1) infection and some transient presumably unknown condition in the case of infection with the postulated leukemia agent.

An interesting consequence of this view of the data is that the association between Australia antigen and the disease in question would occur only when the individual is exposed to Australia antigen. For example, Australia antigen occurs in high frequency in lymphocytic leukemias only when the patients are exposed to infection with Australia antigen (as by transfusion) but not when they are not so exposed.

Earlier in the paper we presented the evidence supporting the hypothesis that Australia antigen is an infectious agent; all of the tests so far undertaken of this hypothesis have not rejected it. Australia antigen can also be construed to be a serum protein polymorphism. Australia antigen has many chemical and physical characteristics of a serum protein. It migrates by electrophoresis in the alpha position on agar gel; it stains with protein and lipid stains; its density, about 1.21, is greater than that of low density lipoproteins to which it bears similarities, but its density is less than that of most other serum proteins. Millman and his colleagues have isolated Australia antigen and purified it by column separation, sucrose and cesium chloride density gradient centrifugation and digestion with proteolytic enzymes which tend to hydrolyze any remaining serum proteins. The isolated Australia antigen does not have any detectable serum protein as measured by immunologic techniques; when this isolated material is concentrated 10-fold it does not react with high titer antiserum to human serum components. When purified Au(1) is treated with the detergent Tween 80, it partially dissociates into soluble components. These released products appear to be serum proteins including IgG (both heavy and light chain), complement, beta lipoprotein, transferrin, and albumin. Traces of RNA (about 5%) are also found. The nature of the remaining pellet, which probably is some kind of core material, is not known.

Although it could be argued that these proteins are non-specific contaminants, it appears more likely that the Australia antigen particle itself actually is made up of human serum pro-teins, i.e., "host" material.

The relation of Australia antigen to antibody does not appear to be typical of that expected of a simple infectious agent. The peculiarities of antigen and antibody behavior is most striking in the studies of transfused thalassemia patients we have completed in collaboration with Dr. Vierucci of Florence, Italy. Several of these transfused patients (many of whom have been followed for up to 7 years) consistently have antigen and others have antibody, i.e., a transfused patient may "inherently" have either antigen or antibody. This is analogous to the Ag lipoprotein polymorphism in which transfused patients may have a specific antigen or a specific antibody but not both.

There is no reason to assume that these two hypotheses (a) Australia antigen is an infectious agent, and (b) Australia antigen is a serum protein polymorphism, are mutually exclusive. Since neither has been rejected, they can be combined to make a third hypothesis, namely, that Australia antigen is an infectious agent which causes hepatitis in some people infected with it and that it has the characteristics of an (inherited) serum protein polymor-phism. This concept may generate some interesting hypotheses. For example, since this agent is construed to be a polymorphism one can conjecture that the "host" protein on the agent is not necessarily that of the host which it infects, but could be related to the previous host or hosts, i.e., it could be an isoantigen. If this concept is correct, then we would expect to see inter-actions between the infectious agent and the host which are analogous to transfusion reactions. In blood transfusion, if the patient is blood group A and received type A blood, no antibodies will develop. If the patient receives type B, then antibodies will form and a transfusion reaction can occur. Similarly, if a host is infected by an agent which has the same serum protein specificity as the host, no antibody will form and presumably invasion by the organism can occur. If the specificities are different, then antibodies will form and this may or may not result in invasion and in symptoms of one or more different kinds of disease. This could include antigen-antibody complexes.

Finally, we have to consider the likelihood that Australia antigen is not unique and that other diseases are related to

organisms which might also have properties of polymorphisms; kuru
and scrapie are two diseases which come to mind. Because of the
relationship between leukemia and Australia antigen [316] (see
below) it is useful to consider that the postulated agent for this
disease may fall in this "class" of infectious agents. In order to
distinguish these particular characteristics of Australia antigen
and other agents which might possibly be related to it from other
viral or infectious agents we propose referring to them as "Icrons"
[58] (Icron is an acronym derived from the name of The Institute
for Cancer Research). This does not imply that a new systematics
for infectious agents be established but rather serves as a working
nomenclature to refer to this combination of characteristics found
in Australia antigen.

DISCUSSION AND CONCLUSIONS

It can be seen, therefore, that the simple genetic hypothesis
has not yet been rejected. However, there clearly are other
features that bear on the presence of Australia antigen including
sex, age, and maternal effect. Furthermore, the use of methods
which are more sensitive than immunodiffusion may reveal other
information of a non-genetic or genetic character. If the genetic
hypothesis is supported by further studies, several interpretations
are possible.

The data summarized in the introduction indicate that Australia antigen may also behave as an infectious agent. These
findings are compatible with the explanation that there is an inherited susceptibility to chronic infection with Australia antigen
mediated by the Au^1 gene. In populations where the Au^1 gene is
relatively common and where the infectious agent is also common,
then all those individuals susceptible to the agent would become
infected and the segregation in the families would appear to follow
a pattern of autosomal recessive inheritance.

By analogy with other examples of inherited susceptibility to
infection, and from the data we have presented, there are probably
factors such as age, sex, state of nutrition, etc. which also
affect susceptibility and resistance. Under appropriate circumstances, an individual without the inherited susceptibility
factors could become infected. Most patients in the United States
who contract acute viral hepatitis (usually post-transfusion hepatitis) may have the antigen transiently, but it is only rarely
chronic, since they are not genetically susceptible to the chronic
infection. In these patients, the presence of the antigen is
usually associated with evidence of clinical hepatitis and/or highly
elevated serum glutamic pyruvate transaminase levels. In individuals with chronic Australia antigen, such as the large numbers of

apparently normal individuals in Asia, Oceania, and elsewhere, the effect on the liver is much less striking and may be reflected only in minor elevations of serum glutamic pyruvate transaminase, or in no changes at all. A symbiotic accommodation of the organism with the host could have developed in these individuals over the course of many generations, and even though they become infected, they do not develop severe symptoms of the disease. This may represent a protective value of the Au^1 gene and could be associated with the development of what appears to be a genetic polymorphism in this population [51].

Other interpretations of the data are also possible. None of the findings are inconsistent with concepts of lysogeny which have been developed with lower organisms and this indeed may be operating in this case. In addition, we have suggested that the infectious particle may also behave as if it, itself, were a serum protein polymorphism composed of a variety of serum proteins, which are known to be polymorphic. In this connection we have found that the Au(1) and IgG gamma globulin (Gm) polymorphisms are associated, at least in populations of patients who have received large numbers of transfusions. This relation is described in a recent publication but has as yet not been supported by other published findings. If they were associated, it would indicate a direct connection between the polymorphism of Australia antigen and of the gamma globulins and perhaps help to understand how these polymorphic traits act in terms of resistance to disease.

Acknowledgments. This work was supported by U.S.P.H.S. grants CA-06551, CA-06927 and RR-05539 from the National Institutes of Health, by funds from the World Health Organization, and by an appropriation from the Commonwealth of Pensylvania.

11. Discussion
GENETIC PREDISPOSITION TO HEPATITIS

Nicholas Petrakis

University of California, School of Medicine,

San Francisco, California

I am going to approach my discussion from a genetic epidemiologic viewpoint. Dr. Blumberg has brought out a substantial body of evidence indicating that the persistence of the Australia antigen for prolonged time periods is evidence of genetic susceptibility which is inherited as a simple autosomal recessive trait. However, he wisely treats this as a hypothesis.

The hypothesis is based on several courses of evidence, including familial clustering or aggregation of individuals with persistent Australia antigen. He used segregation analyses of affected family members to test the hypothesis that this is a recessive genetic trait.

As he recognized, and as we all do, familial aggregation may be indicative of common environmental exposure as well as genetic susceptibility. However, the strong familial aggregation is important support of a genetic hypothesis.

At present there are two major groups that have studied the segregation of the trait in families, Dr. Blumberg's group and Dr. Ceppellini in Turin. Dr. Blumberg's data comes mostly from the South Pacific, and that of Dr. Ceppellini, from Sardinia. Dr. Blumberg's families were identified through index persons positive for Australia antigen. Ceppellini used a similar approach and supports Blumberg's hypothesis, but with some distinct qualifications.

Here I would like to point out that when one uses any population screening test, such as that for Australia antigen, there

are certain general considerations which arise involving the validity and reliability of the test. The validity of a test is defined
as the ability of that test to separate those who have the condition
sought, from those who do not. If we apply any diagnostic test to
a population, we will beget four categories of results.

Table 1. deals with the efficiency of any screening test. In
the present situation, the test is for Australia antigen persistence.
There are people who are true positives, always having persistent
antigen with a positive test. Also, there will be people who are
false negatives but who actually have persistent antigen. On the
other side of the table we can have persons who do not have persistent antigen but who have a positive test; they are actually false
positives. Finally, we have true negatives, i.e., those who are
non-persistent with a negative test.

In discussing the genetic analysis in terms of screening
tests, a number of factors trouble me.

In Dr. Blumberg's study, testing for Australia antigen was by
agar immunodiffusion techniques. There are now many newer methods
available which, according to today's newspaper, are much more sen-
sitive--I am not trying to be funny here. The effect of a more sensitive test would be to increase the number of true positives, assuming similar specificity, or if a less sensitive test is employed,
to increase the number of false negatives. Another troublesome
problem is that Australia antigen persistence decreases with age,
dropping from around 20% under the age of 20 down to 1% in old age
in the Pacific Region. In Sardinia it drops from 10% to zero per
cent. This decrease in frequency was assumed by Ceppellini to

Table 1. Efficiency of screening for Australia antigen (Au)

Actual result of Au testing	True classification of persons tested for presence of Au	
	Persistence	No Persistence
Positive (Pos)	True pos	False pos
Negative (Neg)	False neg.	True neg

Sensitivity = (Persons with persistence of Au who have true pos test) / (All persons with persistent Au) = True pos / (True pos + false neg)

Specificity = (Persons without persistent Au who have true pos test) / (All persons without persistent Au) = True neg / (True neg + false pos)

reflect the decreasing penetrance of the gene. This age effect also would have the effect of increasing the number of false negatives. I don't know much about the antigenic sharing between hepatitis virus and different unrelated viruses which might be present in a population, but, if there were any, this might increase the number of false positives. Therefore, if we can accept the assumption that sensitivity and specificity problems are involved in population and family testing for Australia antigen persistence, it seems possible that with different techniques of measurement, different segregation ratios might be found which would not necessarily support the recessive hypotheses. One other epidemiologic caution-- several years ago Lilienfeld noted that the methods of genetic segregation analyses which involve binomial techniques, have low ability to discriminate between genetic and non-genetic hypotheses.

I would like to ask if Dr. Blumberg has analyzed his data with different techniques. I see that Ceppellini used the same technique as Dr. Blumberg but with a correction for penetrance.

An important factor in the determination of the frequency of persistent carriers is that of exposure of presumed susceptible genotype to the Australia antigen. The importance of exposure was seen in the Down's syndrome patients where very high carrier rates were found in institutionalized patients as contrasted with total absence of antigen persistence in patients kept out of the hospital and at home. Dr. Blumberg has suggested that the tropics provide the environment in which the hepatitis virus is most readily transmitted and in which a polymorphism for susceptibility may have developed. In non-tropical areas this polymorphism does not seem prominent. However, this point is difficult to determine since the question of exposure again arises and we have no way of identifying the carrier state except by the presence of Australia antigen.

There are many other factors in the environment, such as nutrition, socio-economic status, et cetera, which could affect exposure and the frequency of persistent carriers, and more epidemiological studies are needed, of course.

I wanted to bring out one other point in Ceppellini's paper. I hate to do this to Dr. Blumberg, but I am certain that he will handle it all right. All of the reported matings, except in one key family, are between parents where only one is positive and one negative, or where both parents are negative for Australia antigen. In the one critical mating that Dr. Ceppellini reported from Sardinia, both parents are positive for the Australia antigen offspring, and yet only two of the seven children are positive. It is assumed that these are legitimate children. This is a critical mating and does not support the simple autosomal recessive hypothesis. I want to ask Dr. Blumberg if there are additional families of this kind known to him, and, if so, what the results are.

12. Discussion
GENETIC PREDISPOSITION TO HEPATITIS

Joshua Lederberg

Stanford University, School of Medicine

Stanford, California

It isn't often that an esoteric "blood group" deserves the critical scrutiny that the Australia antigen is receiving: this is obviously just a manifestation of its crucial importance in this modern era of medicine.

Dr. Blumberg indicated that he makes hypotheses because of their fruitful impact regarding further experimentation; and I think the fruitfulness of this hypothesis needs no further comment. Precisely because of the importance of this area, one is obliged to remark that there are still many open questions about the genetic foundations of the transmission of the Australia antigen.

Now, no one can doubt the general principle that genetic factors are likely to influence predispostion or susceptibility to viral infection. In the present context, e.g., the role of Trisomy 21 in making susceptibility almost inevitable is very well documented. The question is whether the factor that appeared in the families that Dr. Blumberg and Dr. Ceppellini have published do represent the segregation of a simple inherited gene or whether other hypotheses are still equally tenable.

Nothing that has been presented so far is incompatible with a simple genic determination. That is not necessarily saying very much because as soon as you introduce variable penetrance (and the necessary concomitants of other factors--exposure to viruses, and so forth) you might reconcile any volume of data with "a simple genetic hypothesis".

As Dr. Blumberg has pointed out, one crucial contradiction to the hypothesis would be the failure of Au(1) to cluster in families. This is contra factual in that the disease is clustered in families.

I don't think it helps very much to bring in hypothetical polygenic factors. The data should, of course, be scrutinized very carefully to be sure that the apparently discontinuous occurrence of the Australia antigen factor is not a threshold artefact of our assay methods. But a single recessive gene for susceptibility works out as well as any other genetic hypothesis.

This situation is typical of many nurture/nature paradoxes and problems in man, and they are very, very difficult to resolve. In some respects, this one is more sharply focused than the question of nature -vs- nurture influence on such developmental outcomes as intelligence, because we are presented with what appears to be a discontinuous distribution of a biochemically assayable product.

One would like to know the outcome if the level of the postulated gene product could be quantitatively measured over a wider dose range of infective unit particles. Our present assay methods do not enable us to reach that far into subclinical manifestation of viremia which may still be important in the transmission of the disease without being accessible to immunological tests.

The alternative hypothesis is, of course, that there is no genetic factor whatsoever in the families in Sardinia or in the South Pacific, and that the familial clustering is entirely a consequence of opportunity for the virus. It stands to reason that if a parent is excreting the virus, this will augment the chance that any of the offspring will pick it up. This seems to be favored by the greater role of the mother as a transmitter of the factor than the father, and I am left with the rather uncomfortable conclusion that I cannot reject the contradictory hypothesis; namely, that there is no gene difference whatsoever and that all of the data, all of the clustering, is due to the opportunity for environmental exposure.

It would be, then, one of those far-fetched but not impossible coincidences that the ratios that came out in the first studies happened to coincide with those of a simple data segregation. I am sure that if I had seen the data Dr. Blumberg has presented from the earlier studies, I would have reached exactly the same conclusions he did; but, on a more detailed consideration of all the data he has presented, one simply cannot decide between the extreme alternatives; namely, simple Mendelization of the gene with variable penetrance on the one hand, and variable opportunity for infection on the other. That, of course, admits many intermediary positions also.

But then we have to ask, "What can we do next, if that ambiguity is still unresolved?" And I guess the only technique that I can suggest (from the tradition of nature/nurture research) would be the examination of adoptions. If the early family environment is the mechanism for transmission of the antigen to the offspring, then in situations where there have been early adoptions, one might expect to find an incidence of the antigen which follows the characteristics of the adopted parents to a much greater degree than those of the biological parents in question.

Thus, if it were possible to find circumstances where illegitimacy were assured, it seems to me this might be one of the most promising methods of analysis one could chose. Failing such studies to give a sharp confrontation between the chromosome -vs- the virus-contaminated environment as the nexus of transmission, there is very little that we can do to prove either conclusion.

Another possible approach would be the demonstration of a clear-cut genetic linkage. That is to say, if we could establish a correlation in the transmission of the antigen with a genetic marker segregating in a kindred, we would then be in a very much stronger position than we are today.

This is still difficult. It would be greatly simplified if we had a clear-cut manifestation of the Australia antigen factor in cell culture, because we could then take advantage of the newly developed, very elegant techniques of cell fusion for demonstration of linkage of genetic factors in man. We are still some time from that.

Finally, I wish to mention the relationship of the Gm incompatibility with the hepatitis factor. The importance of this correlation in no way depends on the primary genetic hypothesis. Whether or not the Australia antigen itself is transmitted primarily by chromosomal susceptibility or through some other route, the interaction of that phenomenon with other clear-cut genetic factors like Gm is a very important aspect regarding the genetic basis of the susceptibility.

The studies that Dr. Blumberg reported are a considerable, albeit not yet conclusive, indication that Gm incompatibility protects against infection with the hepatitis virus. This is a theoretically plausible conclusion if we accept the data indicating that the hepatitis virus uses proteins from the infected cell, and from which it has departed, in building its own cell code. There are precedents, of course, for this with many other viruses.

This would suggest, then, that the likelihood of infection, when transmitted to the new host, would be diminished if the new

host were distinctive in its Gm characteristics and not tolerant
to the Gm factors in the coating of the virus particle. The potential significance of such correlation is not attenuated in
any way by uncertainties about the distribution of the Australia
antigen itself.

Chairman, Dr. Schmid: Dr. Blumberg, would you like to
respond to these two discussions?

Dr. Blumberg: I am honored to have my paper discussed by
Drs. Petrakis and Lederberg. The work described in the paper
which I have just presented was done in collaboration with Drs.
London, Sutnick, Millman, Scott, Melartin, Coyne, Levene and
others.

Dr. Ceppellini has told me that they were not able to retest
the family in which both parents were Au(1). However, he has no
reason to disbelieve his initial findings. The argument certainly
is valid--that with the exception of Dr. Ceppellini's paper, there
are no published critical matings (i.e., Au(1) x Au(1)) to test
the genetic hypothesis.

I want to emphasize the point made early in the paper, that
is, that one makes hypotheses to generate experiments in an
attempt to disprove them. We followed this plan to test the infectious agent hypothesis. I believe this strategy has revealed
many interesting aspects of Australia antigen that are not
characteristic of a virus. Similarly, the genetic hypothesis was
stated in the most simple and demanding form. We then designed
studies that could reject it. We have not quite done that yet but
the investigations have revealed characteristics of the system
which are atypical for simple genetic traits. We're prepared to
abandon the genetic hypothesis any time it is clearly rejected,
particularly since the alternative hypotheses are likely to be
even more interesting.

Now, to answer some of the other points raised by Dr. Petrakis.
The postulated inherited susceptibility factor, if our views are
correct, would be manifest only when people are exposed to the
infectious agent. As a consequence, the Down's syndrome patients
who live in large institutions where they have massive exposure,
are likely to get the Australia antigen, but if they live at home
or stay in small institutions where they are less likely to be
exposed, they are less likely to develop chronic hepatitis with
persistent Au(1). It is as a consequence of this concept that we
believe that the chronic hepatitis found in the Down's syndrome
children is a preventable disease. One cannot assume that all
individuals admitted to an institution for the mentally retarded
are bound to develop hepatitis. By the use of proper sanitation

measures in the large institutions (if this is possible), or (preferably) by maintaining the patients in small institutions, or at home, hepatitis can be prevented. It is also possible that this form of chronic hepatitis can be treated by removing the affected children to an environment where they will not be exposed as readily; and this is discussed in more detail elsewhere [55].

We have completed a family study using the complement fixation method. The complement fixation method is more sensitive than immunodiffusion, and has the advantage of providing quantitative information. These studies still must be critically reviewed and, therefore, they have not yet been published; but I can comment on them tentatively by saying that the simple genetic hypothesis using the immunodiffusion method was rejected by these findings. However, a new hypothesis which is similar to the old hypothesis was supported, namely, that the amount of persistent Australia antigen is to a large extent under genetic control. Age, sex and maternal effects are also factors in determining the amount of Australia antigen present.

The interesting study suggested by Professor Lederberg is feasible. In some primitive populations people often adopt other children, sometimes in an informal way. People who have a small number of children (or none) will adopt some from families who have many. I think that this is an excellent suggestion for a critical study.

There have been some studies on genetic linkage. As far as I know, linkage of Au(1) has not been established for any of the traits. In particular, Professor Ceppellini did not find linkage with the HLA locus.

I am pleased that Professor Lederberg emphasized the importance of the Gm association. Our finding has not been confirmed by other laboratories, but, if it is true, it means that we have a probablistic method of identifying people who are going to react in different ways to infection with Australia antigen. That means that that we may be able to determine before infection who will develop antibody, who will develop persistent antigen, and who will get acute hepatitis. I am, of course, extrapolating a great deal from the meager data, but the nature of this evidence is such that it shows how we may define the reaction that people will have to a particular infection before they get infected. If this were possible, preventive methods could be taken on a rational basis.

DETECTION
OF HEPATITIS B ANTIGEN

Chairman: J. R. Krevans

13. SEROANALYSIS BY IMMUNODIFFUSION:
THE SUBTYPES OF TYPE B HEPATITIS VIRUS

George Le Bouvier

Yale University, School of Medicine

New Haven, Connecticut

Synopsis. This review discusses certain aspects of the antigenic analysis of Australia particles by means of immunodiffusion.
It describes the 3 main surface determinants: the "group" antigen,
a; and the 2 mutually exclusive subdeterminants, d and y. These
subspecific determinants define the two antigenic subtypes - D and
Y - of Australia antigen (Au, or HBAg). It is postulated that the
d and y determinants are the phenotypic expression of 2 distinct
genotypes of type B hepatitis virus, provisionally referred to
as HBV-D and HBV-Y. Those rare individuals, in whom the d and y
antigens are present together, are probably examples of concurrent infection with both viral subtypes. The technique of
immunodiffusion is discussed, with which all the first steps have
been taken, up to now, in characterizing new antigenic components
of the Au particles. The method has recently brought forward 2
further candidates, w and r, as potential new HBV-specified antigens of the Au-particle surface. Several workers have independently identified different Au determinants: their findings are
compared, and their respective terminologies correlated. Brief
reference is made to other methods of seroanalysis, more sensitive and sophisticated than immunodiffusion, that have been
pressed into service in the quest of the subtypes. The existence
of 2 separate subtypes of HBV implies potentially important differences in their behavior--in the community; in their natural
hosts; and in experimentally infected animals and cultured cells.

Introduction. Australia antigen [49] (Au, or HBAg) appears
in the serum during the course of infection with the virus of type
B hepatitis (HBV) [162, 384]. The antigenic reactivity is associated with 20 nm-diameter spherical and tubular particles [37,
39]. It is also present on the outer membrane of the rarer, 42 nm,

"Dane" particles which are found in certain Au-positive (Au+) sera [123]; but Au antigen is apparently not detectable on the "rhinovirus-like" internal component of these Dane particles [8].

Although the elaboration of Au particles during the later part of the incubation period of type B hepatitis is evidently dictated by the infecting virus, the precise nature of these particles and their relationship to the HBV virion have yet to be defined. The most probable explanation is that they represent specifically modified fragments of host-cell membrane, similar in antigenic structure to the viral envelope, and churned out in huge excess by the infected cells.

The Surface Antigens of Australia Particles. The finding of multiple antigenic specificities within the Australia system was first described by Levene & Blumberg in 1969 [290], and has since been independently reported by several groups of investigators [181, 186, 243, 283, 284, 304, 317, 319, 399, 402, 418, 468]. The correspondences between their respective determinants will be discussed later. It is now well established that the surface of Au particles is antigenically complex. This complexity is reflected in the "spurs" of precipitate which are produced by certain combinations of antigen and antibody reactants in tests of 2-dimensional, double immunodiffusion. Analysis of these reactions has led to the recognition, on the Au particle, of a common specificity, or "group" antigen, called a, which is shared by all Au-positive sera; and of 2 subsidiary specificities, called d and y, which are not equally shared by all such sera. Though at present apparently homogeneous, each of these 3 antigenic configurations may well be susceptible to further analysis, when appropriate antibody reactants come to hand.

Various other specificities have been described, and these will be touched upon later. At this point, I might just mention the one designated x, in order to dismiss it [283]. Although it is carried on the Au particle, it now seems very likely to be, in fact, a component of the human host, which either becomes integrated into the membrane of the particle, or else quite tenaciously attached to its surface [285].

As for the 2 subsidiary determinants, d and y, practically all the evidence from our own and other laboratories over the past 18 months indicates that they are mutually exclusive [107, 163, 174, 176, 212, 283, 304, 335, 386, 468]; with a few interesting exceptions, which will be considered later, they have not been found together in the same serum, nor even separately in sera taken at different times from any one individual. This observation suggested an initial grouping of Au-positive sera into 3 sets--D (or "ad"), Y (or "ay"), and A (or "plain a")--depending on the detection of the d̲ or the y̲ antigen, or of neither. The antigenic constitutions of the sera in these 3 categories are shown in Figure 1:   D = {ad̲+y̲-}; Y = {ay̲+d̲-}; and A = {a+dy̲-}.

The Hypothesis of Two Major Antigenic, and Viral, Subtypes. Thanks to the active gathering of data by many colleagues during the past year, it has become increasingly evident that most, if not all, Au-positive sera possess either the d̲ or the y̲ determinant; and it now seems justified to regard the sets D and Y as real and distinct classes, which may legitimately be dignified by the name of anti-genic subtypes. On the other hand, the 3rd category, "set A", though still a convenient repository for unsubtypable individual Au-positive specimens, may in the future become an 'empty set', with the advent of more refined methods for detecting the d̲ and y̲ deter-minants. At present, it appears to be a heterogeneous collection of odd, weakly positive sera, many of them afflicted with heavy bacterial contamination. Most of these sera probably came from individuals harbouring either ad̲ or ay̲ antigen, but in whom the synthesis of the d̲ or y̲ determinant was temporarily suppressed, or in whom the subspecific antigen was being "masked", or destroyed, or made in concentrations too small to be detectable by immunodif-fusion. Nevertheless, despite everything, one still hopes to en-counter, somewhere in the world, examples of a true third subtype, with its own new subspecificity; but it must be admitted that the chances of doing so seem to be dwindling.

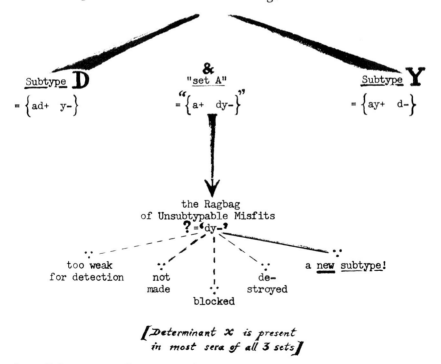

Figure 1.   Subtypes of Australia antigen (and, by inference, of HBV).

This, then, is the present position: a growing body of
evidence now supports the hypothesis that the d and y determinants
are the phenotypic expression of 2 distinct genotypes of hepatitis
B virus, and not the expression of different genotypes of the infected host. These viral subtypes are provisionally referred to
as HBV-D and HBV-Y.

The Genetic Individuality of HBV-D and HBV-Y. So far, the
viruses of type B hepatitis appear to "breed true", in the sense
that a given strain of HBV gives rise to Au antigen of only one
kind, either ad or ay. Some of the data leading to this conclusion are presented in Table 1. They include the results of 2
transmission studies, in which the MS-2 [259] and J.W. [309]
"strains" of HBV were used as inocula. Every recipient of MS-2
who became Au+, i.e., 23 children and 1 adult, acquired antigen
which was consistently and exclusively of subtype Y: ay+ and d-.
In the general population of the same institution, there were more
than twice as many D's as Y's. In the other transmission study,
only ad antigen appeared in those receiving the J.W. virus; while
in 2 cases who developed antibody, but no antigen detectable by
immunodiffusion, the agglutinins were both anti-a and anti-d.

Table 1. Distribution of Au (HBAg) subtypes in different populations.

Population	Total number of persons studied	Number with Au antigen of subtype	
		D	Y
Willowbrook:			
MS-2 recipients [259]	28	0	24
General population	45	31	14
Connecticut:			
J.W. recipients [309]	9	6	0
North Carolina:			
acute hepatitis cases in a military camp [488]	108	0	48
Iowa:			
patients and staff of hemodialysis unit [232]	47	8	0
London:			
1. hepatitis patients in 4 dialysis units [110]	18	1	16
2. patients in the RPMS "spilled-blood episode" [371]	7	0	7
Edinburgh:			
patients and staff in the 1969 dialysis-unit outbreak [286]	25	0	17
Au-positive controls	33	15	18

The other surveys are of populations within which one or
another individual strain of HBV might be expected to spread.   In
the military camp, all cases of acute Au+ hepatitis during 1970
had antigen of subtype Y.   The proportion of patients giving a history of repeated parenteral drug abuse was similar in the Au+ and
Au- groups: 23 of 48, and 29 of 60, respectively [488].   In the
dialysis-unit outbreaks of HBV infection, one was a "pure D", 5
were "pure Y", while one appeared to be mixed, with a single D
carrier among 3 Y's [7, 110, 232, 286].   In the study of the high-
mortality Edinburgh outbreak of 1969-70 [68], it was possible to
include as controls "sporadic" hepatitis patients and other Au+
carriers unconnected with the epidemic: among the renal-unit cases
only ay antigen was found, but 8 of them could not be subtyped by
immunodiffusion; among the controls, both Y's and D's occurred with
similar frequency [286].   These findings are compatible with the
idea that most of the outbreaks were caused by the spread of single
strains of HBV.   One subtype per dialysis unit seems to be the
rule: of 8 outbreaks studied by other authors, 3 were Y, 1 was
mixed, and 4 (all in Holland) were D [243, 335, 468].

Methodology: the Analysis of Au (HBAg) Antigen by Immunodiffusion.   Having outlined the present status of the principal
surface determinants of the Au particles, I would like to consider next the method by which this information was obtained,
that of 2 dimensional double immunodiffusion (ID) [371].   This
procedure has very definite vices, but also some counterbalancing
virtues.   It has been stigmatized by its detractors as "tedious",
"cumbersome" and "onerous".   But its worst faults are its insensi-
tivity, and its requirement that antigen and antibody reactants
be not only sufficiently potent, but at the same time of roughly
equivalent concentration.   Imbalance between the reactants can
produce false negative results, which may be total, or may affect
particularly one or the other of the determinants; such disproportion can also lead to the spurious doubling of precipitates,
and to consequent confusion.

As a compensation for these weaknesses, the ID method has
certain positive attributes: it is simple; it can discriminate
between the components of complex mixtures; and it offers a direct
demonstration of identity, partial relatedness, or non-identity
between different antigen or antibody reactants, provided these
are of adequate, and proportionate, strength [371].

Attempts have been made to increase the sensitivty of ID.   One
may cite, for example, the concentration of weak reactants by
freeze-drying or treatment with Lyphogel [23]; the unexplained
effect of pre-adding some of the antiserum to the antibody cups
4 hours before setting up the test [244]; the use of templates or
matrices to permit relatively large volumes of reactant to diffuse

into very thin layers of gel [191]; the method of rheophoresis, in which the extent and direction of the diffusion is modified by a flow of liquid into the gel [217]; and even such homely devices as reducing the concentration of the agarose, using outsize cups for the weaker reactants, and pre-filling cups 1/2-1 hour before re-filling them at the time of putting up the test.

The antibody reactants used in the analysis of Au antigen were initially derived from multitransfused patients, such as hemophili-acs. Subsequently, they have included antisera from hyperimmunized guinea-pigs, rabbits or goats; and sera from naturally or experimen-tally infected chimpanzees. The antibody molecules taking part in these reactions are in most cases IgG [397].

The Criterion of "Spur" Formation. A "spur" of precipitate is the one sure and essential sign, in ID, of a difference in reac-tivity between 2 reactants placed in adjacent cups. In the case of Au antigen, the relevant antigenic determinants are carried to-gether on the surface of the same particles, which possess either a+d, or a+y [283]. This physical linkage of the antigens causes the formation of a particular kind of "one-way spur", as illus-trated in Figure 2. In such systems, the "spur" will only develop

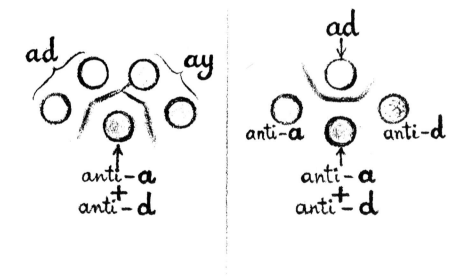

Figure 2. Surface antigens of Australia particles. Key: the "one-way spur" formed between different antigen reactants, but not between different antibody reactants.

between adjacent, partly dissimilar antigen reactants, and not between adjacent antisera, even though these contain antibody molecules of different specificities.

When the ad+ serum and the ay+ serum are placed side by side, and confronted with an antiserum containing anti-a and anti-d antibody, a "spur" is formed, which consists of particles aggregated only through their d antigenic sites by anti-d agglutinins. The precipitate on one side of the "spur" is mixed, being composed of particles linked through their a or their d sites, or through both; beyond the "spur", the continuous band of identity is made up of particles joined only through their common determinant, a.

The events taking place at the growing-point of such a "one-way spur" are depicted diagrammatically (though not to scale) in Figure 3. Passing beyond the developing combined precipitate, which is formed cooperatively by ad and ay particles agglutinated by anti-a antibody, the IgG molecules of anti-d encounter both ad and ay particles, but can only interact with the ad, thus generating the d "spur".

The entire analysis rests on this fact--that the different antibody specificities are carried on separate, and for the most

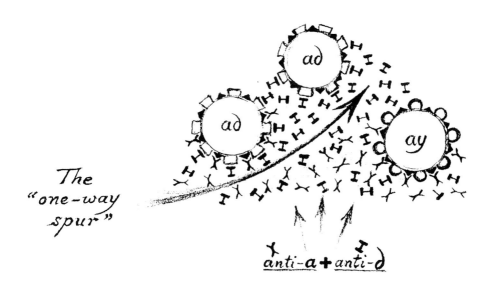

Figure 3. The basis of the Au antigenic analysis: the antigens are on the same particle, but the antibodies are separate molecules.

part separable, molecules of immunoglobulin. This permits the
preparation of unispecific anti-d and anti-y reactants, by adsorption of anti-a molecules with antigen of the converse subtype.

   Up to now, all the original findings of defined antigenic
differences within the Au system have been made by means of ID.
These have now been confirmed and extended by other, more sophisticated methods, following the trail already blazed (see below).
But in the first stages of certain kinds of analyses, it would
seem that a rather sensitive technique, such as complement fixation [399, 418], can furnish so continuous a spectrum of minor
variations in reactivity, that interpretation falters: the woods
cannot be seen for the trees. One should hasten to add that ID,
too, can be used in such a way as to yield similarly complex results, as when comparisons are made of the types and degrees of
interactions observable between large collections of antigen and
antibody reactants. This "population" approach [402] can evidently
reveal a remarkable variety of minor, as well as major, similarities and differences, though their delineation and assessment may
be difficult. It is undoubtedly of interest to scrutinize the
individual trees; but one also wants to stand back a little, and
see the shape of the woods.

   The New Au-Particle Determinants, w and r. To conclude this
discussion of ID with a fresh example of its rewards, I should like
to allude to some as yet unpublished work, which is being done by
Drs. Bancroft, Mundon and Russell, at the Walter Reed Army Institute of Research [30]. I am indebted to them for permission to
refer to their data. They prepared 2 antisera in rabbits, one
against an ad+ serum from Thailand, the other against an American
ay+ serum. With the help of these 2 antisera, they have been able
to define 2 new determinants on Au particles, which they designate
w and r. So far, the combinations adw, adr and ayw have been found,
but not ayr. All Au+ sera tested have contained either w or r.
The w and r appear to be mutually exclusive, in much the same way
as d and y. These new determinants show a strikingly uneven geographical distribution, as indicated in Table 2. The big question

Table 2. Frequency of the "regional" Au-particle antigens, w and
r, in hepatitis patients and asymptomatic carriers.

Country	Ratio		
	r	:	w
U.S.A.	1	:	40
Thailand	7	:	1
Korea (U.S. Army)	1.33	:	1

Data kindly made available by Major W.H. Bancroft, USA (MC), Walter
Reed Army Institute of Research [30].

is whether or not they are virus-specified. If they are, they will constitute a useful criterion for subdividing the D, and perhaps also the Y, subtype. Could the finding of an unusually high frequency of r among Americans in Korea be a straw in the wind? Time, and more data, should tell.

"Multicentric" Characterization of the Au Antigenic Determinants. As indicated above, the analysis of Au antigen and anti-Au antibody has been the subject of independent study in a number of laboratories. Different investigators have introduced their own, sometimes contradictory, terminologies. To acknowledge their independent findings, and to try to reduce any incipient confusion, the correspondences between the various determinants, insofar as they have been worked out, are presented in Table 3. I am indebted to my colleagues, namely Doctors Blumberg, Espmark, Gust, Tilles, and van Kooten Kok-Doorschodt for sending me the reactants for comparative tests.

As regards Levene & Blumberg's specificities b and c [290], the supply of antibody reactants has unfortunately been exhausted. It would appear, however, from the pattern of their ID reactions, that these antigens are not situated on the Au particle; and it has been possible, in comparative tests with known b+ and c+ reactants, to show that they are serologically distinct from determinants d and y [283].

Kim & Tilles' specificity b [243] was initially believed to be possibly identical with x [283]. But later tests have failed to substantiate this; and here too, the stock of characterized b+ serum appears regrettably to have run dry.

Magnius & Espmark [144, 304] have recently adopted the letter y as the designation for their determinant b; and they have now also identified d. Their antigen c, now re-named e, is one of a new group of antigens that only occur in Au+ sera, but are apparently not carried on the Au particle. The Swedish workers found a high frequency of antigen e among patients on hemodialysis (18/23), and a rather low frequency in patients with acute hepatitis (6/43); both groups studied possessed Au antigen which was predominantly ay. By contrast, in 17 Au-positive blood donors, 16 of whom were ad+, antigen e was not seen at all. Instead, however, antibody against e, or against other members of the new antigen complex, was present in 13 of the 17. In 151 blood donors and 24 dialysis patients who were Au-negative, e antigen was not observed. It seems to be unrelated to the Milan antigen [132, 499], as it was not detected in 37 cases of Au-negative, presumptive type A hepatitis [144]. The authors speculate that e may signal an infection with a relatively "contagious" strain of HBV [304].

Table 3. Correspondences of the different, HBV-specific, Au antigenic determinants, independently identified by means of immunodiffusion.

Levene & Blumberg [290] 1969 (Philadelphia)	Kim & Tilles [243] 1971 (Boston)	Le Bouvier [283] 1971 (New Haven)	Magnius & Espmark [304] 1972 (Stockholm)	van Kooten Kok-Doorschodt et al. [468] 1972 (Utrecht)	Gust [186] 1972 (Melbourne)
a	a	a	a	A	1
-	c	d	-	B	2
-	-	y	b	C	-
b?	b?		c?		
c?					

(The determinant x has been omitted from the table, since it appears to be an Au-particle component which is specified by the human host.)

Double Infections With HBV-D and HBV-Y? This may be a suitable point at which to take up again the question of the concurrent
presence of ad and ay antigens in the same serum. The mutual ex-
clusiveness of the d and y determinants has been emphasized. Yet
there have been a few instances where both determinants have been
found together in the same specimen. Dr. van Kooten Kok-Doorschodt
and her colleagues have one such case which they have studied in
some detail [468]. The patient, a woman, was being treated with
hemodialysis. She was carrying Au antigen of AC (=ay) subtype.
Over the course of a few months, it was noted that determinant B
(=d) had appeared in her serum, whereas the y had fallen to about
1/24 of its former level. Meanwhile, the concentration of the
common antigen, a, had only declined by 1/2 to 1/4. Addition of
anti-y antibody to the serum abolished the y reactivity, but left
the d unaffected, showing that the d and y determinants were present on different particles, and not being carried together on any
hypothetical new population of d+y+ particles. These findings
suggest that this patient was already infected with HBV-Y, and
producing ay antigen, and then acquired a second infection, this
time due to HBV-D, while she was attending for hemodialysis [468].

Unless proved otherwise, a double infection seems to be the
most likely explanation for cases exhibiting antigen of both subtypes, whether concurrently or in sequence.

Subtyping by Serological Techniques other than Immunodiffusion.
Workers in laboratories employing techniques other than ID have
begun to apply these effectively to the problems of Au subtyping.
Those concerned will no doubt be discussing their findings in this
area during the course of the Symposium. I will merely give some
indication, in Table 4, of the seroanalytical methods that have
been used. None of this information has yet been published, as
far as I know. It is derived from personal communications, for
which I am greatly indebted to the colleagues concerned. The list
displayed may well be incomplete, and I apologize in advance for
any names or procedures that may unwittingly have been omitted.

For large-scale diagnostic and survey work, the low-voltage
counterelectrophoresis technique of Dr. Holland and his co-workers
would seem to be well suited: more sensitive than ID, it has
detected either d or y antigen in over 900 serum samples, leaving
not a single Au-positive serum unsubtypable in their hands [212].
For this purpose, the authors used anti-d and anti-y reactants that
had been made by blocking the anti-a of the starting antisera with
an excess of antigen of the opposite subtype. The absorbed antisera
could be used without any further treatment, since the residual
unbound absorbing antigen migrated away from the reaction area,
and the antigen-antibody complexes were not dissociated in this
type of test.

Table 4. Serological methods, other than ID, that are being used for the determination of Au (HBAg) antigenic subtypes.

Procedure	Workers
Counterelectrophoresis	Holland, Purcell, Smith & Alter [212]
Hemagglutination-inhibition	Prince [386]; Vyas [474]
Radioimmunoassay:	
1. double-antibody system	Purcell [397]; Shorey [429]
2. solid-phase { coated beads	Goldfield & Black [174], Aach [2]
coated tubes	Ginsberg, Bancroft & Conrad [163]
Immune electron microscopy (for detecting the internal-component antigen(s) of the "Dane" particles)	Almeida, Rubenstein & Stott [8]

Hemagglutination-inhibition [386, 474] and radioimmunoassay [163, 174, 397, 429] are more elaborate and more costly, but they do take the fullest advantage of valuable standard reactants that may be available in limited quantity. Using absorbed, unispecific anti-d and anti-y, these supersensitive techniques should be able to give unequivocal determinations of subtype with all specimens found to be positive for Au antigen by the method concerned--unless, of course, there do indeed exist some rare examples of Au antigen that are genuinely negative for both d and y, and that remain so, consistently, in successive sera from the same individual.

To my knowledge, the methods of complement fixation, charcoal- and latex-particle agglutination, immune-adherence hemagglutination, and immunofluorescence have not as yet been adapted to the detection of Au antigen or antibody subspecificities; but one need not stress the potential value, for their intracellular identification, of such tools as determinant-specific immunofluorescent reagents.

Although it has not yet been used to identify the different antigenic determinants of the Au-particle surface, immune electron microscopy has been added to the list in parenthesis [8], for it has opened up the interesting prospect of analysing the internal-component antigens of the Dane particle, the most credible current candidate for the role of HBV virion.

Conclusion. The known epidemiological relevance, and possible clinical and immunoprophylactic significance, of the D and Y subtypes of HBV are questions that will undoubtedly be taken up by other speakers. And since this Symposium is primarily concerned with blood transfusion, they will certainly be discussing the striking general predominance of subtype D among donors and asymptomatic carriers, but the peculiar preponderance of Y in one or two special places.

In concluding, I would like to emphasize again the ostensibly dual nature of type B hepatitis virus, and of the Au antigenic particles whose proliferation it induces. One can no longer speak simply of Australia antigen--or HBAg-- as though it were a single homogeneous entity, or even a broadly uniform population of particles exhibiting a continuous spectrum of minor variations in antigenic configuration. There exist 2 major antigenic subtypes-- and, ex hypothesi, 2 principal viral genotypes. These 2 subtypes of HBV presumably code for different polypeptides and thus, directly or indirectly, generate different antigens; and they may also be expected to differ in their interaction with genetically diverse human and animal hosts, and perhaps even in their behaviour (one of these days!) in cell and organ cultures.

Acknowledgments. I am grateful to my colleagues Dr. Robert McCollum, Walter Hierholzer and Gilbert Irwin for their encouragement, interest and advice; I am indebted to fellow investigators, whose names appear in the text and references, for the opportunity of discussing their unpublished work.

The studies reviewed in this article were supported in part by contract DA-49-193-MD-2062, from the United States Army Medical Research and Development Command, Department of the Army, under the sponsorship of the Commission on Viral Infections, Armed Forces Epidemiological Board, Office of the Surgeon General.

14. Discussion

SEROANALYSIS BY IMMUNODIFFUSION: THE
SUBTYPES OF TYPE B HEPATITIS VIRUS

Irving Gordon

University of Southern California, Medical School

Los Angeles, California

Dr. Le Bouvier's work has been cardinal in establishing the
concept that hepatitis B antigen (HBAg) particles possess mutually
exclusive subdeterminants, d and y, plus the common group antigen
a. He has lucidly presented and convincingly analyzed the supporting data, which we owe not only to his own careful immunodiffusion experiments but also to the antecedent work of other
laboratories. The importance of this concept for future investigations is obvious; our ability to discriminate between the d or
y subtypes is presently the most important criterion by which different HBAg's can be distinguished from one another, and this criterion has already become the basis for fruitful epidemiologic
studies of the spread of hepatitis B. In turn, the subtyping data
collected in epidemiologic surveys has led to a further deduction
of germinal significance. Le Bouvier has postulated that the mutually exclusive d and y determinants are phenotypic expressions
of two corresponding virus genotypes. In outbreaks of hepatitis B
spread by contact amongst unrelated individuals of different genetic
constitution, one would then expect to find only a single HBAg subtype; a demonstration that this is so would constitute unambiguous
evidence in favor of the hypothesis that the genotype of the HBAg
particle is determined by hepatitis B virus (HBV), and not the
host. This is the case. Accordingly, it appears that there are
at least two genotypes of HBV, which Le Bouvier terms HBV-D and
HBV-Y; and that HBAg is, by a still unspecified mechanism, a virus-
coded product or byproduct.

I should like to give additional data consonant with this deduction. They corroborate the twin premises on which it is based,
namely, that the distribution of the d and y subdeterminants is

mutually exclusive, and that only a single subdeterminant type
occurs in a common-source outbreak of hepatitis B. In our laboratory the typing of the HBAg's was done by immunodiffusion, utilizing monospecific antisera from groups of guinea-pigs immunized
respectively with the HBAg from a single patient. The criteria
discussed by Dr. Le Bouvier were employed to determine the antigenic subtypes, and tests by him of our typing antisera and prototype antigens agreed with our determinations.

These data, Table 1, show that both the d and the y subtypes
occur in acute, persistent, and chronic active hepatitis patients,
all of whom were under the care of our colleague, Dr. Redeker, with
whom we collaborated. The pertinent fact is that there were no
instances in which both subdeterminants were found in a single
HBAg specimen. Our results are thus concordant with those from
Le Bouvier's and other laboratories. (Le Bouvier has discussed
the rare instances of concurrent d and y subdeterminants as probably due to double infection.) However, the results of a study
(led by our colleague, Dr. Mosley) of a hemodialysis-associated
outbreak of hepatitis B (Table 2) are in striking contrast to our
data given in Table 1.

None of the patients exhibited HBAg of the d subtype; all
possessed y. In a more extended and detailed analysis of this
outbreak [335], classifying the HBAg's from 16 epidemiologically
related but genetically unrelated cases, 13 out of 16 were found to be
d-negative. In transfusion-associated nondialysis patients, 14

Table 1. Distribution of d and y determinants by clinical form
of hepatitis [176].

	d	y	Both	Totals
Acute	29	18	0	47
Persistent	5	3	0	8
Chronic active	17	4	0	21
				76

Table 2. Hemodialysis-associated hepatitis [335].

	Source of antigen	Type	
		a+y	other
22	hemodialysis patients	22	0
11	staff members of unit	11	0
1	secondarily infect tech.	1	0
5	members of families of hemo- dialysis patients	5	0

of 32 HBAg's were $\underline{d}$-negative, **while none of** those from 23 trans-fused hemodialysis patients were $\underline{d}$-negative; and the HBAg's from 17 of 28 medical or paramedical patients not working in the hemo-dialysis unit were $\underline{d}$-negative, whereas each of the 13 from those who did work in the hemodialysis unit was $\underline{d}$-negative. These data indicate that the subdeterminant phenotype of these HBAg's must have been directed by the infecting HB virus.

There are still further analyses of the HBAg to be made. Of special importance is the identification of the antigenic com-ponent(s) involved in virus neutralization. Its isolation in pure form might provide a basis for both active and passive immunization. In the meantime, ongoing investigations, discussed by other par-ticipants in this symposium, will reveal whether immunity to hepatitis B virus infection is correlated with the $\underline{d}$ and $\underline{y}$ subde-terminants. _____

Dr. Blumberg: Dr. Krevans asked me if I would comment on Dr. Le Bouvier's paper on specificities in order to stimulate some further questions.

The work which preceded the Australia antigen involved lipo-protein specificities, as I mentioned earlier. One of the first things which became apparent in that study was the presence of multiple specificities of the lipoproteins. This subsequently led to a considerable amount of work, particularly in Europe, in which a complex system of alleles segregating at three (or more) loci was determined. When we discovered the Australia antigen system, we more or less followed a similar plan of investigation. In the first paper on Australia antigen we noticed that there were specificity differences in the human antiserum, and this now has been very much more ordered by the work of Dr. Le Bouvier and others.

The initial studies on multiple human antisera specificities were published by Dr. Raunio, and his colleagues, working in our laboratory. He identified seven classes of antisera which could be determined by a smaller number of antigenic specificities. An experimental finding by Dr. Raunio was the existence of several sera which contained what appeared to be both Australia antigen and antibody, detected by the immunodiffusion methods.

Dr. Raunio and his colleagues then examined these more care-fully and found that in these sera the antigen and antibody had different specificities. A person could have antigen of one specificity and antibody of another specificity. This may have a bearing on the use of vaccines or of antibody to treat hepatitis. Very specific antisera or antigens may be required for different antigenic varieties of the infective agents.

15. DETECTION OF HEPATITIS-ASSOCIATED ANTIGEN: ELECTROPHORETIC ASSAY PROCEDURES

David J. Gocke

Columbia University, College of Physicians & Surgeons

New York, New York

This discussion will describe the application of immunoelectrophoretic principles to the detection of Australia antigen (Au) and relate our experiences with clinical applications of this method. The counterimmunoelectrophoretic (CEP) technique as employed for detection of Au takes advantage of the fact that the antigen and its homologous antibody have differing electrophoretic mobilities. When the antigen and antibody are placed in wells cut into a thin layer of agarose on a glass slide and properly oriented in an electrical field, the antigen and antibody migrate towards each other and a visible precipitation reaction occurs in the zone between the wells where the antigen and antibody meet.

The advantages of the CEP technique are twofold. First, the speed of the reaction is much greater than conventional immunodiffusion since it is possible to obtain a positive reaction with 30-90 minutes of electrophoresis. Secondly, the reagents move in one direction rather than diffusing radially from the wells so that there is a consequent gain in sensitivity. Figure 1 illustrates a typical positive reaction and demonstrates the configuration of wells employed. A standard 3 1/4 x 4 inch lantern slide can be prepared with three sets each containing three rows of opposing wells. The unknown specimen is placed in the central well and a known standard antiserum is placed in the well toward the anode. It is also possible to test for antibody in the unknown by placing an antigen-containing specimen in the well on the cathodal side.

Table I summarizes the various conditions of the reaction which we now consider optimal in our laboratory [168]. A standard lantern slide (3 x 4 inches) is covered with 10 ml of a 0.85%

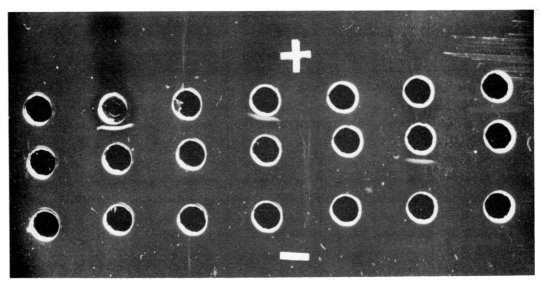

Figure 1.   An example of a typical counterelectrophoresis slide.
The center wells contain the unknown specimens.   The wells on the
anodal side contain a known anti-Australia antigen antiserum and
the wells on the cathodal side contain known Australia antigen.

Table I.   Conditions

Agarose: 0.85%   (10 ml per 3 x 4 in. slide)
Buffer in Agarose: Veronal 0.05 M, pH 8.2
Buffer in Chamber: Veronal 0.05 M, pH 8.2
Well Size: 5 mm
Well Distance: 3 mm
Amperage: 20 mAmp/3 x 4 in. slide
Time: 60 minutes
Temp: ambient (20 - 25° C)

---

agarose solution dissolved in Veronal buffer, 0.05 M, pH 8.2.   It
is important to be aware of the fact that variations in the composition of agarose are frequently encountered both from one manufacturer to another and in between lots from the same manufacturer.
It is important, therefore, to find and work with a batch of agarose which performs satisfactorily.   The agarose with which we have
had best success is supplied by Fischer Chemicals.   It is possible
to obtain reactions in Ionagar or in Noble agar, and it is also
possible to mix agarose and Noble agar in varying proportions.
However, we have not found these to be advantageous.   In addition,
we have attempted many variations in the buffer composition and
pH and find the conditions noted above to be optimal.   Other workers have employed Tris buffer at slightly different pH and ionic
concentrations and report good results [15].   In addition, the
technique of discontinuous immunoelectrophoresis, consisting of the

use of a different buffer system in the chamber from that employed to dissolve the agarose, has been advocated [481].

We have also experimented with different well sizes and distances between the wells and find that for our antibody a well size of 5 mm in diameter, separated by an inter-well distance of 3 mm edge to edge, is optimal. When a 3-well configuration is employed for simultaneous detection of anti-Au in the unknown, it is helpful to place the well containing known antigen at 5 mm from the center well (edge to edge) to prevent the antigen from overrunning into the center well.

The voltage or current which is applied across the slide can also be varied. In our experience the so-called high voltage IEOP technique [388] gives no better results than the use of relatively low voltages and currents, as described here. We routinely employ constant current at 20 mAmps per lantern slide, although it is possible to achieve satisfactory results over the range of 15 to 40 mAmps. This is equivalent to about 1/3 or 1/4 of voltage employed in the high voltage system. The optimal time of electrophoresis in our experience is 60 minutes. Although it is possible to see positive reactions in as little as 20-30 minutes, it is not advisable to shorten the running time, especially when dealing with weaker reactions. It may be necessary with weaker antibodies to allow 90 minutes of electrophoresis but the run should not be extended beyond that time in order to avoid the hazard of artefacts produced by overrunning the center well. By employing the low voltage technique, regulation of the temperature for these short periods of time is not necessary and the reaction can be run at room temperature. Routinely, reactions are read immediately upon completion of electrophoresis. Allowing further diffusion to occur overnight does not increase the yield of positives and if a 3-well system is being employed may introduce confusing reactions. Staining of the slides with various protein stains does not really enhance the positive reaction beyond that which can be recognized by an experienced observer with proper lighting, and it does prolong the time required significantly.

In the final analysis, the single most important determinant in obtaining good results with the CEP system is the availability of good reagents, especially a potent antibody. If one employs a good antibody, minor variations in buffer, agarose composition, voltage, etc. are relatively insignificant.

There are several hazards and artefacts which may be encountered with this system. In most cases these artefacts can be recognized with experience and need not obscure the true positive reaction. The most common artefact is produced by turbidity of the serum specimen which causes a halo of precipitation completely around the well.

This problem may be due to bacterial contamination of the specimen, improper storage, use of plasma rather than serum or by hyperlipemia. We routinely collect sera in 0.01% Na azide and store specimens at -25° C. Turbid sera are clarified by centrifugation before use. The halo type of artefact is easily recognized, however, and should not be confused with a truly positive reaction. Another artefact may occur if the slide is allowed to electrophorese for an excessive period of time or if it is allowed to incubate overnight in an attempt to enhance weak reactions. In this case the antigen positive control serum in a 3-well configuration may overrun the center well and react with the standard antibody creating a precipitin line which may be misinterpreted as a positive reaction between the unknown and the antiserum. Thus, it is not advisable to save the plates overnight in an attempt to enhance the reaction as this has been shown to be unfruitful and potentially confusing.

Table 2.   Current methods of detection of Australia antigen.

	Absolute Sensitivity	Speed
Two-Dimensional Immunodiffusion	1	1-2 days
Counterimmunoelectrophoresis	10-15	1-2 hours
Complement fixation	20	1-2 days
Hemagglutination Inhibition	20-50	1 day
Radioimmunoassay	?100-1000	3-6 days

Table 2 summarizes the comparative sensitivity of various methods for the detection of Australia antigen in our experience. If the two-dimensional immunodiffusion system is assigned a relative sensitivity of 1 and used as the basis of comparison, then CEP is found to be from 10-15 fold more sensitive, in addition to having the advantage of requiring only 60-90 minutes for completion. Complement fixation [287] is slightly more sensitive for the detection of antigen than CEP but has the disadvantage of requiring an overnight incubation period for optimal sensitivities and is technically more difficult to perform. Hemagglutination inhibition [477] is also somewhat more sensitive but again has the disadvantage of requiring greater technical skill and the availability of highly purified antigen with which to sensitize the erythrocytes. Hemagglutination is an excellent test system for detection of antibody. Finally, radioimmunoassay techniques have been described and are currently being further developed [277,483]. These techniques are much more sensitive for the detection of small amounts of antigen but are time consuming and require expensive radioactivity counting equipment.

Table 3. Comparative Sensitivity of Different Test Methods

Method	Range of Percent Positives
ID	25-77
CE	32-96
CF	69-98
HA	90-94
RIA	97-99

Table 3 demonstrates the usefulness of these various test systems in a practical field trial type of comparison. The study summarized here represents the findings obtained on the panel of 120 coded unknown specimens supplied by the NRC-CDC to a number of laboratories throughout the country [246]. It will be noted that even at best the immunodiffusion reaction was distinctly inferior to the other techniques, regardless of the experience of the laboratory in which it was performed. The CEP method scored poorly in some laboratories, but in other more experienced laboratories was found to yield a total number of positive specimens comparable to that obtained with the more sensitive complement fixation, hemagglutination, and radioimmunoassay methods. Thus, it should be noted that when carried out properly and with good reagents the CEP technique is able to approach the yield of positives which can be obtained by techniques with much greater absolute sensitivity.

Another way of comparing the clinical usefulness of these various methods is to consider what happens in patients. We have previously reported that the presence of Australia antigen in donor blood is indicative of infectivity [166]. Table 4 presents obser-

Table 4.

Au-Positive Recipients	Au-Positive Donors By Gel Diff.	CEP	HAI
45	30	34	34

vation on some of our transfusion recipients from a different point of view. These 45 transfusion recipients developed hepatitis which was Australia antigen-positive during the acute phase. It can be seen that the gel diffusion technique detected only 30 of the 45 positive cases. CEP and hemagglutination increased the yield slightly, but not by a great deal. There were still 11 cases which could not be shown to be related to a positive donor.

One must consider the possibility that the infection was acquired from sources other than the transfusion, but it may be that some donors contain such small amounts of virus that it cannot be detected even by the most sensitive techniques. The point to be made is that the CEP gave as good a yield as the more sensitive hemagglutination technique and is much less time consuming and cumbersome to perform. Thus, in terms of practical, clinical utility, we believe the CEP system has much to offer.

16. Discussion

DETECTION OF HEPATITIS-ASSOCIATED ANTIGEN: ELECTROPHORETIC ASSAY PROCEDURES

Herbert F. Polesky

Minneapolis War Memorial Blood Bank

Minneapolis, Minnesota

Counterimmunoelectrophoresis (CEP) [120], which was developed as a more rapid and sensitive screening test for HBAg, has been clearly described by Dr. Gocke, one of the investigators who pioneered the method [168,388]. I would like to reemphasize one of the points he has made, i.e., good results with CEP depend on the availability of a potent antibody.

In a series of tests on 100 normal donors found to have antibody by agar gel diffusion [377] only 20% reacted when tested by CEP and many of these could only be detected when the pool of antigen-positive sera was diluted 1:4. This is not surprising since antibodies in most normal donors are not potent and in routine CEP test systems will not be detected because of antigen excess. The same problem occurs in licensed test systems when a strong antigen is not detected unless the donor's serum is diluted. This rare phenomenon resembles prozoning as seen in some agglutination systems.

The second problem encountered in CEP systems is antibody specificity. Figure 1 shows the percentage of positive sera detected by six "potent" antibodies when tested under identical conditions against a panel of twenty reactive sera (defined by radioimmunoassay [85,295] and complement fixation [399]). These results can be partially explained by subtype differences between HBAg-positive sera. An additional cause of false negative results and limitation of the sensitivity of the test system is antibody excess. If the serum to be tested contains only a minimal quantity of antigen the CEP test may be negative though, as seen in Table 1, more sensitive methods such as RIA will be positive.

DETECTION OF HB Ag. BY CEP

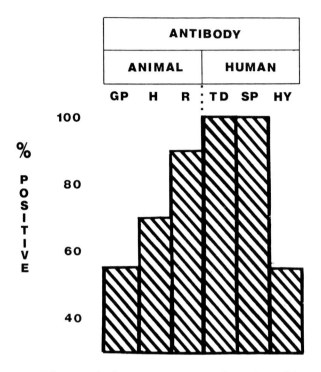

Figure 1. Twenty HBAg-positive sera tested under identical conditions using six potent antibodies. All antibodies gave 100% con-
cordance on eleven samples that included antigens known to be ad
and ay positive. (GP-guinea pig, H-horse, R-rabbit)

Table 1. Detection of HBAg: Comparison of CEP with other more
sensitive methods.

	No. Tested	No. Positive			
		AGD CEP	CF	HAI	RIA
Donors	2,125	0	0	0	4
Kidney Pts.	44	5	5	6	8
Hepatitis Pts.	56	36	35	34	45

Thus in CEP as in other precipitin systems, the concentration
of antigen and antibody can be critical and the zone of equivalence
will vary depending on the source of antibody.

Unlike Dr. Gocke, we use a 2-well pattern, testing only for antigen and have found it useful to re-read CEP plates after overnight incubation. Occasionally additional positive samples are identified by this procedure, though it is possible that the precipitin band was present but not seen immediately after the electrophoretic run.

Acknowledgements. The technical assistance of Miss Carol Olson, M.T. (ASCP) and Mrs. Margaret Hanson, M.T. (ASCP) BB, for HBAg testing and Miss Margaret Helgeson, M.T. (ASCP) BB, and Mr. Tom Hoff for art work is gratefully acknowledged.

17. COMPLEMENT FIXATION TESTS FOR DETECTION OF ANTIGEN AND ANTIBODY ASSOCIATED WITH VIRAL HEPATITIS, TYPE B

Nathalie J. Schmidt and Edwin H. Lennette

The Viral and Rickettsial Disease Laboratory, California

State Department of Public Health, Berkeley, California

The complement fixation (CF) technique has been used increasingly in the past few years for detection of hepatitis type B antigen (HBAg) in blood products, for diagnosis of type B viral hepatitis infections, and for monitoring HBAg at sequential steps of purification and after physical or chemical treatments.

This discussion will consider the relative advantages and disadvantages of the CF technique as compared to other assay methods, and also some of the problems and pitfalls in performing CF tests for detection of HBAg and antibody (anti-HBAg).

Comparative sensitivity of complement fixation, counterimmunoelectrophoresis and gel diffusion tests for detection of HBAg, anti-HBAg. CF tests are more sensitive for detection of HBAg than other procedures such as gel diffusion (GD) and counterimmunoelectrophoresis (CIEP) which are generally available to blood bank and diagnostic laboratories. However, they are more cumbersome and expensive to perform, and they require more highly-trained personnel.

Table 1 summarizes the results of several studies [15,35,218, 417,436] which have been reported on the comparative sensitivity of CF, CIEP and GD tests for detection of HBAg in sera from various sources. Overall, the CF test detected a greater number of positive sera than did the CIEP and GD tests, but with 3 groups of sera, viz, the hepatitis patients studied in this laboratory [417], sera from a state hospital [218] and sera from a group of commercial blood donors [218], an equal or greater number of antigen-positive bloods was detected by CIEP. In the case of the hepatitis

Table 1. Comparative sensitivity of complement fixation (CF),
counterimmunoelectrophoresis (CIEP) and gel diffusion (GD) for
detection of HBAg.

Ref #	Source of sera examined	Number of sera examined	Number of sera positive for HBAg by		
			CF	CIEP	GD
[35]	Hepatitis patients	180	90	75	9
[15]	Hepatitis patients	118	102	88	38
[417]	Hepatitis patients	353	162	168	160
[436]	Hepatitis patients	341	201	137	85
[436]	Renal transplant recipients	95	49	46	44
[436]	Blood donors	3,574	84	2	2
[218]	Clinical laboratory specimens	760	89	82	74
[218]	State hospital staff and patients	362	46	46	46
[218]	Commercial blood donors	7,140	29	31	21
Totals		12,923	852	675	479

patients studied in this laboratory, the sera which were positive
by CIEP and negative by CF were collected toward the end of the
antigenemia when CF titers had declined to <1:4. Thus, in some
instances the CIEP test may be more sensitive than CF tests by
virtue of the fact that sera are examined undiluted in this test
system and at dilutions of 1:4 and higher in CF tests.

Table 2. Relationship between CF titers of HBAg and ability to
detect antigen by CIEP and GD tests.

CF titer of HBAg	Number of sera	Number of sera positive for HBAg	
		CIEP	GD
1:4	16	12	5
1:8	2	2	1
1:16	4	4	3
1:32	13	13	13
1:64->1:2048	40	40	40
Totals	75	71	62

Table 2 relates the CF titers of 75 positive sera to ability of the CIEP and GD tests to detect antigen. All three types of tests were performed with the same antiserum. It is seen that the CIEP test failed to detect antigen only in sera which had low CF titers of 1:4, while the GD test was negative with some sera having CF titers of 1:4 to 1:16. Additional studies in this laboratory [420] have shown that antisera to HBAg may differ in their sensitivity for detection of HBAg in CIEP tests, and some may fail to detect antigen in sera having CF titers of 1:8 and 1:16.

It appears that the sensitivity of the CF test for detection of HBAg is only slightly greater than that of the CIEP test using antisera and procedures of maximum sensitivity, and that neither test will invariably detect antigen in all of the sera positive by the other.

Table 3. Comparative sensitivity of complement fixation (CF), gel diffusion (GD) and counterimmunoelectrophoresis (CIEP) for detection of antibody to HBAg (anti-HBAg).

CF titer of HBAg	Number of sera	Number of sera positive for HBAb by				
		GD	CIEP with antigen diluted			
			≥1:10	≥1:20	≥1:40	≥1:80
1:32	2	2	2			
1:16	1	1	1			
1:8	5	5	5			
1:4	13	13	5	6	2	
1:2	6	6	2	1	2	1
<1:4*	5	5	0	2	3	
No. positive	32	32	15	9	7	1

* Sera anticomplementary at lower dilutions

It is seen in Table 3 that the CF test is generally the least satisfactory of the three methods (CF, CIEP and GD) for detection of antibody to HBAg [417]. This is a reflection of the fact that anticomplementary (AC) activity at 1:2 serum dilutions may mask low levels of antibody. The GD test using an "enhancement pattern" is a more sensitive method for demonstrating antibody in such sera. The CIEP test is less useful than GD for detection of anti-HBAg because of the greater inhibitory effect of an antigen excess in this test system; some antibody-positive sera can be detected only through the use of very dilute antigen.

Comparative sensitivity of the complement fixation technique, hemagglutination test and radioimmunoassays for detection of HBAg, anti-HBAg. Both the hemagglutination test [477] and radioimmuno-assay procedures [214,275,483] have been found to be markedly more sensitive than CF tests for detection of antibody to HBAg, and antigen titers obtained by these techniques are also higher than CF titers. However, the tests have not been appreciably more sensitive than CF tests for detection of antigen in sera.

The hemagglutination technique described by Vyas and Shulman [477] gave antibody titers 100 times higher than those obtained in CF tests, and antibody was demonstrable in a number of sera which were negative by CF. The sensitivity of CF and hemagglutination inhibition tests was found to be comparable, however, for detection of antigen in sera from hepatitis patients.

Similarly, the radioimmunoassay (RIA) technique developed by Walsh, et al. [483], the radioimmunoprecipitation (RIP) test developed by Lander, et al. [275] and solid phase radioimmunoassay techniques [214] have been 100 to 1000 times more sensitive than CF tests for detection of antibody to HBAg, and these procedures have detected antibody in a high proportion of sera from non-ill blood donors and laboratory personnel who were negative for antibody by CF. The RIP test has also demonstrated seroconversion in viral hepatitis type B infections [276]; previously, using the CF technique, it had not been possible to demonstrate conclusively the development of antibody following primary infections [418]. Although HBAg titers obtained with radioimmunoassay techniques are generally higher than those seen in CF tests, the procedures have demonstrated antigen in only a low proportion of sera negative by CF tests.

Hemagglutination inhibition and radioimmunoassay techniques are not generally applicable at this time for routine screening for HBAg, but the CF test is almost as sensitive for this purpose and it does not require highly purified antigen or potentially hazardous radioisotopes.

Problems in the use of CF tests for detection and assay of HBAg. One impediment to the widespread use of the CF test has been the limited availability of suitable antisera for use in this system. The sera must be of relatively high titer and free from AC activity or anti-human serum reactivity at dilutions which contain 4 to 8 units of antibody. Antisera of human origin rarely have high CF titers, and satisfactory antibody levels tend to be transient. Further, sera from multiply-transfused individuals are often AC at the lower dilutions at which they would be used as a source of antibody for CF tests. Many human sera which are highly satisfactory for CIEP or GD tests are not suitable for use in CF tests. Antisera produced in animals generally contain antibodies to normal human serum proteins, and absorption to remove these antibodies may make the antisera anticomplementary. However, antisera free from antibodies to human serum proteins have been produced by immunization of guinea-pigs with highly purified antigen [398], or by immunization of guinea-pigs rendered immunologically tolerant to normal human serum proteins [303]. Antisera prepared by immunization of chimpanzees with partially purified HBAg have also been satisfactory for use in CF tests [307].

In the CF test system an excess of antigen may result in a prozone of negative fixation [111,399,418,432], and it is necessary to test serial dilutions of each serum against the standard dose of antiserum to avoid "false negative" results. This requires more antiserum than is needed in CIEP or GD tests in which only a single sample of undiluted test serum is examined, or for HAI or radioimmunoassay techniques which utilize very dilute antiserum. The need to test multiple dilutions of serum also makes the CF test more cumbersome and time-consuming to perform than CIEP or GD tests.

One objection to the use of the CF procedure in routine testing for HBAg in blood banks is the fact that most standard test procedures use an overnight incubation period for fixation of complement, and thus the test requires 2 days for completion. Studies have been conducted in our laboratory comparing the sensitivity of a 1-day CF test with that of the standard overnight procedure for detection of HBAg [419]. Although the shorter test tended to give slightly lower antigen titers than the overnight test, it was comparable in sensitivity for detection of antigen. The CF test can be automated, and with the wider availability of suitable antisera, the 1-day CF test may become feasible for large-scale use in the detection of HBAg in blood banks and clinical laboratories.

Perhaps the biggest limitation to the widespread use of the CF method in testing for HBAg is the need for experienced and well-trained personnel who are thoroughly familiar with the principles of of CF. Table 4 illustrates the variation which may occur in the ability of different laboratories to detect HBAg by the CF procedure. These data are from the National Research Council's comparative study on methods for detection of HBAg (Kissling, R. E. and Barker, L. F., personal communication). Twelve different laboratories using the same antiserum performed CF tests on a panel of 120 sera which contained 78 known positive and 42 known negative sera. It is seen that the percent of positive sera detected by CF tests ranged from 94 percent to 62 percent in the different laboratories. The ability of the laboratories to detect HBAg by CF could not be related to the basic procedure employed (all micro methods). It is likely that the amount of experience which a

laboratory has in CF testing is the most important factor in determining the reliability of their tests for detection of HBAg.

Table 4. Variation in the ability of different laboratories to
detect HBAg by complement fixation tests. Tests conducted by 12
different laboratories using the same antiserum.

Percent of positive sera detected	Number of laboratories	Basic CF method employed*
94	2	A, B
93	1	C
92	1	A
90	1	B
87	2	A, D
85	1	A
75	1	?
69	1	C
67	1	A
62	1	C

*A -Lennette, E. H. in Diagnostic Procedures for Viral and Rickett-
   sial Infections, 4th Ed. Amer. Pub. Health Assoc., 1969, p.52.
 B -Sever, J. L., J. Immunol. 88:320, 1962.
 C -Casey, H.L., Pub. Health Monograph No. 74, 1965.
 D -Kent, J. F. and Fife, E. H., Amer. J. Trop. Med. and Hyg.
   12:103, 1963.

     A modified complement fixation method has been described [252]
which may prove to be suitable for large-scale screening. It utilizes gels in which sensitized sheep erythrocytes are imbedded. Mixtures of test serum, antibody and complement are incubated and then
added to wells in the gel. After incubation at 37°C for one hour,
negative reactions are detected by a halo of lysed erythrocytes
around the well, while positive CF reactions are indicated by lack
of hemolysis. This procedure does not require daily standardization of reagents or as much technical experience as do conventional
CF techniques.

     Occurrence and significance of anticomplementary activity in
sera from hepatitis patients. Anticomplementary (AC) activity of
test sera, i.e., fixation of complement by the serum alone in the
absence of antibody or antigen, may mask low levels of HBAg or anti-

HBAg, as was illustrated above in the case of sera containing low levels of antibody, and this may limit the value of the CF test in some instances.

In certain studies, a high proportion of hepatitis patients have shown AC activity in their sera during the course of their illness, and AC titers have been higher than those seen in routine CF testing [432,462]. It has been suggested that the activity is due to the presence of immune complexes of HBAg and anti-HBAg [432], and that the demonstration of AC activity in sera from hepatitis patients may have diagnostic significance.

Table 5. Occurrence of anticomplementary (AC) activity in sera from hepatitis patients.

Ref. #	Patients studied	Number	HBAg	#	AC activity #	%
[432]	Hepatitis patients	130**	+ 0	98 42	123	95
[399]	Hepatitis patients	32**	+ 0	4 28	1 4	16
[399]	Patients without hepatitis	32**	0	32	1	
[418]	Hepatitis patients	86**	+ 0	47 39	6 5	13
[80]	Hepatitis patients	28	+	28	4	14
[358]	Hepatitis patients	43	+ 0	23 20	5	12
[358]	Patients without liver disease	50	+ 0	2 48	7	14
[462]	Hepatitis patients	46	+	46	4	9
[462]	Cirrhosis patients	22	+	22	10	46
[462]	Healthy carriers of HBAg	39	+	39	3	8

** Serial specimens examined

Table 5 summarizes the occurrence of AC activity in sera from hepatitis patients in various studies. In the first study [432]

AC activity was observed in 95 percent of the patients at some
time during the course of hepatitis. The concept that AC activity
in these sera was due to immune complexes was strengthened by the
demonstration that the activity was reversible by incubation with
excess antigen (purified) or antibody. Ross and Pringle [412] have
also suggested that AC activity may be due to immune complexes of
HBAg and antibody, and they reported that antigen and antibody may
be dissociated by heating the sera at 85°C for one hour, which
apparently destroys the antibody and results in the disappearance
of AC activity and the demonstration of higher CF titers of antigen.

     In the next two studies shown in Table 5, which also examined
serial serum specimens from hepatitis patients, AC activity was
noted in a much smaller proportion of the patients (13 and 16 percent), and levels of AC activity were low. In the study conducted
in this laboratory [418] attempts were made to reverse the AC
activity of hepatitis patients' sera by incubating with an excess
of HBAg; however, of 22 sera tested, only one showed specific
reduction in AC activity after incubation with excess antigen;
the other sera showed either no change in AC titer, or a similar
reduction after incubation with either antigen-containing or negative sera.

     In the next three studies, which dealt with single serum spe-
cimens, the percent of hepatitis patients showing AC activity in
their serum ranged between 9 and 14 percent. Newman, et al. [358]
found a similar proportion of AC sera in patients with hepatitis
and in those without liver disease. Thiry, et al. [462] noted a
much higher incidence of AC activity in sera from patients with
cirrhosis than in hepatitis patients or healthy carriers.

     These findings indicate that the demonstration of AC activity
in sera from hepatitis patients must be interpreted with caution,
and it should not be considered to represent immune complexes of
HBAg and antibody unless this can be confirmed by electron microscopy [9] or by the specific reversal of the activity with excess HBAg
or anti-HBAg [432]. AC activity in human sera may be the result
of other antigen-antibody systems such as the coronavirus immune
complexes demonstrated by Zuckerman, et al. [500], and it may also
be produced by prolonged storage of sera, even in the frozen state,
by repeated freezing and thawing of sera, or by a variety of other
conditions which cause denaturation of serum globulins.

18. Discussion
COMPLEMENT FIXATION TESTS

N. R. Shulman

National Institutes of Health, National Institute of

Arthritis and Metabolic Diseases, Bethesda, Maryland

I think Dr. Schmidt has presented an excellent, accurate and realistic summary of the complement fixation procedure among various procedures that are available for routine screening of samples for the hepatitis antigen and/or antibody. I would like to offer an opinion concerning some of the complications, and perhaps an explanation for some of the observations that seem a bit obscure about the complement fixation procedure.

I will first speak with respect to speed of reaction. I have never had the patience to wait overnight for a complement fixation procedure result, so our tests have all been done with a one-hour incubation, at most; within two or two and a half hours I think one can get the accuracy that was depicted on one of Dr. Schmidt's figures. This is, I think, comparable to the sensitivity available by overnight incubation procedures.

I think also with respect to radioimmunoassay we tend to put down "one" or "two" or "five" days, when comparing with another technique, but the times are getting shorter and I think a matter of hours will be permissible for any of the techniques that we have discussed so far, or probably will discuss.

With respect to simplicity, I think there is also no argument there. Anyone attending this Symposium, I think, would be insulted if it were said that he couldn't do a complement fixation test. On the other hand, it may not be worth doing if it is a little more complicated than some other technique and does not give you any more information. We ourselves, when we screen, use the counter immunoelectrophoretic test for antigen, because to use

a complement fixation test does not give us that much more information. We find the complement fixation test a valuable tool,
particularly for research procedures; however, sometimes when we
have a complement fixation test set up, we use it for screening
blood donors rather than electrophoresis, because they are both
comparable in terms of numbers of positives that they pick up.

With respect to sensitivity, I think that is a very important
consideration, and I think it is becoming apparent that the techniques of counterimmunoelectrophoresis and complement fixation and
hemagglutination inhibition for antigen are going to be roughly
comparable. Even immunodiffusion, a sensitive technique in some
laboratories, is going to give the same number of percent positives
in a donor population.

On the other hand, I don't think there is any argument at all
that hemagglutination and radioimmunoassay are 100 or 1,000-fold
times more sensitive for antibody. I won't talk further about that
because it will be discussed soon. I will dismiss complement fixation as a technique for measuring antibody routinely, say in the
post-infectious period of hepatitis, and now talk about the measurement of antigen.

I think what we are dealing with is probably a skewed concentration of antigen in a population, and each of the techniques
that is a little more sensitive for the antigen measurement just
does not allow us to pick up that many more positive individuals.

In some work with archeological sera, in which I aided Dr.
Barker and Dr. Murray, it was found that serum could be diluted a
million-fold, e.g., down from 10^8 or 10^9 particles to 10^3 particles
and still cause infection (as determined by the presence of HBAg
or jaundice developing in the recipient). Yet, if the particular
serum that was used for inoculation was diluted perhaps 100 times,
we would lose the ability to detect antigen, by any of the sensitive
techniques. Therefore, only the top fraction of HBAg carriers can
be detected in the population. This would be true with the complement fixation procedure and probably counterelectrophoresis,
which would be a portion less sensitive, but not sufficiently different in sensitivity that it would pick up many fewer or more
carriers.

I believe the "guesstimates" are that a third of the positives
are being picked up now. It has not yet been reported but suppos-
ing it were possible to sensitize the test another one or two logs,
as probably will be possible by radioimmunoassay; then, with one
log additional sensitivity, it may be possible to pick up another
few positives. The detection system would have to be pushed perhaps two logs more sensitive before 2/3 of the positives would be

detected, and there would still be many, as Dr. Gocke implied, un-measurable with that increased sensitivity.

One word about anti-complementary activity. I think I have to say something about that, because of the very high frequency of anti-complementary reactions in one group of patients that we stud-ied. This was in our report several years ago, and one group of 130 patients that Dr. Schmidt referred to was a group among the more than 300 we studied, and this group was from Dr. Murray's collection. We had 4,000 individual blood samples on that group, roughly 30 apiece, after inoculation. In that group we found an unusual pattern of anti-complementary activity. We noticed in six of the patients that there was a peculiar pattern of anti-complementary activity developing, sometimes before antigen appeared, and then again sometimes in the recovery period. The sera that showed anti-complementary activity of that type were analyzed thor-oughly by electron microscopy and by neutralization with excess antigen and antibody, as referred to by Dr. Schmidt; we did not analyze the sera from all 130 patients. On the basis of the fact that the anti-complementary activity was associated with particles in the plasma; and that it did disappear in the presence of anti-gen excess during this acute disease; and that it reappeared again, sometimes, in a few patients in the recovery period; we proposed that this represented antigen-antibody complexes.

19. DETECTION OF HEPATITIS B ANTIGEN AND ANTIBODIES BY HEMAGGLUTINATION ASSAY

G. N. Vyas, M. A. Mason, E. W. Williams

University of California, School of Medicine

San Francisco, California

More than 30 years ago the immunochemical basis of serologic specificity was, conceptually and experimentally, elucidated by Landsteiner [278]; more recently the investigation of biochemical aspects of human blood group substances [327] has extended these concepts and enhanced the usefulness of hemagglutination procedures in immunochemistry and molecular biology. For more than half a century, the inhibition of ABH hemagglutination by water soluble salivary blood group substances, their haptens and simple sugars has been routinely used in serial dilutions for their quantitation. The passive adsorption of proteins on erythrocytes treated with tannic acid, and subsequent hemagglutination with antiprotein sera, described by Boyden [70] provided an unlimited scope for this simple serologic procedure. Passive hemagglutination or indirect hemagglutination (HA) is an antigen-antibody reaction causing agglutination of inert indicator red cells coated either with an antigen or infrequently with an antibody of sufficient immunochemical purity [202]. Most antigens can be coated on the surface of the red cells by means of a variety of chemical agents; cells thus coated are among the most sensitive means of detecting minute amounts of antibodies which are incapable of causing immunoprecipitation in agargel [155,202]. Inhibition of minimal amounts of such antibodies has been most advantageously used for detection of homologous antigens by hemagglutination inhibition (HAI). The simplicity, convenience, rapidity and sensitivity with which HA and HAI can be carried out make them important serological procedures in laboratory medicine.

While studying the effects of metallic cations on human erythrocytes, Jandl and Simmons discovered chromic chloride as an agent

for coupling human plasma proteins to red cells [233]. This method
has been extensively applied to a variety of immunological assays
by Fudenberg, et al. [156]. The principles of competitive binding
between antigen and antibody form the conceptual basis for the
hemagglutination assay [477] and the radioimmunoassay (RIA) for
detection of antigens and antibodies associated with viral hepatitis type B [86]. However, for a successful HA or RIA, highly purified monotypic HBAg and/or anti-HBAg are essential.

Anti-HBAg-coated red cells.   Juji and Yokochi used HBAg-anti-
HBAg complexes for dissociation and chromatographic separation of
IgG anti-HBAg [238]. They coated the antibody onto formalinized,
tanned human erythrocytes and detected HBAg by direct agglutination of antibody-coated red cells. This system, termed reversed
passive hemagglutination, was found to be more sensitive than the
gel-diffusion method. In a well carried-out study they found that
50 out of 54 HBAg-positive sera were specifically detected by anti-
HBAg-coated cells. With four sera, the agglutination was considered non-specific because normal human IgG-coated control erythrocytes were also agglutinated and hence indistinguishable from the
specific agglutination reaction. The fact that 94% of the patients
with HBAg are positive for rheumatoid factor [493] necessitates a
reevaluation of the Japanese work with improved affinity-chromato-
graphic separation of anti-HBAg, and taking into account the heterogeneity of the HBAg [12]. This question is currently being looked
at in our laboratory and we hope to get the results in the not-too-
distant future. A latex-agglutination test employing an identical
approach has been evaluated and the results will be presented by
Dr. Perkins in his discussion later in this session.

Purified HBAg coupled to red cells for HA and HAI.   Plasma
from normal blood donors positive for HBAg can be obtained in
large amounts by plasmapheresis. Two-unit plasmapheresis per week
can be carried out for several months, without significant drop in
titer of the antigen. A large amount of such plasma obtained from
an apparently healthy normal young adult has been distributed to
several investigators as NBRP HBAg Control #1. This donor is type
ad [283]. Isolation of the HBAg from plasma proteins is accomplished by two successive isopycnic bandings in cesium chloride gradients. A final rate sedimentation in a cesium chloride gradient
resolves the HBAg into its three morphologic forms [67,158]. The
details of the isolation will be covered at some length by Dr.
Gerin and Dr. Bond in their topics later in this Symposium. The
first peak consisting exclusively of 20 nm particles is taken as
the purified antigen which is devoid of detectable human plasma
proteins. Because of the high cost of purification of HBAg, it is
not yet available for extensive experimental work on HA and HAI
using HBAg-coated cells.

The extinction coefficient, $E_{1\ cm}^{0.1\%}$ = 3.73, serves as a useful
guide for measuring protein concentrations. A 0.35 mg/ml solution
giving an optical density of 1.3 at 280 nm wavelength is found
optimal for coating red cells stored for 2 - 10 days at 4°C. Although an enhanced coupling of HBAg could be accomplished by using
cells stored for less than twenty-four hours, in our experience
this only enhances the titer of anti-HBAg without an increase in
the ability to detect additional HBAg-positive sera in the HAI.
Indeed, the detection of anti-HBAg in normal and patient sera is
increased to a level where several serial two-fold dilutions are
required to detect excess antigen in the sera showing presence of
weak anti-HBAg. In our laboratory we have chosen to truncate this
level of antibody detection to make detection of HBAg less cumbersome without sacrificing the primary objective of detecting the
HBAg by HAI. Conventionally four agglutinating units of antibody
are used in the inhibition assay for detection of an antigen; this
ensures that the results are unequivocal since a threshold dose
of antibody may cause failure to agglutinate the cells, a result
indistinguishable from a true inhibition reaction. However, Dr.
Prince successfully uses two agglutinating units of anti-HBAg for
the modified HAI assay using overnight incubation at 4°C. Since
the methods used in Dr. Prince's laboratory and our laboratory
are essentially similar it would be redundant to detail the
assay when Dr. Prince has described it in his discussion. The
steps involved in the hemagglutination assay for detection of
antigen and antibodies related to HBAg are outlined as follows:

1. <u>HBAg coating of cells with CrCl$_3$</u>

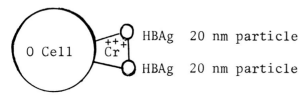

2. <u>Antibody detection</u>

Test Serum (T.S.) + HBAg-cells → Aggln. = Anti-HBAg in serum

3. <u>Antigen detection</u>

T.S. + 4 units anti-HBAg + HBAg-cells
    (incubated at 25°C for 60 minutes)

Aggln. = T.S. -ve

No Aggln. = T.S. +ve

Kinetics of HBAg binding to red cells. The checkerboard method, using various dilutions of a given antigen and chromic chloride [476], was adapted by Vyas and Shulman [477] for serologically determining the optimal conditions for coating HBAg onto red cells. Since the mechanism and the role of various factors controlling the binding of HBAg is poorly understood, the kinetics of protein binding were studied by using ^{125}I-labelled HBAg and ^{51}CrCl$_3$. The labelling of HBAg was carried out by the method of Hunter and Greenwood [225] using a reaction time of only 15 minutes [1]. The labelled material was mixed with concentrated HBAg so that the mixture had an O.D.$_{280}$ of 2.0. Radiolabelled ^{51}CrCl$_3$ was added to 1% CrCl$_3$ and used with ^{125}I-HBAg in a representative checkerboard experiment (Table 1) for determining the amount of ^{51}Cr and ^{125}I-HBAg bound to red cells which had been stored for four days at 4°C.

Table 1. Coating red cells with HBAg and CrCl$_3$. The serial numbers in the table denote the coat number

		1% CrCl$_3$ Dilutions		
HBAg	1:10	1:20	1:30	1:40
O.D. 2.0	1	2	3	4
" 1.0	5	6	7	8
O.D. 0.5	9	10	11	12
" 0.25	13	14	15	16
O.D. 0.1	17	18	19	20

The results of the serologic reaction (Table 2) show that there is a threshold of cell-bound HBAg below which it is serologically undetectable. It was also shown that, depending upon the age of the red cells, there is considerable variation in the amount of HBAg bound to the red cells. Because a large proportion of HBAg remains unbound, Dr. Prince uses the unbound HBAg in two or three consecutive binding procedures. The maximum amount of cell bound HBAg (∿30%) is found when red cells less than 24 hours old are used. The freshly drawn,well oxygenated, red cells usually get too strongly coated. Such strongly coated cells detect antibodies in 10 - 15 percent of normal sera tested and about 50 - 80 percent of the sera from persons with a history of hepatitis during the period two-years preceeding testing (author's unpublished observations). The titers of antibody detected with heavily coated cells approach those obtained with RIA. There remains little doubt that HA is the most sensitive, simple and rapid method for detection of anti-HBAg [394,430,456], irrespective of the d and y subtype specificities (author's observations).

Table 2. Counts per minute (C.P.M.) for cell-bound ^{51}Cr and ^{125}I-labelled HBAg. The normal cells coated with HBAg and titrated with human anti-HBAg show that the threshold for detection of cell-bound HBAg is around 10,000 C.P.M. (10% binding)

Coat #	^{51}Cr C.P.M.	^{125}I C.P.M.	Ratio of $^{51}Cr/^{125}I$	Anti-HBAg Titer
1	36,357	9,108	3.992	1280
2	18,045	10,215	1.766	1800
3	11,918	9,685	1.231	1800
4	4,018	2,262	1.776	0
5	16,312	5,782	2.821	0
6	13,238	5,110	2.591	0
7	3,865	2,050	1.884	0
8	6,910	4,960	1.393	0
9	32,555	11,835	2.750	1800
10	13,992	7,190	1.950	0
11	16,322	6,192	2.636	0
12	3,220	968	3.326	0
13	23,498	6,880	3.410	0
14	3,172	2,082	1.523	0
15	6,507	2,342	2.779	0
16	5,968	890	6.70	0
17	27,565	7,005	3.935	0
18	21,228	4,732	4.486	0
19	8,142	1,408	5.780	0
20	4,768	2,092	2.279	0

Storage of HBAg-coated red cells. HBAg-coated red cells in glycerol can be frozen at -20°C in glycerol, stored for at least three months, or frozen in liquid nitrogen without alteration of their reactivity. The method for freezing cells in glycerol and recovering them is described by Mollison [325]. The recovery of glycerolized-frozen cells is poor (~35%). However, HBAg-coated cells have been frozen in liquid nitrogen using the method of Huntsman, et al. [226] and the recovery has been about 70 percent of HBAg-coated cells. Several investigators find that storage of HBAg-coated cells in liquid nitrogen is convenient and practical. Frozen cells offer a great advantage of uniformity of test reagents over a period of time.

Chemical fixation of red cells. Since storage in liquid nitrogen for transportation was found rather impractical for HBAg-

coated red cells and freshly-coated cells start deteriorating
after about a week, an improved hemagglutination assay should have
red cell membranes chemically stabilized to permit uniform and
successful coating with HBAg and long term storage of the coated
cells. After several failures with aldehyde fixed cells, we decided to use difluorodinitrobenzene [40]. A 20 mg percent concentration of 1,5-difluoro-2,4-dinitrobenzene was found adequate in
fixation of red cells so that they were totally resistant to lysis
by distilled water.

Cells stored under refrigeration for 24 hours were washed
free of plasma proteins and 0.5 ml of the packed cells was suspended in 100 ml of freshly made buffer (pH 7.8) containing 90 ml Hart-
mann's lactate ringer solution, 5 ml of 0.1 M phosphate buffer,
4 ml of 0.3 M dextrose, 1 ml 0.15 M magnesium sulfate and 0.5 g.
sodium bicarbonate. 20 mg/ml of difluorodinitro-benzene dissolved
in absolute methanol was gradually added to the cell suspension.
After 4 hours reaction at room temperature with constant sti. ring
the cells were fixed. The suspension was centrifuged and the sediment of fixed cells was washed four times. The washed packed cells
were used in studying the kinetics of ^{125}I-HBAg binding using
^{51}CrCl$_3$. The results are depicted in Table 3. The data indicate
that binding of ^{51}Cr and HBAg to fixed cells is more uniform than
that with the untreated cells (Table 2).

Table 3. Red cells fixed with 20 mg percent DFDNB followed by
coating with ^{125}I-HBAg in the presence of ^{51}CrCl$_3$, C.P.M./ml

Coat #	^{51}Cr C.P.M.	^{125}I C.P.M.	Ratio of ^{51}Cr/^{125}I	Anti- HBAg Titer
1	1,975	4,508	0.4381	1280
2	2,178	2,612	0.8336	640
3	1,550	2,228	0.6957	320
4	1,422	2,230	0.6379	80
5	1,720	4,848	0.3548	320
6	2,022	3,245	0.6233	640
7	2,028	3,148	0.6442	80
8	1,588	2,900	0.5474	80
9	1,425	5,048	0.2823	10
10	758	3,592	0.2109	10
11	1,585	3,645	0.4348	10
12	1,425	3,605	0.3953	10

In a limited number of tests the cell coat #1 stored up to 30 days
at refrigeration temperature was suitable both for HA and HAI for

HBAg. Although still in the developmental stage, this procedure shows promise of being a stable, reproducible system for the detection of HBAg.

Evaluation of HA for detection of HBAg. The first report of a hemagglutination assay by Vyas and Shulman [477] demonstrated that HA is a simple, sensitive, specific and rapid method for detection of the antigen and antibodies associated with viral hepatitis type B. HA was shown to be 2,000-fold more sensitive for the detection of antibody and HAI was shown to be 100-fold more sensitive for the detection of the antigen than the standard immunodiffusion test [430]. In the first large-scale coordinated trial of various test procedures and reagents (conducted in 1970 by the C.D.C., N.R.C., N.I.H), limited results from HAI indicated it was the most specific and most sensitive procedure for HBAg.

A comparison of the standard counter-current electrophoresis (CEP) and HAI, using the same antiserum for testing sera of hepatitis patients, revealed the failure rate of CEP to be five-fold more than HAI for the detection of the HBAg (Table 4).

Table 4. Comparison of CEP and HAI for HBAg testing on sera of 700 patients with clinical hepatitis. The same goat anti-HBAg was used for both CEP and HAI.

	CEP+	CEP-
HAI+	201	50
HAI-	9	440

A similar correlation was also found by Shaffer et al. in the case of concurrent testing of 8,000 normal healthy blood donors [427]. The data of Shaffer et al. indicated that besides the relative sensitivities of the test procedures, the antibody specificity was the most significant cause of discordant results [427]. Depending upon the antibody used, the hemagglutination assay can detect 1-60 ng amounts of HBAg [478]. Purely on conceptual and pragmatic grounds we assumed that the best possible HA system should employ antibodies against the common determinant "a" of ad and ay subtypes. Selection of suitable antisera was based on tests with a battery of antisera. The ad type HBAg isolated from N.B.R.P. HBAg #1 was used as the coat material. The results are represented in Figure 1. The antibodies most successful in detecting maximum number of selected discrepant samples happen to be of human origin. Subsequent tests by Dr. Le Bouvier showed that these antisera had anti-a specificity. What we do not know about the specificities of anti-HBAg became more apparent when

CELLS COATED WITH HAA #1

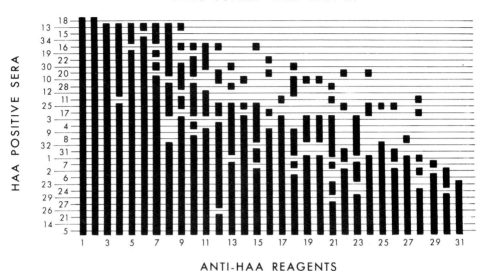

Figure 1. Hemagglutination inhibition of 31 antisera by a panel
of 32 HBAg-positive human sera selected for discrepancy in previous results. These 32 sera included both ad and ay subtypes.
Antisera 1, 2 and 3 were of human origin and typed as anti-a by
Dr. Le Bouvier. Antiserum 1 was an antibody from a dialysis
patient in France and kindly provided in large amount by Professor
J. P. Soulier of the National Blood Transfusion Service, Paris.

CELLS COATED WITH HAA #2

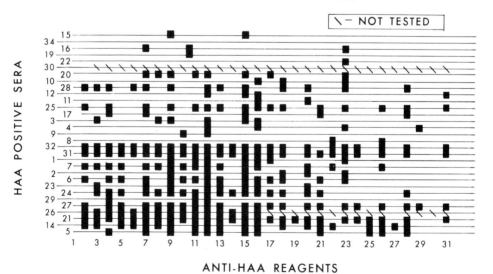

Figure 2. Results of hemagglutination assay performed on the antisera and HBAg-positive sera shown above (Figure 1) using another
HBAg, purified and provided by Dr. Brumelhuis of Amsterdam. The
results are not consistent with the hypothesis of anti-a having
the ability to detect HBAg in an unfailing manner by hemagglutination assay, irrespective of the HBAg subtype used for coating
red cells.

another HBAg coat was used and the results with the same human
anti-HBAg of subtype "a" specificity were not consistant with the
concept that anti-a may form an unfailing HAI system (Figure 2).
A further revelation came in a more recent trial conducted by Dr.
Goldfield for the group of contractors of the National Blood Resource Program. We found that in using the routine system in our
laboratory we were missing certain ay type HBAg-positive sera which
were picked up in Dr. Prince's laboratory indicating that the antibody used by Dr. Prince has performed better than the selected
human antibody from France that we have been using in our laboratory. I am sure Dr. Prince will discuss his accumulated data and
experience in HAI, particularly with regard to the subtypes of
HBAg.

An outstanding advantage of the HAI is the unequivocal specificity of HBAg-positive results, which are possible to accomplish
with the current state of the art in conceptual and technical
immunochemistry. The question of specificity may be of national
value particularly in blood donor screening since a false positive
laboratory test for HBAg can stigmatize the voluntary blood donor
who forms a valuable human resource for our country.

In conclusion, from the author's personal experience, it seems
that HAI and RIA are experimental methods most suitable for detection of HBAg. Until the subtleties of the antibody specificity
and the nature of the antigen and its subtypes are adequately understood, HAI may be held in abeyance as the method of choice. In my
opinion, HAI lends itself to versatile serologic engineering and
experimental manipulations to yield a system best suited for large
scale rapid and successful testing of HBAg. Our efforts are directed towards a careful development of such a system and its
automation.

Acknowledgments. Original investigations reported in this
review were supported in part by the U.S.P.H.S. Research Grants
AM-14514, CC-00578 and Contract N.I.H. 71-2355. We cannot adequately acknowledge our debt to Dr. George Le Bouvier of Yale
University, for helping us with subtyping of selected sera and
for getting us started with subtyping work.

20. Discussion

HEMAGGLUTINATION ASSAY: SUBTYPING BY
HEMAGGLUTINATION INHIBITION, AN ULTRA-
SENSITIVE IDENTITY TEST FOR HB ANTIGEN

A. M. Prince, B. Brotman, and H. Ikram

The New York Blood Center and Cornell Medical Center

New York, New York

It is not often that people working in different parts of
the country on a highly competitive problem with the same techniques become close friends. However, anyone who has had the experience of working with a technique that is relatively insensitive
knows the degree of gratitude one feels when someone develops a
technique which is more sensitive. The development by Vyas and
Shulman of a hemagglutination assay for detection of the hepatitis
B antigen (HBAg) and antibody (anti-HBAg) and their willingness to
make this technique available to all investigators has been appreciated by all of us.

I would like to discuss very briefly several aspects of the
hemagglutination technique. The question that is perhaps most
germane to the blood banking community is whether this technique
is likely to be useful for routine screening of donor blood, and
if so, when? I agree entirely with Dr. Vyas that this technique
has great potential and that it is a marvelous research tool.

However, many laboratories, including our own, have had difficulty both in preparation for and execution of this technique.
Not all red cells are adequate, and, as Dr. Vyas has clearly indicated, not all batches of antigen are suitable for coating. Some
lots of antiserum are not suitable for agglutination inhibition
tests. These problems require additional study on a research
level. It thus seems unlikely, at least for the present, that
this technique will be employed as a routine screening method.

Hemagglutination and hemagglutination inhibition assay
methods. We have relied heavily on a modification of the passive
hemagglutination method first described by Vyas and Shulman [477].
As our method appears to be more sensitive than that described by
these authors, we describe it here in detail:

1. Group O Rh-negative red cells are collected in ACD or EDTA and
used for coating 12-24 hours after collection. Prior to use, red
cells are oxygenated to arterial blood color by gentle shaking or
magnetic stirring.

2. Cells are washed four times >10 volumes of normal saline,
packed with a final centrifugation of 20 minutes at 4,000 rpm,
and made up to 40% v/v.

3. For coating we mix in order:

    a. 3 volumes purified (>90% purity) antigen in normal saline
    b. 1 volume, 40% washed rbc
    c. 1 volume chromic chloride, 33 mg/100 ml saline
       ($CrCl_3$-$6H_2O$)

We have usually employed purified antigen obtained from Electro
Nucleonics Laboratories, 4921 Auburn Avenue, Bethesda, Maryland
20014. This is first concentrated (if necessary) to an $O.D._{280}$
of 0.7 or greater by ultrafiltration with an Amicon PM30 filter.
The antigen is then dialyzed overnight vs. 2 changes of 100 volumes of normal saline. Preliminary coating is then carried out
with 25 µl rbc, 75 µl antigen and 25 µl chromic chloride using
dilutions of antigen. These are tested to determine the lowest
concentration of antigen giving optimal antibody titers in the
HA test, with clear negative patterns in control wells receiving
no antibody. Optimal antigen concentrations with different batches
of purified antigen which we have used, have varied in $O.D._{280}$
between 0.31 and 0.72 (0.1 - 0.2 mg/ml assuming $E^{0.1\%}_{1\ cm}$ = 3.73 [478]).

4. The coating mixture is held for 5 minutes at room temperature
with gentle mixing and then centrifuged. The supernatant fluid is
immediately placed in 1/4" diameter dialysis tubing and rapidly
dialyzed against 2 x 100 volumes of saline overnight. The solution is then concentrated to 80% of the volume of the antigen
added to the first coating mixture, and used for a second coating.

5. The coated cells are washed four times with saline and finally
suspended in Vyas and Shulman's TAP buffer: 0.01 M phosphate-
buffered normal saline, pH 7.2 containing 0.0025% PVP (40,000 Mol.
weight), 1/20,000 Tween 80, and 0.01% sodium azide. Bovine serum
albumin (Armour, Fraction V̄) is added, 0.5% v/v concentration, to the
solution used for a day's work only. When large batches of cells

are being prepared for routine use, they are suspended in TAP buffer to a volume corresponding to half the volume of antigen used for coating. The cell suspension is then diluted with an equal volume of the cryoprotective additive solution described by Rowe et al. [413]. This solution is prepared by adding 70 ml of glycerol, (Fischer high purity grade, 99%) to 180 ml of 4.2% mannitol in 0.9% sodium chloride.

The cell suspension is then sealed in pyrex ampoules (Wheaton Glass Co.) in amounts suitable for one day's work. 1 ml of frozen cells provides about 280 ml of final suspension.

6. For each day's use, one ampoule is removed from liquid nitrogen storage, and thawed rapidly by immersion in a 42°C water bath. The red cells are diluted in 10 volumes of 16% mannitol in 0.9% saline and centrifuged for 5 minutes at 1000 rpm. The cells are then washed in 0.9% saline by 2 to 3 additional centrifugations for 2 minutes at 5000 rpm until no hemoglobin is visible in the supernatant. The cells are finally resuspended in TAP buffer to a concentration of about 0.05% v/v, i.e., 1 ml frozen cells to 280 ml of TAP buffer.

7. Hemagglutination (HA) and hemagglutination inhibition (HAI) titrations are carried out with an automatic dilution apparatus (Autotiter II, Canalco Instruments, Rockville, Maryland) using disposable V-shaped plastic depression plates having 8 rows of 15 depressions. Each serum is thus tested at 15 dilutions. Each plate includes as a control, a) TAP buffer and, b) Standard antiserum or antigen of known titer which had been stored at -70°C.

Hemagglutination inhibition (HAI) titrations are carried out by simultaneous addition of 2 HA units of antibody to the antigen dilution. Coated red cells are then added after a one hour incubation period.

8. For logistic reasons, and because we find plates easier to read by this method, we hold our plates overnight at 4°C, then 1 hour at room temperature prior to centrifuging in special carriers (Canalco) in a PR-2 International Equipment Co. Centrifuge for 30 seconds at 1000 rpm at 20°C. The plates are then held at an angle of 60 degrees for 30 minutes prior to reading on an inclined viewer of the type used for reading X-rays, i.e., white glass transilluminated with white fluorescent bulbs.

In hemagglutination titrations the end point is taken as the highest dilution showing complete agglutination, i.e., all cells are confined to a clear button with no streaming.

In hemagglutination inhibition titrations, the end point is taken as the highest dilution showing no agglutination, i.e., cells stream uniformly in a line to the edge of the well.

9. To test for specificity of HA tests we dilute the specimen in parallel in TAP buffer and in TAP buffer containing 1000 HAI units per 0.025 ml of HBAg. An eight-fold or greater reduction of HA titer is taken to indicate inhibition. To test for specificity of HAI tests we test in parallel with 2 HA units of anti-HBAg and with 100 units. An eight-fold or greater reduction in titer is taken to indicate specific inhibition.

Coated-red cells may be preserved at 4°C for several weeks in the following maintenance solution: (Personal communication, W. J. M. Duimel and H. G. J. Brummelhuis, Central Laboratory Netherlands Red Cross): 0.02 M Na_2EDTA, 0.02 M $Na_2HPO_4 \cdot 2H_2O$, 0.5% w/v glucose, 0.1% w/v chloramphenicol, 0.75% human serum albumin (added in the form of 1/5 volume 3.5% albumin in 0.004 M Na caprylate, 3% dextrose in normal saline).

Comparative sensitivity of the hemagglutination inhibition (HAI) assay for detection of HBAg. At the AABB meeting in Chicago [391], we reported, as did Dr. Vyas, that HAI detected 20% more HBAg carriers than counter electrophoresis (CEP) (Table 1).

Table 1. Comparison of sensitivity of IEOP and HAI techniques for detection of HBAg carriers.

Population	# Tested	# IEOP/ AGD +	# HAI Additional +		# IEOP + Missed by HAI
			≥1:128	1:8-1:64	
Donors-volunteer	680	0	2	3	0
paid	462	2	1	1	0
Drug Addicts	340	4	0	3	0
Senegal Army	227	35	5	8	4
Mentally Retarded in large institutions	1300	158	26	10	15

I think this was an underestimate of the comparative sensitivity of HAI. Initially, we compared CEP and HAI by testing sera drawn from different populations. Included in these populations were children from institutions for the mentally retarded, persons from Africa, paid and volunteer blood donors. We now know that the mean quantity of antigen present in serum of retarded children and Africans is much higher than that found in U.S. blood donors.

If the comparison is restricted to volunteer or paid blood donors, 2 to 3 times as many HBAg carriers are detected by HAI.

Why do different antisera that seem to have anti "a" specificity differ so widely in their ability to detect sera containing HBAg? It is possible that detection of the common "a" antigenic specificity may be related to the affinity of a particular antibody; and may also depend upon how much of the "a" locus is seen by the particular collection of antibodies that we call an antiserum. Whether or not an antigen is suitable for use in coating red cells may also depend on how much of the "a" locus is exposed.

Use of HAI for subtyping of HBAg. Sera to be tested for subtypes a, y and d are tested by use of cells coated with either ad or ay antigen and tested versus absorbed antiserum that is more than 90% monospecific for A, Y or D (Table 2).

Table 2.   Subtype analysis

| Serum # | Titer of HAI with Lot 17a Cells (ad) vs | | | | Titer of HAI with Lot 18a Cells (ay) vs | | | Con-clu-sion |
	Pool #1 1:100,000 (8 units)	GP anti-d 1:6,400 (2 units)	d	Pool #1 1:100,000 (2 units)	RK/D 1:2,400 (4 units)	y	
69- 352	128	<2	-	1024	512	+	ay
69- 459	256	<2	-	1024	1024	+	ay
69- 350	256	2048	+	64	<2	-	ad
69-4730	1024	4096	+	512	<2	-	ad
68-1534	128	<2	-	<2	<2	-	? a
68-1782	64	<2	-	64	<2	-	? a

Monospecific Y antibody can, for example, be obtained by absorption of an AYX antiserum with adx antigen in the region of antigen excess [392]. HAI is ideally suited for subtyping since only 2 to 4 units of antibody are employed in the inhibition tests.

We have investigated possible associations between subtype antigens and virulence. Initially it appeared that subtype ay was more frequently associated with acute illness. However, this interpretation has not been supported by additional subtype analysis: 64% of cases of fulminant hepatitis from France and no cases from the U.S. were found to be ad; asymptomatic chronic HBAg carriers with a past history of illicit drug use were almost all ay, as were acute cases of hepatitis arising from that population; 80% of blood donors from New York City were found to be ad; cases of chronic active hepatitis and post-transfusion hepatitis from the U. S. were found to be equally associated with ad and ay (Table 3).

Table 3.   Distribution of subtype antigens in disease sera.

		HAI Test Results		
Category	Number Tested	AD %+	AY %+	? A % +
1. Acute Hepatitis				
Fulminant Hepatitis				
USA	6	0	NT	0
France	11	64%	NT	0
Shared Needle Hepatitis	92	7%	86%[1]	5%
Post-Transfusion Hepatitis	20	45%	55%	0
Unknown Exposure	70	30%	NT	0
2. Chronic Liver Disease				
Chronic Active Hepatitis	18	61%	NT	0
Cirrhosis	8	75%	0[2]	0[2]
Polyarteritis Nodosa				
France	10	40%	NT	0
3. Asymptomatic Carriers				
NYC Volunteer Donors, Chronic Carriers				
SGPT <25	61	80%	18%	2%
SGPT >50	59	78%	22%	0
Drug Users	24	8%	92%	0

   NT denotes not tested
[1] 86% of 73 patients tested for AY
[2] 1 patient tested for AY, 7 tested for ? A

Also, in cases of post-transfusion hepatitis there does not appear to be a relationship between subtype and development of clinical versus subclinical illness (Table 4). Our preliminary data suggest that the distribution of subtype antigens reflects the population from which the sub-population under study is drawn.

Table 4. Distribution of subtype antigens in post-transfusion hepatitis.

Category	HAI Test Results D Subtype	
	Number Tested	Percent Positive
Cases:		
Icteric Hepatitis	5	60%
Anicteric Hepatitis	3	67%
HB Antigenemia Without Hepatitis	3	33%
Donors to Cases of:		
Icteric Hepatitis	8	100%
Anicteric Hepatitis	8	88%
HB Antigenemia Without Hepatitis	15	87%

Subtyping: An ultrasensitive identity test for HBAg. When a positive test result is obtained by CEP, it is always possible to carry out an "identity test" to assure that the substance detected is the hepatitis B antigen [283]. A blood donor whose serum is found by CEP and agar gel diffusion (AGD) to contain HBAg can be notified of this finding without fear of an error in test specificity.

There is now much evidence to support the possibility that HBAg can be transmitted nonparenterally. The blood donor whose serum is found to contain HBAg is cautioned against making future blood donations and is also informed of the medical significance of being a chronic HBAg carrier (including the possibility of transmission to his close contacts). It would, of course, be highly undesirable to notify a donor of positive test results if the specificity of these results could not be confirmed.

If ultrasensitive tests such as HAI or radioimmunoassay (RIA) are to be used for routine screening, positive results will be obtained which cannot be confirmed by conventional, less sensitive methods such as AGD or CEP. The more sensitive tests can however, be made subtype specific by use of appropriately prepared monospecific antisera. This property makes possible a new form of "identity test", i.e., complete subtype characterization. There appear to be 2 "allelic" loci, d/y [283] and w/r (Bancroft, Personal

Communication), that are mutually exclusive. In addition, there
are two specificities that appear to be almost universal in human
strains of HBAg: a and x. If a positive serum is found by subtype analysis to contain d but not y, w but not r, or vice versa,
and if it also shows the presence of a and x subtype antigens, it
may be assumed that the substance detected is the hepatitis B
antigen. Any laboratory which can carry out RIA or HAI assays can
also subtype by these methods if suitable monospecific antisera
are made available.

        Acknowledgments. These studies were aided by Grant HE 09011
and AI 09516 from the National Institutes of Health, Contract 70-
2236 from the National Heart and Lung Institute and Grants in Aid
from the Kresge Foundation and from the Strasburger Foundation.
Dr. Prince is a Career Scientist of the Health Research Council of
the City of New York under Contract I-533.

        We are grateful for the technical assistance of B Clinkscale,
E. Echenroth and A. M. Moffatt.

21. RADIOIMMUNOASSAY FOR DETECTION OF HEPATITIS-ASSOCIATED ANTIGEN (HBAg) AND ANTIBODIES TO HBAg

R. A. Aach, E. J. Hacker, Jr., C. W. Parker

Washington University School of Medicine, Department of

Medicine, St. Louis, Missouri

Recognition of the association of Australia antigen with long incubation hepatitis [52,384] has provided an invaluable immunological marker to study this disease. Perhaps the most important clinical application of this association to date has been the screening of potential blood donors for antigenemia. There is now ample evidence that transfusion of blood containing this antigen (also known as the SH, hepatitis-associated (HAA) and hepatitis B (HBAg antigen) carries a significant risk of transmitting viral hepatitis to the recipient [166]. This observation, along with the findings of clinical trials [36] that long incubation hepatitis can occur following the administration of infectious plasma, negative when tested by immunodiffusion or counterimmunoelectrophoresis, has resulted in efforts to develop more sensitive test systems for antigen recognition. At the present time, radioimmunoassay appears to be the most sensitive method of antigen detection [214].

A number of radioimmunoassay techniques now have been described. All utilize a radio-iodinated marker, usually HBAg labelled with ^{125}I. Purified HBAg prepared by rate zonal ultracentrifugation is radiolabelled by the chloramine-T method of Hunter and Greenwood [225]. Prior to use, it is necessary to separate ^{125}I and radiolabelled trace serum protein and/or amino acid contaminants by column chromatography with Sephadex G-25, G-50, or G-200. The most immunoreactive antigen preparation, at least 80% immunoprecipitable, is obtained by subsequent passage through a Sephrose 4B column. Presumably because of HBAg's low tyrosine content and probable inaccessibility of tyrosine to oxidation [478] this reaction yields radiolabelled antigen of relatively low specific activity of about 1 microcurie per microgram of antigen protein. Despite its low specific activity, iodination of 50 micrograms of HBAg

with 2 millicuries of ^{125}I and 100 micrograms of chloramine-T produces enough labelled antigen to permit the screening of at least
1,000 samples. In our laboratory ^{125}I-HBAg has been stored in phosphate buffered saline containing 0.5% bovine serum albumin at -20°C
for as long as 2 months without significant loss of antigenic
activity.

Regardless of the specific method used, virtually all radioimmunoassays are based on the competition of HBAg, if present in
test material, with the antigen marker ^{125}I-HBAg for anti-HBAg
binding sites. The major difference in the systems described to
date, is the manner in which antibody-bound antigen, that is, the
immunoprecipitate, is separated from free antigen after incubation.

The method of Walsh, et al. [483] utilizes paper chromatoelectrophoresis for separation. This technique takes advantage of the
differences in mobility of free and antibody-bound antigen in an
electric field. This procedure is sensitive and reproducible for
antigen but identifies antibody less well than other radioimmunoassays and requires the handling of paper strips.

Several different groups including our own [1,100,214,275]
have applied double antibody radioimmunoassay for detection of HBAg
and anti-HBAg (Figure 1).

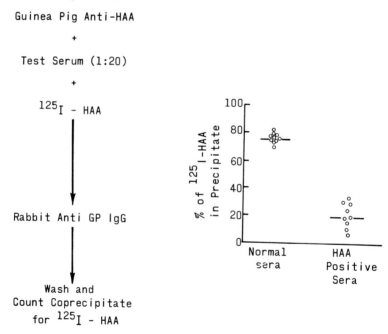

Figure 1. Schematic representation of double antibody radioimmunoassay used for detection of HBAg.

The standard double antibody procedure is performed over a 4 - 6
day period. In this method, incubation of the test specimen with
sera containing anti-HBAg antibodies (first antibody) and ^{125}I-HBAg

is followed by addition of sera containing heterologous anti-gamma globulin antibody (second antibody) to coprecipitate the antigen bound to first antibody. In our laboratory, guinea pig anti-HBAg serum serves as the first antibody and rabbit anti-guinea pig gamma globulin acts as the second antibody. The coprecipitate after incubation is isolated by centrifugation and counted in an automatic gamma counter. HBAg, if present in the test specimen, competes with ^{125}I-HBAg marker for first antibody binding sites thereby lowering the amount of radioactivity in the coprecipitate as compared to simultaneously run antigen-negative sera.

Double antibody radioimmunoassay is a particularly sensitive method of recognizing circulating antibodies to HBAg in human serum (Figure 2). For anti-HBAg detection, the test specimen is first

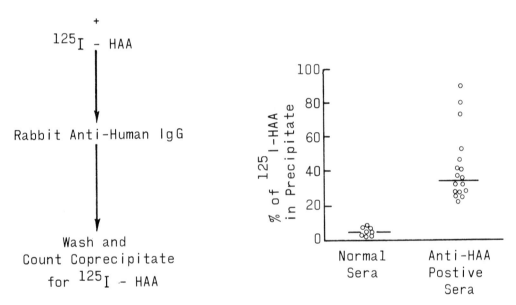

Figure 2.   Double antibody radioimmunoassay procedure for detecting antibodies to HBAg in human serum.

incubated with ^{125}I-HBAg. Rabbit or goat antibodies to human gamma globulin are then added and the incubation is continued to allow formation of insoluble immune complexes which are isolated and counted as for antigen. Anti-HBAg, if present in the test sample, binds ^{125}I-HBAg resulting in markedly increased recovery of radioactivity in the coprecipitate compared to control sera.

Recently several different solid phase radioimmunoassays have been developed to shorten the time required for screening samples. Solid phase systems can be completed within a 6 - 48 hour span but as presently designed they do not readily detect human antibodies to HBAg. In one method anti-HBAg is conjugated to solid particles such as Sepharose [86]. After incubation of test sample

and antigen marker, separation of antibody-bound HBAg is accomplished by brief centrifugation. In another system, polystyrene reaction tubes are coated with anti-HBAg prior to the addition of test
material and labelled antigen [214]. Repeated washing after incubation removes unbound ^{125}I-HBAg. These methods, although more rapid at present are also less sensitive and less reproducible than
the double antibody radioimmunoassay [214]. An interesting variation of this solid phase system, presently under evaluation, has
recently been described. In this method labelled anti-HBAg rather
than antigen serves as the labelled marker [164]. Test serum is
added to propylene reaction tubes which have been coated with
guinea pig anti-HBAg. After 16 hours of incubation the tubes are
washed and ^{125}I-labelled anti-HBAg is added. The incubation is
continued for 1 1/2 hours following which the contents are aspir-
ated, the tubes washed, and counted for radioactivity. In contrast
to other radioimmunoassays, in this "sandwich" technique, HBAg-
bound by unlabelled anti-HBAg is identified by increased recovery
of radioactivity (^{125}I anti-HBAg which combines with antibody-
bound antigen). Another "sandwich" solid phase system of promise
has been developed by Dr. Goldfield and his colleagues [172].
Glass beads, rather than reaction tubes, are coated with purified
anti-HBAg derived from human serum. Test samples are incubated
over night with the antibody adherent beads. After washing, ^{125}I
anti-HBAg is added and the incubation is continued until the next
day. HBAg in test samples is detected after isolation of the beads
by an increase in radioactivity (^{125}I anti-HBAg) as compared to
control sera. This method has the advantage of minimizing the
problem of non-specific sticking of radiolabelled marker to the
reaction tubes.

Radiolabelling anti-HBAg antibodies, rather than HBAg, results
in a labelled marker of much higher specific activity. Theoretically this should increase the sensitivity of HBAg detection and
will increase the number of samples which can be screened after a
single radioiodination [372]. The advantage of increased sensitivity by use of an antibody marker of high specific activity may
be offset to some extent in the "sandwich" techniques, in that not
all antigenic sites in the HBAg particles are available for binding
to radiolabelled antibody.

At the present time it would appear that the double antibody
radioimmunoassay is the most sensitive method of detecting both
HBAg and anti-HBAg [1,214]. Based on comparative studies of the
same sera, it is 1000-5000 times more sensitive than agar gel diffusion in recognizing antigen. Hollinger and his associates [214]
observed titers of HBAg by this procedure that were 5 - 10-fold
greater than that found by hemagglutination inhibition. Double
antibody radioimmunoassay is even more sensitive in recognizing
antibodies to HBAg. Analyses in several laboratories [1,214,275]

indicate a 20,000 - several million-fold increase in sensitivity over the results of testing by immunodiffusion.

Although comparison of the relative sensitivity can serve as a guide to the potential application of the radioimmunoassay, its usefulness as a method of screening for antigen and antibody must be based upon the study of sera obtained from patients with well-documented disease (i.e., type B hepatitis) and healthy individuals with no history or evidence of disease. We have now compared double antibody radioimmunoassay (RIA) to counterimmunoelectrophoresis by studying the sera of over 500 individuals, including 200 randomly selected, healthy volunteer blood donors (Table 1).

Table 1. Results of screening the sera of 200 volunteer blood donors and 35 patients with parenterally transmitted hepatitis by counterimmunoelectrophoresis (CEP) and double antibody RIA.

NUMBER OF POSITIVE INDIVIDUALS

Population	Number	CEP		RIA	
		HAA	anti-HAA	HAA	anti-HAA
Volunteer Donors	200	0	1	3 (1.5%)	36 (18%)
Type B Hepatitis	35	18	–	32	6*

CEP = Counter immunoelectrophoresis
RIA = Double antibody radioimmunoassay

*4 patients had both circulating HAA and anti-HAA.
In all, 34 of 35 (97%) hepatitis patients were positive

None of the 200 had HBAg when their sera were screened by CEP and only one had detectable antibodies to HBAg*. When the same specimens were screened by RIA, three donors (1.5%) were found to have circulating HBAg. Thirty-six of the two hundred donors, or 18 percent, had detectable anti-HBAg, an incidence comparable to the 14.4% frequency observed by Lander, Alter and Purcell [275] in a similar population of volunteer donors using a modified double antibody RIA.

---

* On a larger scale of screening by CEP (4,125 donors) this population has an incidence of HBAg of 0.2% and anti-HBAg of 1%.

    The sera of thirty-five patients acutely ill with long incu-
bation hepatitis also have been studied. Twenty-five of the thirty-
five patients had antigenemia by CEP; none had detectable anti-
HBAg. When screened by radioimmunoassay, thirty-two of the thirty-
five (91%) had circulating HBAg. Six were found to have antibodies
to HBAg, four of whom were also antigen positive. In all, thirty-
four of thirty-five (97%) had detectable HBAg and/or anti-HBAg. It
should be emphasized that these were single determinations and not
part of a prospective study. Rather, each patient's sample was
drawn at different times during the acute phase of disease. Thus,
the sera of essentially all patients with long incubation hepatitis
are positive by radioimmunoassay when studied during clinically
active disease.

    Presently the major drawback of double antibody radioimmuno-
assay as a practical method of screening is the 2 - 6 day period
generally required to complete the procedure. The effect in antigen recognition of varying the incubation times is shown in Figure 3.

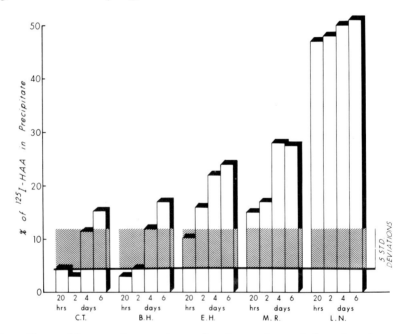

Figure 3.   The effect of varying the lengths of incubation on
antigen recognition by double antibody radioimmunoassay.

Five sera with widely different HBAg levels were subjected simultaneously to four different incubation conditions: 1) a 20 hour
incubation [1 hour at 37°C and then four hours at 4°C with guinea
pig anti-HBAg and ^{125}I-HBAg (first reaction); 15 hours incubation
at 4°C with second antibody, rabbit anti-gamma globulin (second
reaction)]; 2) 48 hour incubation at 4°C (24 hours first reaction;
24 hours second reaction); 3) 4 day incubation at 4°C (48 hours
for both first and second reactions); and 4) 6 day incubation at
4°C (4 days first reaction and two days second reaction).

The degree of inhibition produced by HBAg in the test sera was generally greater after 4 and 6 days, but the difference was quite small. All samples were positive after incubation for only 20 hours including very weakly antigen-positive sera. Thus, despite increased precipitation of ^{125}I-HBAg with increasing length of incubation the percent inhibition of unlabelled HBAg was almost unchanged. Obviously these observations would not necessarily apply to all antisera since equilibrium should be approached by both the first and second antibody reactions in order to obtain near maximal sensitivity. However, similar results have been obtained with four other guinea pig anti-HBAg sera and two other second antibody (rabbit anti-guinea pig gamma globulin) preparations. These observations indicate that with appropriate antisera, blood can be screened in less than 24 hours by double antibody radioimmunoassay with little or no sacrifice in sensitivity.

In detecting serum antibodies to HBAg different results are obtained (Figure 4). With an incubation time of 20 hours antibody may remain undetected, even in patients late in the covalescent phase of type B hepatitis infection.

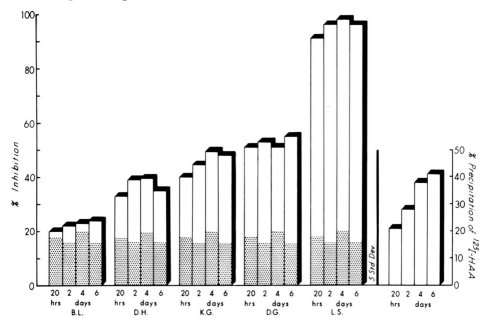

<u>Figure 4.</u> The effect of varying the length of incubation on the recognition of human antibodies to HBAg.

This is demonstrated by study of antibody-positive sera from five different individuals under the four incubation conditions (20 and 48 hours; 4 and 6 days) used in the antigen study. Whereas the one sample containing high-titered antibody was strongly positive by radioimmunoassay within 20 hours, sera containing very low levels of anti-HBAg required at least 4 - 6 days of incubation for definite antibody recognition.

Utilizing the radioimmunoassay we have been able to confirm and extend the recent observations of Le Bouvier on antigenic subtypes to HBAg [283]. As is true with other test systems used in subspecificity characterization (e.g., immunodiffusion) radioimmunoassay requires antisera which recognize different HBAg determinants. Such antisera has been produced by repeated immunization of guinea pigs with HBAg of subtypes D and Y*. ^{125}I-HBAg of either D or Y specificity is used as the radiolabelled antigenic marker. Because all HBAg share a common determinant, a, all antisera should contain anti-a antibodies. One might expect than, that test samples positive by immunodiffusion would be strongly positive by radioimmunoassay using any anti-HBAg antisera in combination with radiolabelled antigen of either D or Y specificity. Characterization of subtypes then would not be possible without the use of monospecific anti-d or anti-y antisera as first antibody. However, we have observed that the proportion of anti-a to anti-d or anti-y antibodies varies in different guinea pig antisera following immunization. In certain antisera, anti-a is present in relatively low amounts. Further, different preparations of purified HBAg appear to have variable representation of antigenic determinants. Thus, purified HBAg of D subtype, after radioiodination may react strongly only with antisera which contain anti-d antibodies; anti-a are recognized poorly and anti-y antibodies not at all. Therefore, subtypes of HBAg can be readily detected by radioimmunoassay provided appropriate combinations of anti-HBAg (first antibody) and radiolabelled antigen marker are used. This is shown in Figure 5 which compares the results of analysis of different radioimmunoassay systems. The sera of 12 antigen-positive hepatitis patients were studied; 5 were representative samples of antigenic subtype D, 5 were subtype Y and 2 were set A by immunodiffusion. Guinea pig anti-a, anti-d sera used in radioimmunoassay system I had relatively low titered anti-a as compared to anti-d and the antigen marker had much greater d than a antigenicity. Sera containing HBAg of D subtype were strongly positive in this system whereas sera with HBAg of subtype Y exerted no or only weak inhibition. Radioimmunoassay system II, using guinea pig anti-a, anti-y antisera (predominantly anti-y) with ^{125}I-HBAg marker of subtype Y (primarily y antigenicity) produced converse results. The test samples with subtype D antigen were negative or only weakly inhibitory whereas the samples containing HBAg of subtype Y were strongly positive.

---

* Confirmation of antigenic determinants was accomplished by immunodiffusion using antisera and sera containing HBAg of subgroups D ($a^+d^+y^-$), Y ($a^+y^+d^-$) and set A ($a^+d^-y^-$) kindly supplied by NIAID-NIH; Dr. H. E. Bond, Electro Nucleonics, Bethesda, Maryland, and Dr. James W. Mosley, Liver Service, U.S.C. Medical Center, Los Angeles, California.

	System I	II	III	IV
Guinea Pig Anti-HAA Antibodies	anti-a,d	anti-a,y	anti-d	anti-y
^{125}I-HAA Marker Antigenic Specificity	a^+,d^+	a^+,y^+	a^+,d^+	a^+,y^+
Determinants Recognized	a,d	a,y	d	y

12 Hepatitis Sera Subtype	PERCENT INHIBITION OF ADDED ^{125}I-HAA MARKER			
D (a^+,d^+) Patients 1-5	95(90-97)	23(9-30)	80(71-85)	6.2(0-13)
Y (a^+,y^+) Patients 6-10	13(4-23)	92(88-97)	12(2-19)	92(85-96)
A (a^+) Patient 11	9	89	3	88
Patient 12	50	28	58	0

Figure 5.   Detection of antigenic determinants by double antibody radioimmunoassay.

To confirm these results, monospecific anti-d and anti-y anti-sera were prepared by repeated absorption with sera containing crossreacting HBAg. Thus, absorption of anti-a, anti-d antisera with excess subtype Y antigen resulted in first antibody monospe-cific for anti-d. First antibody monospecific for anti-y was pro-duced by crossreacting anti-a, anti-y antisera with excess subtype D (a^+d^+) antigen*. Results virtually identical with radioimmuno-assay system I were obtained when the same 12 samples were tested by monospecific anti-d antisera and radiolabelled a^+d^+ antigen (system III). Radioimmunoassay with monospecific anti-y, first antibody, and ^{125}I-HBAg of subtype Y (system IV) yielded results quite similar to radioimmunoassay system II. These studies indi-cate that D and Y subtyping can be performed by radioimmunoassay with antisera that do not have to be rendered monospecific by prior absorption with antigen provided the proper combinations of first antibody and labelled antigen marker are used.

To date, we have not been able to identify the x^+ determinant by radioimmunoassay. However, radioimmunoassay of the two sera with set A antigen has yielded interesting results. By immuno-

---

* Complete absorption was shown by the failure to find coprecip-itation of crossreacting ^{125}I-HBAg when incubated with absorbed first antibody. Excess second antibody, rabbit anti-guinea pig gamma globulin was added in each case to assure maximal coprecipi-tation.

diffusion these two sera have HBAg with only $\underline{a}$ determinants. By radioimmunoassay, however, one serum had in addition $\underline{d}^+$, whereas the other was found to have $\underline{y}^+$ specificity. These results were consistently obtained, regardless of the radioimmunoassay system used. Obviously, additional set A positive sera need to be studied, but the radioimmunoassay results suggest that all HBAg can be subtyped as either D or Y (that is all HBAg have $\underline{d}^+$ or $\underline{y}^+$ determinants in addition to $\underline{a}^+$). Although the proportion of $\underline{a}$, $\underline{d}$, or $\underline{y}$ antigenicity may vary from sample to sample, these results confirm the original observations of Le Bouvier that $\underline{d}+$ and $\underline{y}+$ specificity is mutually exclusive even with a test system of considerable sensitivity. As yet, no antigen has been characterized as being totally free of the $\underline{a}$ determinant including one sample which by immunodiffusion demonstrated only $\underline{d}^+$ specificity.

These studies emphasize that the selection of first antibody and antigen marker (or the antibody marker in the "sandwich" technique) can markedly influence the efficacy of antigen screening. Radioimmunoassay systems favoring recognition of one subtype over another will be less effective in the general screening of HBAg-positive sera even though they may be highly sensitive for detecting $\underline{d}$ or $\underline{y}$ determinants.

Our most effective screening system at the present time is one in which guinea pig antisera with anti-$\underline{a}$ in high titer is used with radiolabelled antigen of predominantly $\underline{a}^+$ specificity (Figure 6). In contrast to the radioimmunoassay systems demonstrating subtypes, all 12 sera were strongly antigen positive when screened by this system. On more extensive screening, no serum samples HBAg-positive

	System V
Guinea Pig Anti-HAA Antibodies	anti-a
^{125}I-HAA Marker Antigenic Specificity	a^+, y^+
Determinants Recognized	a

12 Hepatitis Sera Subtype	PERCENT INHIBITION OF ADDED ^{125}I-HAA MARKER
D (a^+, d^+) Patients 1-5	87 (80-92)
Y (a^+, y^+) Patients 6-10	90 (87-93)
A (a^+) Patient 11 Patient 12	85 80

Figure 6.   Screening of sera for HBAg by radioimmunoassay.

by other test procedures (immunodiffusion, CEP, complement fixation, and hemagglutination) have been negative by this radioimmunoassay system to date. Alternative approaches under study for the general screening of HBAg include the use of antisera containing anti-a, -d, and -y antibodies in high titer with a combined marker composed of radiolabelled HBAg of both D and Y subtypes.

The eventual acceptance of a test system as "the" best method of antigen (and antibody) screening must be based on consideration of a number of factors. These include sensitivity, reproducibility, and ease of performing the procedure as well as the time required for screening samples, the number of samples that can be screened at one time and the cost per sample. Indeed, different methods may better satisfy different needs. For example, a large blood bank requires rapid large scale screening of donor sera whereas an investigative laboratory may demand quantitation and subtyping capability

All HBAg detection systems developed to date have both advantages and disadvantages and this is true of each of the different types of radioimmunoassays as well. Few properly controlled studies have been performed as yet in which coded samples have been independently analyzed by different techniques. The results of these limited comparisons in such a rapidly progressing area are difficult to evaluate. Clearly, radioimmunoassay is an extremely sensitive method of detection which permits precise quantitation, if desired. As a whole, radioimmunoassay requires more time and is less simple to perform than other methods of screening, although advances in technology may minimize these shortcomings in the near future. Reproducibility with radioimmunoassay varies with each procedure and indeed for any given method, from lab to lab, as is true of other sensitive techniques as well. This should be less of a problem as more experience is gained, judging from the success of radioimmunoassays of various circulating peptides, drugs, etc. Ultimately, the basis for adopting the most effective method of screening for antigen must not rest solely on relative sensitivity or reproducibility alone, but rather the ability to reliably and selectively recognize sera capable of transmitting viral hepatitis. This information can only be gained by evaluating test systems in prospective studies of blood donors and recipients. Such studies are underway.

Acknowledgement. This study was supported by National Heart and Lung Institute Contract NIH-71-2353 and Public Health Service Grants AM-05280 and AI-04646.

22. Discussion

RADIOIMMUNOASSAY FOR DETECTION OF HEPATITIS-ASSOCIATED ANTIGEN (HBAg)

F. Blaine Hollinger

Baylor College of Medicine, Department of Virology

and Epidemiology, Houston, Texas

Since publishing our initial studies on a double-antibody radioimmunoassay (RIA-DA) procedure [214], several modifications have been instituted which have resulted in enhanced precision and sensitivity without altering specificity. Recent comparative tests in our laboratory have revealed hepatitis B antigen (HBAg) titers which are 100-fold greater than those obtained by the passive hemagglutination (PHA) method and 1000-fold greater than those obtained by complement fixation (CF). Hepatitis B antibody (anti-HBAg) titers are 20-fold greater than those obtained by PHA, but 50,000-fold greater than those obtained by CF. This enchanced sensitivity has been achieved primarily by increasing the incubation period of the first reaction to 2 - 3 days for HBAg and to 4 - 5 days for anti-HBAg.

As reported by Aach et al. in their paper, incubation of the initial reactants (unknown + anti-HBAg + labeled HBAg) for periods up to four days prior to the addition of immunoprecipitating antibody (second antibody) failed to significantly enhance the sensitivity of their test. However, the ratio of bound to free labeled HBAg (B/F ratio) increased from 0.25 to 0.7 as the incubation period lengthened (derived from their Figure 3), which may have resulted in the smaller differences observed between the shorter and longer incubation periods. Kinetic analysis of RIA-DA studies in our laboratory have demonstrated that improved sensitivity can be achieved by allowing unlabeled HBAg to react with anti-HBAg (step 1) 18 - 24 hours before addition of radiolabeled HBAg (step 2). A similar observation has been made by Rodbard et al. [411] and Midgely [314]. Increasing the incubation temperature from 4°C to 37°C for step 1 results in a more rapid reaction rate permitting earlier addition of labeled HBAg without sacrificing sensitivity.

Another approach toward enhancing the sensitivity of the RIA-DA technique concerns the production of labeled HBAg of high specific activity. As Dr. Aach indicated, the low tyrosine and histidine content of purified HBAg or the possible inaccessibility of these amino acid residues to oxidation may be important factors which limit effective iodination of this antigen. Recently, however, my colleagues and I have been able to increase the specific activity of purified HBAg 20- to 40-fold by utilizing either a lactoperoxidase-catalyzed procedure [328] or a modified chloramine-T procedure [182], in which optimal quantities of protein were reacted with an excess of chloramine-T at an elevated pH. These preparations resulted in increased yields of radio-ligand and in HBAg and anti-HBAg titers which were 2- to 4-fold greater than those obtained using comparable counts per minute of a conventionally prepared label.

Over the past four months we have used this modified RIA-DA procedure to examine approximately 3000 donor units for the presence of HBAg (Table 1). In this donor population, HBAg was detected in 15 units by the counterimmunoelectrophoresis (CIE) technique,

Table 1.   Radioimmunoassay results of donor units collected at Ben Taub Blood Bank, Houston, Texas.

No. Units Tested (CIE Negative)	RIA-DA Results		
	Negative (<2 S.D.)	Positive	
		(3-4 S.D.)	(>5 S.D.)
2970	2745	44 (15)*	181 (61)

* Rate per 1000 units   S.D. = standard deviations from normal
                                          (HBAg-negative) control panel.

an incidence of five positive units per 1000 units tested. In contrast, an incidence of 61 positive units per 1000 units tested was observed using the more sensitive RIA-DA procedure (>5 standard deviations from a control panel of sera negative for HBAg and anti-HBAg). This high frequency is similar to the reported incidence of anicteric and icteric hepatitis cases occurring in recipients of transfused blood derived from a comparable donor population.

The risk of contracting viral hepatitis type B following infusion of RIA-DA positive, CIE negative blood is presently unknown.

In a recent prospective post-transfusion hepatitis study conducted at the Providence Veteran's Administration Hospital in Rhode Island [165], 1155 donor units were administered to 161 recipients who were followed at 2 - 4 week intervals for six months. Seven of these recipients (4.2%) developed biochemical and histological evidence of viral hepatitis, three anicteric and four icteric. Sera collected from these seven recipients during the study period were tested, under code, for HBAg by CIE, CF and RIA-DA. HBAg was not detected in any of the seven pre-transfusion blood specimens (Table 2). The post-transfusion sera from two recipients were positive for HBAg by the CIE technique. Further examination by the more sensitive RIA-DA technique revealed significantly elevated levels of HBAg in the sera of three other recipients.

Table 2. Serologic results of 7 recipients who developed biochemical and histological evidence of viral hepatitis during a prospective study involving 1155 donors and 161 recipients.

	Serologic Results*						
	Pre-trans. Specimen		Post-trans. Specimen		Donor Units		
Case #	CIE	RIA	CIE	RIA	CIE	RIA	Interpretation
1	-	-	-	+	-	+	Hepatitis type B
2	-	-	-	-	-	-	Hepatitis type A ?
3	-	-	-	-	-	-	Hepatitis type A ?
4	-	-	-	+	-	+	Hepatitis type B
5	-	-	+	+	-	+	Hepatitis type B
6	-	-	-	+	-	+	Hepatitis type B
7	-	-	+	N.D.	+	N.D.	Hepatitis type B

* -, all specimens negative
+, at least one specimen contained HBAg
N.D., not done.

Of the 101 donor units administered to these seven patients and tested under code, only 1 unit was positive for HBAg by CIE or CF. In contrast, the RIA-DA technique detected HBAg in 10 additional specimens. Following decoding and analysis of these results it was concluded that the administration of RIA-DA positive, CIE negative blood was associated with the development of viral hepatitis type B in four recipients while an additional case was associated with transfusion of a CIE positive donor unit.

A final comment should be made regarding the specificity of the solid phase radioimmunoassay technique employing labeled antibody ("sandwich " solid phase system [164]). Alter et al. (personal communication, June 1971) have observed antibodies to ruminant sera in blood donors at a frequency similar to that of HBAg. Similar antibodies to guinea pig globulin may also exist. If this occurs, false positive tests will result (Figure 1), since the hetero-antibody will bind not only the guinea pig globulin adsorbed on the tube but also the ^{125}I-guinea pig globulin subsequently added.

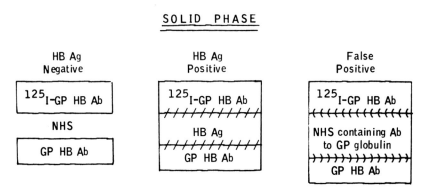

Figure 1. Diagrammatic representation of solid phase radioimmuno-assay, using a "sandwich" technique. This illustrates the mechanism by which false positives can occur.

Such false positives would not occur in the RIA-DA procedure since this method depends only on competitive inhibition between unlabeled HBAg and purified labeled HBAg for specific antibody. Indeed, separation of the bound complex in the RIA-DA method is by addition of immunoprecipitating antibody directed against the globulin fraction of the first antibody, e.g., guinea pig globulin.

    Acknowledgement. Studies from the Baylor laboratory were aided by Research Contract NIH-2231, from the National Heart and Lung Institute, National Institutes of Health.

23. Discussion

RADIOIMMUNOASSAY FOR DETECTION OF
HEPATITIS-ASSOCIATED ANTIGEN (HBAg) AND ANTI-
BODIES TO HBAg

John H. Walsh

Veterans Administration Center

Los Angeles, California

As Dr. Aach and Dr. Hollinger have indicated, radioimmunoassays for detection of Australia antigen and antibody are beginning to realize their potential as highly sensitive and specific
methods which offer significant increases in sensitivity over other
detection systems. Two general methods have been applied to antigen
detection. The first, of which the chromatoelectrophoresis separation was the prototype, is an inhibition reaction in which unlabelled
antigen in unknown or known specimens competes with labelled antigen
for a finite amount of antibody. The limiting factors in the sensitivity of this type of assay are the affinity of antibody for antigen
and the specific activity of labelled antigen. Until recently, the
specific activity has been a major stumbling block, but Dr. Hollinger
and his associates have described promising modifications of the
iodination technique which have allowed them to achieve greater incor-
poration of radioiodine into the HBAg particle. Several workers have
confirmed our observation that repurification of the labelled antigen
by Sephadex or Sepharose chromatography permits isolation of a fraction of the labelled material which exhibits optimal binding
characteristics.

Two major problems with the inhibition systems have been the
necessity for prolonged incubation times to achieve optimal binding between labelled antigen and antibody and nonspecific inhibition
of binding by serum components. The time required for optimal binding varies inversely with the concentration of antibody in the incubation mixture. Maximum sensitivity requires use of the greatest
dilution of antibody which will bind 30 - 50% of labelled antigen.
However, this also requires the greatest incubation time. By increasing the specific activity of labelled antigen, smaller amounts
of antigen can be added to the incubation to achieve the number of

counts necessary for accurate counting and more dilute antibody
can be used. We have calculated that a concentration of labelled
antigen of 5000 counts/min/ml corresponds roughly to 80 ng/ml unlabelled antigen. The sensitivity of the assay is approximately
20 - 40 ng/ml with this concentration of labelled antigen. If the
specific activity of labelled antigen is increased ten-fold, the
same number of counts per ml would contain only 8 ng/ml HBAg and
potential sensitivity would therefore be increased considerably,
consistent with what Dr. Hollinger has reported. The problem of
incubation time is not helped by increasing specific activity. In
fact, since more dilute antibody could be used, longer incubation
times would be anticipated. Dr. Aach has offered a partial solution to the problem by not carrying the reaction to equilibrium.
In our own hands we have found that shorter incubation times increase the variability of results.

The problem of nonspecific inhibition by serum components is
a major difficulty in all inhibition-type radioimmunoassays for
HBAg. Concentrations of normal serum of greater than 5 to 10% in
the incubation mixture interfere with the antibody-labelled antigen
reaction. This problem can be circumvented by performing assays
with unknown sera diluted 1:10 or higher but the necessity for performing such dilutions means that the working sensitivity of the
assay is not as good as the theoretical sensitivity obtained with
purified antigen diluted in buffer alone. Thus an assay capable
of detecting HBAg in a concentration of 5 ng/ml in which an initial
serum dilution of 1:20 is required can detect a concentration of
100 ng/ml in the serum specimen. We have been able to control the
nonspecific inhibition to some extent by use of 1:5 dilutions of
normal serum as controls for 1:5 dilutions of unknown samples, but
the degree of nonspecific inhibition among normal sera varies somewhat and requires that a greater degree of inhibition be obtained
to be confident that antigen is present. The component of serum
which causes this nonspecific inhibition is unknown. We have preliminary evidence that gamma globulin may be at least one inhibitory
factor.

The double antibody separation method appears to be superior
to chromatoelectrophoresis for detection of antibody to HBAg. Use
of double antibody systems has been reported previously by Lander
et al. and by Millman et al. It has been possible to detect anti-
HBAg in the serum of 10 - 20% of normal adult subjects. Experiments
by Dr. Krugman have suggested that the presence of antibody indicates immunity to the long-incubation hepatitis agent. It will be
important to determine whether subjects with low titers of anti-
HBAg are immune to transfusion-induced hepatitis. We (Holland et
al.) observed hepatitis in three patients whose serum contained antibody prior to transfusion. It was not determined whether the
hepatitis was caused by the agent related to HBAg or to another

hepatitis agent. Such information should be obtained from prospective studies of transfusion hepatitis by use of the sensitive techniques now available for antibody detection. Another question which should be answered is whether naturally acquired infections associated with circulating HBAg are followed regularly by detectable antibody responses and whether antibody can be demonstrated over long periods of time.

The recent introduction of a radioimmunoassay for HBAg which utilizes labelled antibody to HBAg provides an independent method for antigen detection. There are several advantages to a system utilizing labelled antibody. It should be possible to achieve much higher specific activities of labelled antibody than of labelled antigen since the molecular weight of antibody is approximately 20 times less than that of the antigen. A direct system should circumvent some of the problems of nonspecific inhibition which interfere with the inhibition type assays. Other apparent advantages include the possibility of using undiluted serum specimens, short incubation time, and the ability to add excess quantities of labelled antibody as the indicator reagent since the second reaction is not an equilibrium reaction. It remains to be determined whether the sensitivity of labelled-antibody "sandwich" technique will prove superior to the sensitivity of the inhibition methods. It is necessary that the labelled antibody be immuno-specific and retain good reaction energy after labelling. Contamination with antibodies directed against normal human serum proteins could lead to false positive results.

Both inhibition and labelled-antibody assays can be used for subtype identification. Dr. Aach has demonstrated the efficacy of the inhibition system for this purpose. The solid state labelled-antibody system should be very satisfactory for subtype determination if immunospecific anti-d and anti-y antibodies can be prepared. The optimal detection system probably would include a screening test in which antibodies directed either against the common antigenic determinant or against all the major antigenic components were utilized. The specificity of the test then could be determined by demonstrating that positive sera exhibited either d or y specificity.

Until it is possible to grow the hepatitis B virus in tissue culture, radioimmunoassay probably will be the most sensitive in vitro technique for identification of HBAg in human serum and will probably remain the most sensitive test which can be applied to the testing of donor blood prior to transfusion. The ultimate objective of the sensitive tests is the detection of the minimum dose of antigen which is associated with the transmission of hepatitis. Serum obtained from prospective studies in which donor blood is collected and stored while transfusion recipients are monitored carefully for hepatitis will provide the critical evidence of whether any of

the tests have achieved this level of sensitivity. The preliminary
evidence we have heard is encouraging, but we must keep in mind the
possibility that a considerable proportion of transfusion hepatitis
even of the longer incubation variety, may be caused by agents not
associated with HBAg.

Evaluation of the sensitivity and specificity of the various
sensitive tests should be performed periodically among the various
laboratories performing these procedures. Distribution of serum
pools which contain varying dilutions of both of the major subtypes
of antigen prepared in normal serum will be helpful for this purpose
Panels of these serum pools, such as the ones prepared and distributed by Dr. Barker, will be useful not only for assessing the
current "state of the art" but for evaluating new generations of
tests as they are developed.

24. AMERICAN NATIONAL RED CROSS EXPERIENCE WITH HBAg TESTING

R. Y. Dodd, J. J. Levin, Louisa Ni, G. A. Jamieson

and T. J. Greenwalt

The American National Red Cross, Washington, D. C.

The incidence of HBAg in the normal, healthy population in the United States is generally given as 0.1% (for reviews, see [430,433,501]): this figure is presumably derived from Blumberg's early studies [49,56]. The incidence of HBAg in the American volunteer blood donor population is also thought to be about 0.1% [95,250,461], whereas blood obtained from paid donors has a much higher incidence of the antigen [95,367,384,452]. However, these studies are based upon relatively small surveys confined to particular cities, hospitals or blood banks [95,250,461].

The American National Red Cross is the largest blood collecting organization in the United States. During the year ending June 30, 1971, 3,405,192 units of blood were collected from 59 Regional Blood Centers situated throughout the country. Individual centers collected between 5,000 and 220,000 blood units in the year from an exclusively volunteer population. Since April 1, 1971, every unit of blood collected has been tested for the presence of the hepatitis associated antigen, type B (HBAg), by a commercially available counterelectrophoresis (CEP) technique (Spectra Biologicals, Oxnard, California). It is the purpose of this paper to present the overall experience of the American National Red Cross in HBAg testing and to provide definitive data on the incidence and distribution of HBAg among the normal volunteer blood donor population of the U.S.A. This study is based upon approximately 2.6 million blood donations made between April and December, 1971.

Incidence of HBAg in the normal donor population. Each of the Red Cross Regional Blood Centers tests every unit of blood drawn for the presence of HBAg. All reactive, or suspected positive, samples are sent to the National Red Cross Headquarters for confirmation, and for further studies. Table 1 records the number of units collected, the number of suspected HBAg-positive units and the incidence of HBAg per 1,000 units, based on the monthly data provided by the individual Red Cross Centers. However, only 82.5% of these samples have been confirmed as HBAg-positive when retested at the National Headquarters Laboratories, so the true overall incidence during the period of this study may be as low as 0.97 per 1,000. On the other hand, it must be recognized that the interpretation of a CEP test is highly subjective and that there is no absolute standard by which the reactivity of a sample may be expressed.

Table 1. Reported monthly incidence of HBAg-positive Red Cross blood donations in 1971

	Number of Units Collected	Number of Units Reported HBAg-Positive	Incidence per 1000
April	294,677	378	1.28
May	295,139	393	1.33
June	290,269	410	1.41
July	252,605	304	1.20
August	275,400	364	1.32
September	288,952	350	1.21
October	301,689	301	1.00
November	306,896	292	0.95
December	290,491	252	0.87
	2,596,118	3,044	1.17

In other words, it is possible that a variable proportion of minimally reactive samples may be overlooked during routine screening or that certain positive samples are unreactive for technical reasons [254]. The results of a Red Cross Proficiency Testing Program when Centers were asked to define the HBAg status of unknown samples, tend to confirm this view.

During the period studied, the incidence of reported positive samples was between 1.41 and 0.87 per 1,000, being relatively constant between April and September but declining thereafter. However, these figures should not be interpreted as indicating a decline in the incidence of HBAg in the normal population. Approximately 80% of Red Cross donors have donated previously so that the exclusion of HBAg-positive individuals from the donor pool should result in a decrease in the incidence of HBAg in donated blood units. Several other points should be considered in interpreting the causes

of this short-term decline in the incidence of HBAg; first, the
sensitivity of the test may vary depending on the batch of antiserum
despite close control by the Department of Biologics Standards
and the Red Cross; second, it is not yet possible to determine
whether this variation could be seasonal. Finally, it is known
that radar operators become fatigued by lengthy periods of negative
sightings and subsequently miss a significant positive sighting; an
analogous situation may apply during HBAg testing, when many thousands of negative samples may have to be observed before a positive
reaction is seen.

Geographical variation in the incidence of HBAg. The incidence of HBAg reported from Red Cross Centers varies from 1 in 5049
(0.2 per 1,000) in Waterloo, Iowa, to 33 in 9590 (3.44 per 1,000)
in Puerto Rico. These are relatively small samples, but the figures are substantiated by an incidence of 0.29 per 1,000 (24 in
81,941) in St. Paul, Minnesota and 3.10 per 1,000 (67 in 21,630)
in Savannah, Georgia (Dodd, to be published).

Table 2. Reported and corrected incidence of HBAg–positive Red
Cross blood donations in the major regions of the U.S.A.

Area	Number of Units Collected	Number of Units Reported HBAg-Positive	Reported Incidence per 1,000	Corrected Incidence per 1,000
Northeast	1,323,348	1401	1.06	0.89
Southeast	436,045	802	1.84	1.70
North Central	453,338	323	0.71	0.38
South Central	55,341	75	1.36	1.28
Northwest	114,978	95	0.83	0.75
Southwest	203,478	315	1.55	1.30
Puerto Rico	9,590	33	3.44	3.44
	2,596,118	3044	1.17	1.01

Table 2 records the incidence of HBAg-reactive donations reported from six major areas of the continental United States as
well as the number of suspected positive samples from each center
which have been confirmed; since some centers did not refer all
suspected positives an estimate number was made from the proportion
of referred samples which were confirmed as positive. In the few
cases where no samples were referred for confirmation, all reported
samples were regarded as positive. Of 3,044 samples reported,
2,547 were referred for confirmatory tests and, of these, 2,102

were confirmed to be positive. Figure 1 maps the reported incidence of HBAg in areas covered by the Red Cross. It may be seen
that the incidence reported from individual centers is in accordance with the broad area breakdown noted in Table 2. For example,
of 29 centers reporting an incidence of less than 1 per 1,000, only
four were from the Southern United States, and all eight centers reporting less than 0.5 per 1,000 came from the Northeastern or North
Central regions. On the other hand, all six centers reporting more
than 2.5 positives per 1,000 were from the Southeastern area.

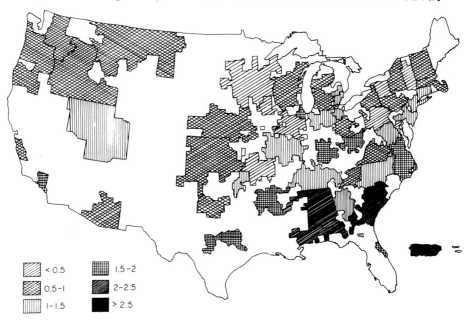

Figure 1. Reported incidence of HBAg amongst Red Cross donors,
April to December, 1971. Blank areas are not covered by the Red
Cross Program.

Further studies. We have established a reference library of
HBAg-positive plasma samples for distribution to interested workers
in the field and we have been performing a number of further studies upon these referred samples, two of which are relevant to this
discussion, i.e., titration studies and subtyping.

Preliminary titration studies were performed by CEP. Samples
of plasma were diluted 1:2, 1:16 and 1:64 in phosphate buffered
saline and applied to the antigen wells of Spectra counterelectrophoresis plates; Spectra antibody was used without dilution. The
majority of samples tested reacted at 1:2 but not at 1:16 (Table 3)
although a different antibody, or a different detection system, may
give markedly different results.

Table 3.   CEP titers of referred HBAg-positive samples

Reciprocal Titer	Number	Percentage
Not read	10	0.7
Negative*	189	12.8
2 - 16	1070	72.3
16- 64	188	12.7
>64	22	1.5
	1479	100.0

*   Negative: no reaction at 1:2 dilution.

With regard to subtyping, Dr. Paul Holland of the National
Institutes of Health has examined samples of HBAg-positive Red
Cross blood for serological subtype (ad or ay) by a CEP technique
(Holland, to be published). Of 670 samples so far examined, 87%
are ad, the remainder being ay. There are some interesting regional
variations in the ad/ay ratio, with a preponderance of ay over ad
in only three geographically adjacent Red Cross Centers (Holland,
personal communication); an observation which may be epidemiologically significant.

Discussion. The overall reported incidence of 1.17 HBAg-
reactive donors per 1,000 is in close agreement with the previously
quoted figure of 0.1% although, as explained above, the initial incidence of around 1.3 per 1,000 is probably a more realistic estimate of the proportion of HBAg carriers in the total volunteer
donor population. It is now apparent that this figure may be regarded as an average incidence for the volunteer donor population
for the United States as a whole, although the regional variations
are considerable. Figures from comparable countries are generally
higher than this; Moore (personal communication) gives an incidence
of 0.26% in the Canadian volunteer donor population and figures
from Northern Europe range between 0.16% for Norway [439] and 0.45%
for France [443]. A preliminary estimate for England is 0.1% [108,
466]. Although the dual volunteer/commercial system in the United
States clearly leads to a selective accumulation of HBAg-positive
donors in the commercial group [384], it is possible that at least
a proportion of this group would still donate in an all-volunteer
environment, accounting for the slightly higher incidence of HBAg
in Canada and in Northern Europe.

The actual incidence of HBAg may be much higher than that described here: a recently developed radioimmunoassay method (Ling

and Overby, personal communication) appears to detect up to ten times as many HBAg-positive carriers in the normal donor population (unpublished).

The geographical variation in incidence within the United States among volunteer blood donors is marked. In general, higher incidences are found in the Southeastern portion of the United States or in large urban areas (Figure 1). It is not clear whether this reflects an actual variation in the overall incidence of HBAg-antigenemia or a variation in the socio-economic structure of the donor population. It is probable that both factors are involved since contact and crowded conditions are known to promote the non-parental spread of hepatitis type B [451].

Titration studies indicate that the majority of reactive samples are of low titer in CEP. Care should therefore be taken to ensure that samples are screened at the maximum available sensitivity

The distribution of subtypes among carriers is of particular interest in view of the suggested preponderance of ay in cases of acute hepatitis type B which may indicate a difference in pathogenicity between the subtypes.

Acknowledgements. We wish to acknowledge the valuable technical assistance of J. A. Kobita, Shari St. Denis, Wendy Quinn and M. McFall. We are also indebted to the Medical Directors and technical staff of the Red Cross Regional Blood Centers who provided samples which are the basis of this report.

Publication No. 245 from The American National Red Cross.

25. A LATEX-AGGLUTINATION TEST FOR HEPATITIS-ASSOCIATED ANTIGEN (HBAg)

H. A. Perkins, S. L. Perkins, E. Chen and G. N. Vyas

Irwin Memorial Blood Bank and the University of California School of Medicine, San Francisco, California

Latex particles coated with antibody to HBAg may be agglutinated in the presence of the antigen, and tests based on this principle have been successfully employed to detect HBAg in several laboratories [154,282,305]. There is general agreement that the sensitivity of the test is as good as or better than those in general use, but that a significant proportion of positive reactions cannot be clearly attributed to the presence of HBAg. The results to be reported are based on tests with antibody-coated latex particles of different origin than that used in previous publications. The results are, in general, similar to those in previous reports; however, a previously unrecognized cause for "false-positive reactions" was identified, and a procedure to eliminate it was developed.

Methods and materials. Latex particles coated with rabbit antibody to HBAg were provided by Hoechst Pharmaceuticals, Inc., together with known reactive and non-reactive control sera. Hoechst also provided latex particles coated with non-specific gamma globulin for the rheumatoid factor test. The HBAg test was carried out on glass plates as used for blood typing. Into the center of each of the inscribed circles, a drop of test serum was placed, followed by a drop of test serum which was followed by a drop of latex particles. The two drops were mixed to an even suspension with a wooden rod. The slide was placed on a VDRL rotator for five minutes, and then inspected for agglutination over the black background and with the indirect fluorescent light of a gel diffusion viewer. As in any agglutination test, the very weak reactions are difficult to see without considerable experience and may result in conflicting reports by different technologists. The known reactive and non-reactive control sera were retested on each plate. Counterelectrophoresis (CEP) was carried out using a number of commercial kits, following the manufacturers' directions. Only results obtained with the Abbott kit will be reported, since this resulted in the fewest number of false-negative results. Hemagglutination inhibition (HAI) tests were carried out by one of us (G.N.V.) by a previously reported method [477]. The antigen used for coating red cells was derived from a healthy HBAg carrier of subtype ad, and the anti-HBAg agglutinator was anti-a from a dialysis patient (kindly supplied by Dr. J. P. Soulier, National Blood Transfusion Service, France). HAI testing was usually done only when positive results were obtained by either the latex test or CEP.

Results. With a panel of sera supplied by the Division of Biologics Standards, the latex test detected four HBAg-positive samples missed by CEP, and missed one which was detected by CEP (Table 1). With a recent panel of test sera employed in proficiency

Table 1.   DBS Panel

Latex	CEP	HAI	DBS	Number of Samples
+	+	+	+	40
+	−	+	+	4
+	−	−	−	1
−	+	+	+	1
−	−	+	+	2 *
−	−	−	−	11
				59

* Panel samples had deteriorated. Gross precipitates evident, which were removed by centrifugation before testing.

testing by the American Association of Blood Banks, the latex test detected two positive samples missed by CEP. There were no latex-negative, CEP-positive results (Table 2). Table 3 lists results with 39 sera in which HBAg had been previously detected by CEP. The latex test was positive with all but one. Table 4 reports on 1000 random hospital patients. The latex test was positive with one sample missed by CEP. Combining results from Tables 1, 2 and 4, there were seven latex-positive, CEP-negative sera and only one CEP-positive, latex-negative serum.

The data presented above indicate that the latex test has a satisfactory degree of sensitivity, but the tables also include

Table 2.   AABB proficiency testing panel #1

Latex	CEP	Known Positives *	Number of Samples
+	+	+	3
+	−	+	2
−	+		0
−	−	+	5
−	−	−	10
			20

* By more sensitive techniques, such as with concentrated test sample.

Table 3.   Previously positive samples

Latex	CEP	HAI	Number of Samples
+	+	+	36
+	+	−	2
−	+	+	1
			39

Table 4.   Sequential patients admitted to a Community Hospital

Latex	CEP	HAI	R.F.*	R.F. 1:20**	# Samples
+	+	+	−	−	1
+	+	−	−	−	1
+	−	+	+	−	1
+	−	−	+	+	9
+	−	−	N.T.	+	9
+	−	−	+	−	25
+	−	−	−	−	20
+	−	−	N.T.	−	32
−	−	N.T.	N.T.	N.T.	902
					1000

N.T. = Not Tested
* R.F. = Rheumatoid Factor with serum tested undiluted.
** R.F. = Rheumatoid Factor with serum tested 1:20

instances in which the latex test has been positive with samples which are not confirmed to contain HBAg by either CEP or HAI. Some of these may well be true positives missed by CEP and HAI, but for purposes of this discussion we will refer to all of them as "false-positives". False-positives were noted in 9.5% of the hospital samples (Table 4) and in 3.6% of normal volunteer donors (Table 5). One possible mechanism for false-positive reactions could be ag-glutination of gamma globulin (antibody)-coated latex by antiglobulin antibodies in the test sera. The rheumatoid factor (R.F.) test, which was developed to detect antiglobulins of significance in rheu-matoid arthritis, is usually run with the test serum at a dilution of 1:20. This test was carried out on all of the HBAg-latex-positive sera. After the study was well under way, testing for antiglobulin activity with undiluted sera was also included, since most of the latex-positive, CEP-negative, HAI-negative reactions were very weak. Table 4 includes these results for the hospital patients.

Table 5.   Volunteer Blood Bank Donors

Latex	CEP	HAI	R.F.	R.F. 1:20	# Samples
+	+	+	+	-	2
+	-	-	+	+	7
+	-	-	N.T.	+	3
+	-	-	+	-	33
+	-	-	-	-	54
+	-	-	N.T.	-	34
-	-	N.T.	N.T.	N.T.	3503
					3636

N.T. = Not Tested

Although only 18 of the 95 "false-positive" HBAg-latex tests were positive in the R.F. test at a 1:20 dilution, 34 of the 54 samples tested with undiluted serum were positive. Similarly, Table 5 shows that only 10 of the 131 "false-positive" donor samples were positive in the R.F. test at 1:20, but 40 of the 94 tested with un-diluted serum were positive. These reactions are summarized in Table 6.

Table 6.   Latex-positive results not confirmed by CEP or HAI

	Hospital Patients			Volunteer Donors		
	# Tested	# (+)	% (+)	# Tested	# (+)	# (%)
Latex HBAg test	1000	95	9.5	3636	131	3.6
RF test, serum 1:20	95	18	19	131	10	7.6
RF test, serum neat	54	34	63	94	40	43

All of the early testing in this study had been carried out with stored serum. When donor serum was tested within a few hours of collection, a new problem appeared. A large proportion of the samples resulted in a faint grainy appearance which would have been interpreted as a weak positive reaction with stored serum. This forced an alteration of criteria for a positive reaction to a level which might have missed some of the previous confirmed positives. Since this type of false-positive reaction was related to the freshness of the serum, it seemed logical that the latex particles might be clumping around fibrin particles still forming after the serum had been separated from the clot. When fresh serum which was causing weak agglutination was stirred with a rod coated with bovine thrombin (5000 units/ml), the positive reactions decreased and in some instances disappeared. The improvement suggested that our hypothesis was correct, but was too inconsistent to be satisfactory for routine use. We considered the possibility that clotting had been completed, but floating fibrin fragments still resulted in some agglutination of the latex particles. We therefore collected a series of blood samples in tubes containing one drop of thrombin to ensure rapid complete coagulation.

Table 7.   Fresh and 24-hour samples with and without thrombin

With Thrombin				Without Thrombin						# of
HBAg		R.F.		HBAg		R.F.				Samples
Fresh	24hr	1:1	1:20	Fresh	24hr	1:1	1:20	CEP	HAI	
-	-	N.T.	N.T.	-	-	N.T.	N.T.	-	N.T.	125
-	-	N.T.	N.T.	+	-	N.T.	N.T.	-	N.T.	36
-	-	+	-	+	+	+	-	-	-	2
-	-	-	-	+	+	-	-	-	-	2
+	+	+	-	+	+	+	-	-	-	2
+	+	-	-	+	+	-	-	-	-	1
										168

N.T. = Not Tested

The effect of thrombin is indicated in Table 7. Thirty-six of the 168 normal donor samples were positive in the HBAg latex test without thrombin when tested with fresh serum, but not with 25-hour serum. When the blood was collected into thrombin, these samples were all non-reactive in the HBAg latex test, even with fresh serum. There were four sera which were positive after 24 hours in the absence of thrombin, but negative with fresh and 24-hour serum in the presence of thrombin. Two of these were R.F.-positive. Three sera were reactive with or without collection into thrombin; two of these were R.F.-positive.

Discussion. The latex test investigated here proved satisfactorily sensitive for detection of HBAg. Its frequency of false-
negatives was less than that of a DBS-licensed CEP kit. The latex-
positive, CEP-positive, HAI-negative results reflected the use of
reagents in the HAI test which did not detect all of the HBAg-related
antigenic determinants. We now know that our HAI test, using ad-
coated cells and anti-a agglutinator misses some of the HBAg-positive
sera of the ay subtype.

The relatively high number of latex reactive results which
cannot be confirmed by any other test are likely to be false-positive
reactions. Some of these may be attributed to antiglobulins in the
test sera which agglutinate the gamma globulin (antibody)-coated
latex particles. In approximately half of the instances in which a
false-positive reaction occurred in the HBAg latex test, latex particles coated with gamma globulin for the rheumatoid factor test were
also agglutinated by undiluted test serum. A positive R.F. test may
thus provide an explanation for a false-positive latex test for HBAg;
however, a positive R.F. test does not necessarily indicate that the
latex HBAg test is falsely reactive. R.F. tests were reactive in a
high proportion of sera confirmed to contain HBAg by multiple tests,
as previously noted by others [493].

When fresh serum was tested, a more frequent cause of false-
positive results was incomplete conversion of fibrinogen to fibrin.
This could be prevented by mixing the freshly-collected blood with
thrombin to ensure immediate and complete clotting. In four instances, this approach also prevented false-positive reactions
which were evident in 24-hour-old serum, even though two of these
sera were R.F.-positive. This indicates that at least some of the
positive R.F. tests are on a non-specific basis rather than a result of antiglobulin antibody.

The occurrence of false-positive results in the latex test for
HBAg could be an obstacle to its adoption by blood banks, but it is
quite simple to retest the samll number of reactive sera with the
more complicated but more specific techniques. Moreover, detection
of antiglobulin activity in sera could be an indication of unsus-
pected disease in some instances, and would thus be for the benefit
of the patient.

The latex test for detection of HBAg appears to have a number
of advantages. It is extremely simple to perform, uses techniques
with which all laboratory technologists are familiar, requires no
special equipment, and can provide an answer in little more than
five minutes. It thus appears ideal for screening donor blood in
an emergency, and could be used for routine screening of blood donors before phlebotomy. It also appears likely that it could be
adapted to a channel of an automatic blood typing machine.

Conclusion.   The latex test for HBAg appears to be highly sensitive.   Its propensity for false-positive reactions, especially with fresh serum, can be overcome to a considerable extent by clotting the test blood samples in the presence of thrombin.

Acknowledgement.   Dr. Lawrence Petz provided the samples of serum from hospitalized patients admitted to the Harkness Community Hospital, San Francisco.

This study was aided by a grant from Hoechst Pharmaceuticals, Inc.

26. IMMUNE ADHERENCE: ITS APPLICATION TO THE DETECTION OF HEPATITIS-ASSOCIATED ANTIGEN IN HUMAN SERUM

R. M. Zarco

Cordis Laboratories, Miami, Florida

Immune adherence was described by R. A. Nelson [354] in 1953 as an in vitro immunological reaction between normal erythrocytes and a wide variety of micro-organisms sensitized with their individually specific antibody and complement. As was expected of a reaction dependent on complement, the adherence to the erythrocyte was temperature dependent, proceeding more rapidly at 37°C than at 0°C.

There are basically four reactants in the immune adherence reaction; namely, the antigen, the antibody, complement, and the indicator particle.

A very wide variety of antigens have been shown to participate in the reaction when sensitized by their specific antibody, allowing the utilization of this reaction in a great number of clinical and research conditions.

The indicator particles for immune adherence have been, by definition, human erythrocytes or non-primate platelets such as rabbit platelets. Human erythrocytes of any blood type are reactive in immune adherence. Most normal human erythrocytes are believed to be reactive, although some difference in degrees of reactivities has been noted. Certain normal individuals have been encountered whose red cells do not react at all in immune adherence. The reason for this has not been explained.

The immune adherence reaction has been employed in various serologic tests. The reaction may be detected by a number of methods. This includes the direct microscope demonstration of the adherent particle on the surface of a red cell in a mixture with specific antibody and complement. Light microscopy is generally adequate for large particles. However, dark field microscopy has been found to be more convenient, especially for bacteria and small particles.

The most frequently used method for demonstrating immune adherence is by hemagglutination of the indicator red cell. The sensitized antigen becomes adherent to 2 or more erythrocytes, causing hemagglutination. This method was first used by Daguet [122] in 1956 with T. pallidum. Since then, it has been used extensively for almost any type of antigen, either particulate or soluble. Originally the tests have been carried out in round bottom test tubes. More recently microtiter plates with "U" or "V" bottoms have been used. This latter procedure utilizes much smaller volumes of reagents and facilitates the performance of a greater number of tests. However, some degree of precision and sensitivity is lost.

Immune adherence tests for antigen, antibody or complement have been described extensively. In all these procedures, the most striking observation is the high degree of sensitivity of the test. Immune adherence is known to be at least ten-fold more sensitive than complement fixation and at least a hundred-fold more sensitive than immune precipitation tests. The sensitivity of immune adherence is given in Table 1.

Table 1. Reported sensitivity of immune adherence for detecting antigen.

Antigen Type	Antigen	Sensitivity	Author
Virus	Poliovirus	Detected 2.5×10^6 Particles	Nelson
	Cauliflower Mosaic Virus	100 x More Sensitive than Immunodiffusion	Nelson & Day
	T2 Bacteriophage	Detected 5×10^6 Particles	Taverne
Soluble Antigen	Ovalbumin	0.005 µg	Turk
	Human Serum Albumin	0.001 µg	Nelson

Because of the high degree of specificity afforded by the immune adherence reaction, the development of a hemagglutination test for the hepatitis-associated antigen (HBAg) was considered, in 1970, under a National Blood Resource Contract (NIH-70-2232).

Antibody against hepatitis-associated antigen was obtained from a hemophilia patient. Serum was dispensed in aliquots, inactivated at 56°C for 30 minutes and stored at -20°C. Antiserum obtained from experimental animals proved to be unsuitable for the test since immune complexes resulting from absorption of contaminating antibodies with normal human plasma reacted with complement and gave positive hemagglutination patterns even in the absence of the hepatitis-associated antigen in the serums being tested.

Complement serum from guinea-pigs was obtained by heart puncture from at least 40 healthy male Hartley guinea-pigs, allowed to clot in separate test tubes at room temperature for 30 minutes and at 0°C for 2 - 4 hours and centrifuged at 0°C. The serum from each tube was pooled and centrifuged at 0°C to remove all cellular elements. The clear pooled serum was dispensed in 100 ml aliquots, frozen in dry ice-acetone mixture and stored at -70°C. Prior to use in immune adherence tests, 100 ml aliquot was thawed and absorbed three times at 0°C with washed, Type O+ human erythrocytes. The absorbed guinea-pig complement was dispensed in 5 ml aliquots, frozen in dry ice-acetone mixture and stored at -70°C.

Human erythrocytes were obtained from a healthy donor, Type O, Rh positive. The blood was collected by vein puncture into twice its volume of Alsever's solution, and stored at 4°C. When required, aliquots were removed aseptically and red cells washed at least 3 times with 0.01 M EDTA, Gelatin-Veronal buffer and standardized to a concentration of 8×10^7 cells per ml in 0.01 M EDTA, GVB. Stored blood was used for periods up to 8 weeks provided it did not become contaminated during storage.

Preliminary to setting up the test assay, a checkerboard titration was performed with varying dilutions of a known HBAg-positive serum, previously inactivated at 56°C for 30 minutes, the human anti-HBAg serum, and absorbed guinea-pig complement. Based on the results of this checkerboard titration, the optimal dilutions of antiserum (1:20) and complement (1:10) to be used in the test were determined. Results from such an assay with varying amounts of HBAg-positive serum and antiserum but with a single concentration of complement previously found to be optimal is given in Table 2.

Unknown sera were inactivated at 56°C for 30 minutes. These were tested for the presence of the hepatitis-associated antigen using microtiter plates with "U" bottoms and reagent volumes of 0.025 ml, as outlined in Figure 1.

Table 2. Checkerboard titration of Australia antigen and human antiserum by the immune adherence test.

Au Antigen dilution	ANTIBODY DILUTION								
	2	4	8	16	32	64	128	256	None
100	+	+	+	+	+	neg	0	0	0
200	+	+	+	+	+	0	0	0	0
400	+	+	+	+	+	+	0	0	0
800	+	+	+	+	+	0	0	0	0
1600	+	0	0	0	0	0	0	0	0
None	+	0	0	0	0	0	0	0	

REAGENTS

Gelatin Veronal buffer (GVB^{++})
Human antibody (Ab)
Guinea pig complement (C_{gp})
Human erythrocytes O+ (E_{hu})

PROCEDURE

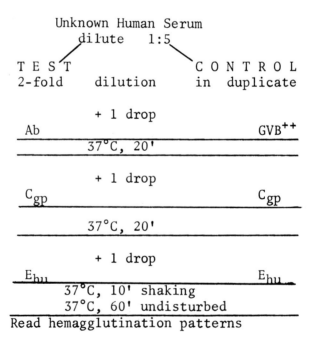

Figure 1. Microtiter plate assay for immune adherence test for Australia antigen in serum.

Results from immune adherence hemagglutination tests on an initial group of 16 serum samples are given in Table 3. At the same time that the immune adherence hemagglutination tests were done, immuno-diffusion in agarose and complement fixation tests using 4 CH_{50} units of guinea-pig complement were done with the same antiserum used in immune adherence tests. Results of both tests are included in Table 3. The immune adherence hemagglutination titers obtained in this group were about 10 times higher than the complement fixation titers and 100 times higher than the immunodiffusion (ID) titers.

Table 3. Comparative measurement of Australia antigen in human sera by immune adherence, complement fixation and immunodiffusion tests.*

Sample	Titers Determined		
	Immune Adherence	Complement Fixation	Immuno-diffusion
1	5,120	160	16
2	1,280	160	8
3	1,280	160	4
4	640	80	2
5	320	20	1
6	320	60	2
7	320	80	2
8	160	40	2
9	0**	0√	neg.
10	0	0	neg.
11	0	0	neg.
12	0	0	neg.
13	0	0	neg.
14	0	0	neg.
15	0	0	neg.
16	0	0	neg.

*   The same human antibody (Britten) was used in all assays.
** Less than 1:10
√   Less than 1:5

The immune adherence hemagglutination and the immunodiffusion tests were repeated in a larger group consisting of 61 human sera. As in the previous group studies, the same antibody was used in both tests. Resulting titers of HBAg in each serum were plotted in a scatter diagram (Figure 2). Good correlation was seen from the distribution of the results. As in the first series of 16 samples, immune adherence titers were about 100-fold higher than immuno-diffusion titers.

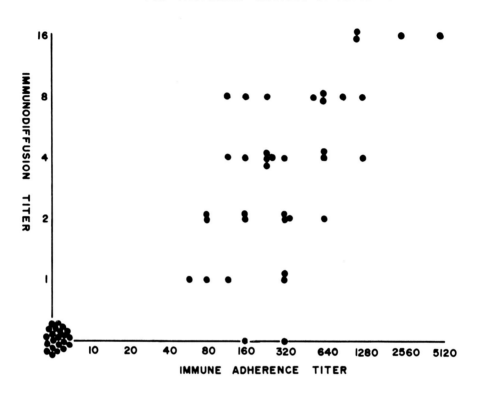

CORRELATION OF IMMUNODIFFUSION AND IMMUNE ADHERENCE TESTS
FOR AUSTRALIA ANTIGEN IN HUMAN SERUM

Figure 2.

Further correlation of the results from the two procedures is given in Table 4. All samples found to be positive by immunodiffusion were likewise detected by immune adherence. However, 2 samples found negative by immunodiffusion showed the presence of HBAg by immune adherence.

Table 4. Correlation of immunodiffusion and immune adherence tests for Australia antigen in human serum.

	IDF Positive	IDF Negative	Total
IA Positive	35	2	37
IA Negative	0	24	24
Total	35	26	61

At the time our study on the immune adherence test for HBAg was in progress, a similar study was reported by Okochi, Mayumi, Haguiro and Saito [366]. The test method employed was similar to the method described above with the exception that they added dithiothreitol in order to inhibit the C3 inactivator normally present in the sera tested. Their results from a series of 5,239 serum samples showed 2% (105) positive reactions. Both immunoelectrophoresis and immunodiffusion detected only half of the IA positive serums. Their study of the immune adherence hemagglutination tests for hepatitis-associated antigen showed the greater sensitivity of the method, which confirmed our results.

The simplicity of the performance of IA hemagglutination; the economy in amounts of reagents required for microtiter tests; the early reading of results coupled with high sensitivity give the workers in the blood transfusion field an added diagnostic procedure to improve the chances of eliminating HBAg-positive blood donors from the transfusion program.

27. STANDARDS FOR HEPATITIS-ASSOCIATED ANTIGEN REAGENTS AND TESTS

L. F. Barker

National Institutes of Health, Division of Biologics

Standards, Bethesda, Maryland

Introduction. In a statement published in January 1970, from a panel of the Committee on Plasma and Plasma Substitutes of the Division of Medical Sciences, National Academy of Sciences-National Research Council (NAS-NRC) a strong recommendation was made for standardization of tests for the Australia antigen (serum hepatitis antigen, hepatitis associated antigen, hepatitis B antigen) [142]. This statement was based on a review of information acquired by using two test methods for HBAg detection: agar gel diffusion and complement fixation. The committee indicated that "......it is clear that the sensitivity and specificity of the tests for Australia antigen vary among laboratories, and there is no agreement on the establishment of a uniform test or tests. Such agreement would be essential before any test could be brought into general use" [142]. Since the publication of this statement there have been many developments in the field of HBAg testing, noteworthy among them being a remarkable increase in the number of methods with potential application to routine testing of donor blood (Table 1) and the introduction of HBAg testing into general use in blood banks. In a statement calling more forcefully for initiating blood donor testing for HBAg as soon as possible, Alter, Holland and Schmidt took the position in mid-1970 that: "While an optimally sensitive, standardised test is highly desirable, it is by no means essential. The cross-match of whole blood has long served as an effective safeguard against the transfusion of incompatible blood despite the fact that there is wide discrepancy in the way this test is performed from laboratory to laboratory. What is essential, then, is not that the test be uniform, but that it be highly specific and perform the function for which it was devised" [17].

Table 1.   Methods for detection of HBAg and anti-HBAg which may
be applicable to large-scale testing.

Agar gel diffusion
Rheophoresis
Counterelectrophoresis
Complement fixation
Platelet aggregation
Passive hemagglutination
Reversed passive hemagglutination
Immune adherence hemagglutination
Latex particle agglutination
Radioimmunoassay

In response to the NAS-NRC recommendation to study test sensitivity and specificity, a series of evaluation trials was conducted
under the guidance of the Center for Disease Control. Antisera and
coded sera positive and negative for HBAg were distributed to a
number of laboratories for comparison of the agar gel diffusion
(AGD), counterelectrophoresis (CEP) and complement fixation (CF)
tests to detect HBAg. Radioimmunoassay (RIA) and hemagglutination
inhibition (HAI) methods were also evaluated in a few laboratories.
The results showed that in order of increasing sensitivity, these
methods could be ranked: AGD, CEP, CF, HAI and RIA [326]. Both
false-positive and false-negative results were obtained with each
of these methods. The wide range of results obtained in different
laboratories with each method appeared to reflect differences in
methodologic details. Based on the results of these studies, the
Committee recommended: "1) That, as soon as practicable, all blood
banks begin routine HAA testing of blood donors with commercial supplies of antiserum licensed by the Division of Biologics Standards
or with locally prepared antisera of equivalent quality, recognizing
that rapid and possibly fundamental methodologic changes may occur
in the next few years. A commercial antiserum should be used only
with the methods for which it is recommended. 2) That, if test
results are required rapidly, blood banks introducing routine screening begin with the CEP test. The AGD test is useful if test results
are not needed rapidly, and it could be used for confirmatory tests
in reference laboratories" [326]. The Committee made a number of
other recommendations to facilitate the implementation of routine
testing as well as to indicate the need for continuing efforts in
the areas of a standardization and quality control of HBAg testing.
At the time of publication of this statement, in April 1971, two
manufacturers had been licensed by the DBS to market Hepatitis Associated Antibody (Anti-Australia Antigen).

Chronology and approach to standards for antibody reagents.
In recognition of the applicability of serum containing antibodies
to Australia antigen to the prevention of serum hepatitis, the
Director of the National Institutes of Health indicated in a statement published in the Federal Register in the fall of 1970 that federal standards to insure the safety, purity and potency of this biological product would be prescribed as soon as feasible [145]. Final
publication of standards for Hepatitis Associated Antibody (Anti-
Australia Antigen) appeared in the Federal Register in January, 1971,
[146] and to date licenses have been issued to seven manufacturers
to produce this antibody reagent for use in four different test procedures (agar gel diffusion, counterelectrophoresis, complement fixation and rheophoresis). Sources of licensed antiserum at the present time include human, guinea-pig, horse and rabbit serum. Antiserum from other sources and additional test methods are currently
investigational. Several important criteria considered in the evaluation of reagents and/or test systems are listed in Table 2.

Table 2. Criteria for evaluating reagents and/or test systems

---

Potency
Broad reactivity
Specificity
Stability
Safety
Efficacy

Potency and specificity of this antiserum are determined by
testing against a Reference Panel of sera which is available from
the DBS. With regard to potency, the standards state that: "To be
satisfactory for release each filling of Hepatitis Associated Antibody (Anti-Australia Antigen) shall be tested against the Reference
Hepatitis Associated Antigen (Australia Antigen) Panel and shall be
sufficiently potent to be able to detect the antigen in the appropriate sera of the Reference Panel by all test methods recommended
by the manufacturer in the package enclosure" [146]. Confirmatory
testing is done at the DBS, using the same Reference Panel. The
panel contains 60 sera with antigen concentrations over a wide range
from high levels which produce troublesome prozones in some systems
to low levels which at present are detectable only by radioimmunoassay. The panel sera were obtained from blood donors over a wide
geographic distribution in this country. There are a number of non-
reactive sera in the panel which are used to examine reagents for
nonspecific activity.

In addition to commercially prepared reagents for HBAg detection
antisera have been prepared for research purposes by the Research

Resources Branch of the National Institute of Allergy and Infectious Diseases (NIAID), at the National Institutes of Health. Thus it is possible to obtain potent, specific guinea pig-antisera and reagent antigens specific for both the AD and the AY subtypes [283] of Australia antigen from NIAID. These antisera have been tested in many laboratories and have been found suitable for use in agar gel diffusion, counterelectrophoresis, complement fixation, passive hemagglutination, immunofluorescence, latex particle agglutination and radioimmunoassay techniques.

Prior to the general availability of commercial reagents, antiserum for use in the agar gel diffusion and counterelectrophoresis methods was made available to state health departments for distribution to blood banks by the National Blood Resources Branch of the National Heart and Lung Institute of NIH. Similar efforts to make reagents available for donor testing have been made in other countries. In each instance the mainstay of standards for potency and specificity has been the empirical use of antigen panels such as the DBS Reference Panel described above.

Future endeavors in HBAg standards. Studies which have shown that viral hepatitis, type B, occurs in recipients of blood in which HBAg cannot be detected by presently available reagents and techniques indicate that there is a need to improve the sensitivity of detection systems. As more sensitive methods such as radioimmunoassay (RIA) are developed, however, specificity becomes an increasingly difficult aspect to evaluate. It is possible that subtyping for the mutually exclusive d and y determinants by the more sensitive methods will be of some assistance in resolving specificity, but at present there is no assurance that these will be the only subtype determinants of HBAg. Almeida et al. have recently indicated that there are other antigenic determinants, probably related to virion cores, which appear to be quite distinct from the Australia antigen [8]. There is a need to prepare standardized specific typing reagents, as has been done by the Research Resources Branch of NIAID for the ad and ay subtypes, for epidemiologic and clinical studies as well as for determining specificity of antigens detected by more sensitive methods.

Recognition of HBAg subtypes and additional hepatitis B virus antigens and their possible significance in passive and active immunization against hepatitis B virus is one of several factors creating a need for standard antigen reagents and test systems to be used for antibody detection. Such antibody detection systems will be of obvious importance in identifying suitable donors for hepatitis B immune serum globulin [394] as well as for eventual evaluation of the potency of active immunizing reagents such as the heated antigen described by Krugman et al [262].

Finally, as standards for both HBAg and anti-HBAg reagents are promulgated and used to assess the potency and specificity of such reagents and test systems which are being used in blood banks and other laboratories throughout the country, it will be of paramount importance that training programs and proficiency testing be continuing activities to ensure that these reagents are performing in a satisfactory manner in the field. To date such programs have been carried on by the American Red Cross, the American Association of Blood Banks, the Center for Disease Control and a number of state health departments and independent organizations.

Conclusion. The optimal HBAg detection system, which may not be practically feasible, is one with a high degree of specificity as well as sensitivity adequate to detect virtually all donors who may transmit viral hepatitis, type B. Although we do not yet know what the distribution of HBAg titers is in the antigen-positive members of the blood donor population, it is already quite clear that the presence of HBAg is not an all-or-none phenomenon for present methods including radioimmunoassays, already have made it possible to detect the antigen over a range of at least five log units. It seems quite possible that there may be an equally wide spread of antigen amounts below the threshold of the most sensitive methods currently available for HBAg detection in carriers of hepatitis B virus [36]; if so, it is unlikely that immunologic methods will ever achieve one hundred percent efficacy in detecting infectious donors. At present, however, this is an area which must be relegated to speculation until such time as more information is available using the most sensitive methods and reagents that can be developed.

CHARACTERIZATION OF HEPATITIS B ANTIGEN

Chairman: E. Lennette

28. ISOLATION AND PHYSICOCHEMICAL CHARACTERISTICS OF HBAg

John L. Gerin

Rockville Laboratory of the Molecular Anatomy Program
Oak Ridge National Laboratory
Rockville, Maryland

The association of HBAg with the etiologic agent (HBV) of long incubation or type B hepatitis has now been well established on epidemiological grounds and there is reason to believe that HBV and HBAg possess common antigenic determinants. The important question as to whether HBAg is itself the virus of type B hepatitis may never be answered satisfactorily until a suitable system for HBV replication is discovered. However, research concerning the nature of the antigen and its definition in physical, chemical and immunological terms will contribute to our understanding of HBV and its pathologic manifestations in man. The purpose of this report is to review our current understanding of HBAg in terms of its physicochemical properties.

The determinants of HBAg are located on particles which, as isolated from serum, present a heterogeneity of morphological forms. Although the relative proportions of the various forms may vary widely between different serum specimens, the bulk of the antigen is usually found associated with a spherical particle, 20-25 nm in diameter. Filamentous forms having the same diameter as the small spherical form (20 nm) and displaying a regular periodicity of 30 nm are commonly observed in HBAg positive serum and are of various lengths. The Dane particle, a larger (42 nm) spherical form of HBAg, possesses a complex structure and is a relatively rare form in most sera.

Dane et al.[123] suggested that the 42 nm form may represent the actual infectious agent (HBV) while the 20 nm and filamentous forms represent excess viral coat lipoprotein released from infected cells. All three particulate forms (20 nm spherical,

filamentous and 42 nm spherical), share common determinants on
their surface as has been repeatedly demonstrated by immune electron microscopy. In addition, Almeida et al. [8] showed that the
27 nm core of the Dane particle possessed determinant(s) not shared
by the outer shell or coat. Detailed descriptions of the morphology
of HBAg and the technique of immune electron microscopy will be
presented in another paper of this Symposium. Since HBAg is defined in antigenic terms, it is imperative to include in any
physical definition all forms which share common determinants
and for this purpose immune electron microscopy is an invaluable
tool. For example, our prototype J.M. serum was found to contain
only 20 nm spherical forms of HBAg when examined by immune electron
microscopy using homologous antibody. However, examination of
certain other sera by this technique reveals all forms of the
antigen in the immune aggregate (Figure 1A). The immune complex
clearly demonstrates the existence of common antigenic determinants
between the 20 nm form of the antigen and the filamentous and
42 nm (Dane) forms. Since the antibody used in this experiment was
produced against the 20 nm form of a different subtype, this complex represents the interaction of antibody with the group specific
or a determinant.

When the serum described above was examined without the
addition of antibody, aggregates of long filaments and 42 nm

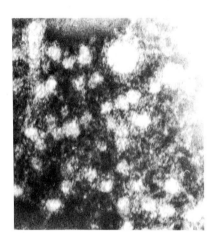 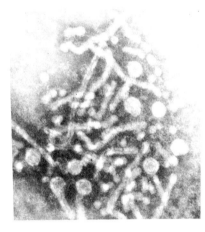

Figure 1. Immune electron microscopy (IEM) of HBAg (ay) positive
serum. Serum was incubated with homologous antiserum (1A) or PBS
(1B) for 1 hr. at 37°C, diluted 1:2 with PBS, and centrifuged for
30 minutes at 21,000 rpm in the SW 50.1 rotor. Pellet was washed
once with PBS, resuspended in distilled water, and examined by e-
lectron microscopy after negative staining with 1% phosphotungstic
acid - (A = 180,000X, B = 100,000X)

particles were observed (Figure 1B) and suggested to us that the filamentous forms and outer coat of the Dane particle possess a common determinant not shared by the 20 nm form.   Fields and Cossart [150] have presented similar evidence to indicate that antigenic differences may exist between the 20 nm spherical and filamentous forms of HBAg.

The proportion of forms observed by immune electron micro-scopy is an accurate estimate of their proportion in serum (J. Almeida, personal communication) and in attempting to isolate the various forms by biophysical techniques, one is well advised to screen by immune electron microscopy in order to select a serum rich in a given morphological form.   Obviously, it is important not only to isolate HBAg from normal serum components, but also to separate the various forms from one another in order to study their antigenic composition.

Fortunately, human serum represents a ready source of high-titered and stable antigen, and centrifugal procedures for the purification of HBAg from human serum are highly developed.   The zonal centrifuge rotors, developed by N.G. Anderson and his colleagues [19] at the Oak Ridge National Laboratories, have been most useful for the large scale isolation of HBAg from serum and at the MAN Program laboratory we presently employ a four-step procedure based on certain biophysical properties of HBAg (buoyant density and sedimentation rate).

As a first-step procedure, isopycnic banding is a useful technique for the concentration and partial purification of HBAg from serum.   The buoyant density of HBAg in sucrose and potassium tartrate is approximately 1.16 g/cm^3 and 1.20 g/cm^3 in CsCl [159]. Since the antigen is very stable to high speed centrifugation in CsCl we have routinely used this gradient material for the first-step isopycnic banding of HBAg.   The distribution of CF reactive antigen on first-step isopycnic banding of a number of different HBAg-positive sera is shown in Figure 2; a broadly reactive hemophiliac serum (R.B.) was used as the source of antibody.   The usual result is complete recovery of CF activity distributed symmetrically about a value of 1.20 g/cm^3 (Figure 2A) although variations of this pattern are occasionally observed (Figure 2B). The skewing of the antigen distribution to the more dense (1.22-1.24 g/cm^3) side of the major peak (Figure 2B, sera j and w) would possibly represent the presence of immune complexes in HBAg excess.   The significance of the high density (>1.39 g/cm^3) (Figure 2B, serum j) and low density (Figure 2B, serum Ytr) CF activity will be discussed later in this text.

Most of our early isolation work was with HBAg from serum (J.M.) obtained by plasmapheresis of a young adult female who developed

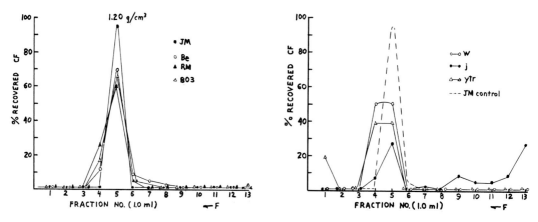

Figure 2. Isopycnic banding of HBAg positive sera in CsCl density gradient, SW41 rotor, 16 hours, at 35,000 rpm and 4°C. 2A, symmetrical distribution of CF activity about 1.20 g/cm^3 peak; 2B, asymmetric distribution.

chronic anicteric hepatitis after accidental exposure to a single unit of blood. J.M. was of the ad subtype according to the nomenclature introduced by Le Bouvier [283]. The B-XXIX zonal centrifuge rotor was used for the first-step isopycnic banding of HBAg from 500 ml of J.M. serum (CF titer = 1:4096) and the antigen was fully recovered at a density 1.20 g/cm^3 in CsCl after centrifugation at 30,000 rpm for 58.5 x 10^{10} ω^2t at 5°C. The peak fractions from this experiment were pooled as JMCs1 and rebanded in CsCl using a B-XXIX zonal rotor at 28,000 rpm for 22 hr. at 5°C (146 x 10^{10} ω^2t) as a second-step purification procedure; additional purification and full recovery of HBAg was obtained in a sharp zone of activity at a density of 1.20 g/cm^3 (CF titer = 1:65,536). Fractions containing peak activity from the second isopycnic banding step were pooled and the CsCl exchanged for phosphate-buffered saline (PBS) using an Amicon cell with an XM-100 Diaflo membrane. Antigen at this stage of purification (JMCs2) was used by Walsh et al. [483] and Landers et al. [275] to develop radioimmunoassays for HBAg and anti-HBAg.

The JMCs2 pool was then sedimented on a preformed "isokinetic" sucrose gradient as a third purification step. A gradient of 5 to 25% w/w sucrose, with a sucrose cushion of 40% w/w was used in a Ti-14 rotor with 29 liner. The sample was centrifuged for approximately 3.5 hrs. (22 x 10^{10}ω^2t), yielding a good separation of the 20 nm spherical form of HBAg from normal serum proteins. Rate separation would be expected to reveal the heterogeneity of morphological forms of HBAg but only 20 nm spherical forms were observed with J.M. in accordance with the results obtained by immune electron microscopy. A marked reduction in CF activity accompanied the rate separation procedure and the reason for this phenomenon is poorly understood. The use of shallow CsCl gradients in place of sucrose did not protect against this loss which seems to be based on the level of purity of the HBAg. The recombination of normal serum proteins and purified HBAg did not reconstitute the CF activity while, in a single experiment, the addition of human serum albumin (0.5%) to the sucrose gradient before sedimentation of the antigen resulted in full recovery. This phenomenon might be explained either by aggregation or slight conformational changes of the antigen upon the removal of a stabilizing protein such as albumin. Despite this loss of CF activity, the purified HBAg remains a potent immunogen and stimulates high levels of CF antibody in guinea pigs [398].

Fractions from the rate separation step were pooled as J.S. Cs2R1 and the material rebanded in CsCl as a fourth-step procedure. A Ti-14 rotor with 29 liner was filled with sample and a shallow CsCl gradient and centrifuged for 19 hrs at 35,000 rpm and 5°C. The density gradient was monitored at 280 nm using an Oak Ridge flow cell (1 cm) and HBAg was recovered in a narrow zone at 1.20 g/cm^3. Additionally, a small amount of protein was recovered in the 1.3 g/cm^3 region of the gradient and probably represents contaminating serum protein, possibly aggregated albumin.

A similar purification procedure was performed using a high-titered serum (Ytr) containing HBAg of the ay subtype and is included in this presentation because it demonstrates the diversity of morphological forms. In a preliminary experiment HBAg (ay)-positive serum was isopycnically banded in CsCl, using the SW 41 rotor at 35,000 rpm for 16 hrs. A large proportion of the CF antigen activity was recovered in the low density region of a CsCl density gradient and, since the flotation of HBAg activity precluded the use of zonal centrifuge rotors, the isopycnic banding steps were performed using polycarbonate tubes in an angle-head rotor. Gradients were fractionated into five discrete density regions and the equivalent fractions from each gradient were combined. The five pools, representing different regions of the initial density gradient, were rebanded in CsCl and all of the initial CF activity was eventually recovered at a density of 1.20 g/cm^3; at this point the combined activity was equivalent to a Cs2 or twice-banded preparation (YtrCs2). We concluded that the low density antigen was either trapped or loosely associated in some manner with the large quantity of lipoprotein in Ytr serum and probably did not represent a distinct morphological or physical form of the antigen.

Rate sedimentation under conditions described for JMCs2, revealed not only the zone of activity associated with the 20 nm form of HBAg but also a considerable quantity of antigen sedimenting at a faster rate. Three pools were made by combining those fractions of the gradient corresponding to the 20 nm form, the antigen peak found on the cushion, and the region intermediate between the other two; each pool was rebanded separately in CsCl as the fourth and final purification step. The 20 nm fraction was centrifuged in the Ti-14 rotor with 29 liner at 40,000 rpm for approximately 24 hrs. ($163 \times 10^{10}\omega^2 t$). The gradient was monitored at 280 nm using the Oak Ridge flow cell revealing a sharp zone at 1.20 g/cm^3, corresponding to the HBAg activity, and a trace amount of protein at a density of 1.31 g/cm^3, presumably a serum contaminant. Similarly, the remaining two pools were separately banded in polycarbonate tubes with CsCl density gradients, and centrifuged in an angle head 30 rotor for 24 hrs. at 28,000 rpm. The HBAg activity was recovered from each pool at a density of 1.20 g/cm^3. Examination of each preparation by electron microscopy revealed the expected results; the 20 nm form, short filaments in the intermediate zone, and long filaments and large spherical forms in the cushion fractions. Rate separation, as well as immune electron microscopy, may therefore be used as a measure of the heterogeneity of HBAg forms. Analysis of a number of fractions from the sucrose gradient established that all forms of HBAg contained both group (a) and subtype (y) determinants. The expression of a given subtype in serum, therefore, is not due simply to the presence or absence of a given morphological form of HBAg. An interesting aspect of the rate separation procedure was the observation of HBAg sedimenting slower than the 20 nm form. Although this population represents only a small proportion of the total antigenic content, it is in a size range which might be expected to play a role in the extrahepatic manifestations of immune complex disease.

Antigens purified by the four-step procedure (Cs2R1Cs1) described above were free of normal serum proteins when examined by sensitive immunological and biochemical techniques. They migrate electrophoretically in the α region and react immunologically with both homologous and heterologous antiserum. The most useful criterion of antigen purity has been the analysis of antibody prepared against the antigen in hyperimmunized animals. When JMCs2R1Cs1 was used as the immunogen, no detectable antibody to normal serum protein were observed in full block CF titration against normal serum; the ay forms have not yet been evaluated by this procedure.

Rate-sedimentation experiments in linear sucrose gradients have yielded widely different values for the sedimentation coefficient of the small spherical form of HBAg ranging from 39S to 110S. In our laboratory, a value of 110S was obtained with JMCs2 samples using internal markers (AAV or 70S ribosomes) in swinging bucket rotors [159] and 54S by computer program analysis from zonal centrifuge experiments [158]. Since there are a number of assumptions which must be made with both of the above techniques we determined the sedimentation coefficient of a highly purified

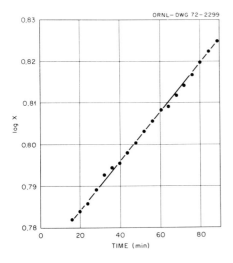
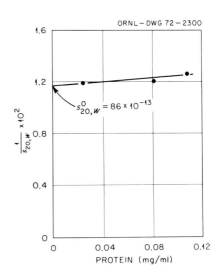

Figure 3. Sedimentation of purified HBAg (JMCs2R1Cs1) in analytical ultracentrifuge. 3A, plot of log χ vs. time at 4 min.
intervals for 20 nm form (0.11 mg protein/ml). 3B, determination
of sedimentation coefficient of HBAg at infinite dilution.

preparation of the 20 nm form of HBAg (JMCs2R1Cs1) in the Model
E using UV optics at 280 nm. The CsCl in the JMCs2R1Cs1 pool
was exchanged with .01M Tris-Cl plus .001M EDTA, pH 7.4 and the
antigen (.11mg/ml) was analyzed in the Model E at 20,000 rpm.
The boundary was sharp and symmetrical and continued to move as
a discrete entity until it reached the bottom of the cell. The
straight line plot (Figure 3A) of log χ vs. time indicates the
precision of the data; the sedimentation coefficient exhibited a
slight concentration dependence (Figure 3B) and at infinite
dilution, a value of $s^o_{20,w}$= 86.1S was obtained. This value,
however, is not in agreement with those obtained from other
laboratories. Schober et al. (personal communication, December
1970) using schlieren optics obtained a value of 35S (+5%) in
good agreement with his earlier estimate (39S) from sucrose zonal
experiments although the ionic conditions were not specified.
Bond et al. (personal communication, August 1971) separated
twice-banded HBAg by sedimentation velocity in a CsCl gradient
using a zonal centrifuge rotor. These investigators noted a
broad and apparently uniformly increasing size distribution
within the population of spherical particles (18-30 nm) and a
linear increase in sedimentation coefficient with increasing
particle diameter. The highest concentration of any form of
HBAg had a diameter of 23 nm and by analytical ultracentrifugation
they calculated a sedimentation coefficient ($s^o_{20,w}$) of 43.6S;
they further suggested that the high values obtained by ourselves
and others might be due to the tendency of purified HBAg to aggregate under certain experimental conditions.

Hirschman et al. [208] reported the presence of endogenous
RNA dependent DNA polymerase activity in particulate fractions of

Table 1.   Inability to Detect RNA-Dependent DNA Polymerase in Purified Australia Antigen.

| | EXOGENOUS TEMPLATE* | | |
	Poly rA-Poly dT	Poly rA-Oligo dT	dAT
AuCs2**			
5 μl	200	0	0
10 μl	50	50	0
AuCs2R1***			
5 μl	0	0	0
10 μl	0	0	0
20 μl	0	0	0
MuLV (suc 1)			
15 μl	20,000	200,000	7,000

  *CPM above No-Polymer control
 **CF = 1:32,768
***.11μg. Au Protein/μl

Table 2.   Inability to Detect DNA Polymerase Activity in Purified Australia Antigen.

| | ENDOGENOUS REACTION | | |
| Reaction* | CPM/Assay | | |
Mixture	60 min.	90 min.	120 min.
Complete	97	158	123
-dATP	72	171	93
+RNase	112	144	136

*40 μl of AuCs2R1/100 μl Rx Mixture

serum obtained from HBAg-positive hepatitis patients; the weak endogenous reaction was much magnified using dAT as a synthetic template.   We examined our preparations at two levels of purity (JMCs2 and JMCs2R1) for the presence of RNA-dependent DNA polymerase activity by methods which have shown this activity in a wide spectrum of viruses.   Both the JMCs2 and JMCs2R1 preparations were tested for exogenous activity against a number of synthetic templates (Table 1) and JMCs2R1 was assayed for endogenous activity (Table 2).   The exogenous templates were fully active for Rauscher and Moloney MuLV preparations and also for a variety of partially purified cellular and supernatant enzymes found in various tissue culture material.   The results clearly indicated the absence of either RNA or DNA dependent DNA polymerases; however, since the JM serum is composed almost entirely of small spherical forms, the possibility that enzyme activity might be associated with another form of HBAg, such as the Dane particle, remains a speculative possibility.   In fact, the centrifugal purification procedure employed by Hirschman et al. [208] would tend to concentrate long filamentous and large spherical (Dane) particles of HBAg.

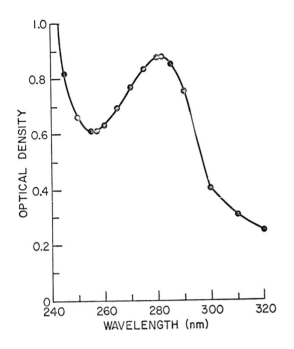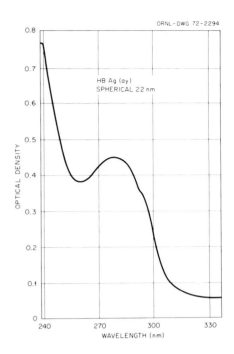

Figure 4.   Ultraviolet absorption spectrum of HBAg.   4A, spectrum
of JMCs2R1 determined manually at 5-10 nm intervals in a 0.3ml
microcuvette against a PBS blank (e = 1cm).   4B, continuous scan
of 20 nm form of HBAg (ay) using Gilford 2400 spectrophotometer
against a PBS blank.

Much effort has been expended in attempts to discover nucleic acid in association with HBAg and most reports have been
negative (Hierholzer, et al., personal communication, June 1970;
Gerin et al. [158]; Brighton, et al., personal communication,
August, 1970).   Ultraviolet (UV) absorption spectra of the small
(20 nm) spherical forms of HBAg (ad) (Figure 4A) and HBAg (ay)
(Figure 4B) are quite typical of protein (O.D. 260/280 = 0.67) and
one would estimate that if nucleic acid were present it must comprise less than 1 to 2% of these preparations; similarly, UV analysis of the filamentous forms of HBAg (ay) yields the same result.
Jozwiak et al. [237] have reported the successful isolation of RNA
from HBAg purified by an entirely different procedure; they were
able to recover 150-250 µg of 9S RNA from 3-5 mg of HBAg specific
proteins.   It is critical that this observation be confirmed by
other laboratories using their purification technique, and since
Jokelainen et al. [236] suggested that the core of the Dane particle contained nucleic acid (based on positive staining with
uranyl acetate), it is again possible that Jozwiak et al.   were
working with preparations particularly rich in the large spherical
forms.

Flotation and staining experiments in early studies revealed the lipoprotein nature of HBAg and, as yet, no carbohydrates other than the ribose associated with nucleic acid have been reported. Kim and Bissell [214] analyzed lipid extracts of purified HBAg for polar lipids by thin layer chromatography on silica gel G. These analyses revealed a preponderance of polar lipids together with cholesterol and small quantities of non-polar lipids. The polar lipids were identified as lecithin and sphingomyelin with phosphatidylethanolamine as a minor component. In their studies on the lipoprotein nature of HBAg, Kim and Bissell [242] found that pretreatment of HBAg with SDS or ether rendered HBAg susceptible to proteolytic attack but did not affect the antigenicity of the particles indicating that the antigenic determinants were protein in nature. Similarly, in our early experiments [159] pretreatment of partially purified HBAg (JMCs2) with ether or deoxycholate (DOC) resulted in a shift in buoyant density from 1.20 to 1.23 in CsCl without loss of CF activity. Treatment with 1% SDS, however, converted the HBAg particle to slow sedimenting components with complete loss of antigenicity. An unusual effect was observed after pretreatment of JMCs2 with 1% Tween 80 for 1 hr at 25°C, in that it released a high density (1.39 g/cm^3) CF reactive antigen, when centrifuged in a SW 40 rotor at 50°C for 18 hr at 111,700 x g. This material had a high O.D. 260/280 ratio typical of nucleoprotein. Almeida et al. [8] have suggested that this antigen may represent the core of the large spherical form. Although the core determinants are not identical to those of the 20 nm form and the outer coat of the Dane particle, broadly reactive human convalescent serum was used in our titration and this serum could contain anti-core antibody. The JM serum, however, does not contain detectable Dane particles and the antigen in our system could possibly represent 10 nm cores of the small spherical forms.

The antigenicity of HBAg is remarkably stable to most physical treatments (heat, pH, freezing and thawing [159]) and proteolytic enzyme treatment [317] and these properties have been used for the successful purification of the antigen from serum in a number of laboratories. Several recent studies [448]; Vyas, personal communication, February 1972; Gerin, unpublished results, indicate that the antigenicity and possibly the morphological constitution of HBAg is dependent upon the presence of disulfide bonds. Vyas et al. reported the complete loss of antigenicity of both the a and d determinants upon reductive alkylation without loss of particulate structure. Sukeno, et al. [448] recovered 80% of HBAg antigenicity by reduction and reoxidation without loss of particulate morphology but did destroy both antigenicity and morphological integrity by reductive alkylation. The extinction coefficient ($E_{1cm}^{1\%}$) of purified HBAg at 280 nm was estimated as 37.26 by Vyas (personal communication) in fairly good agreement to our own estimates. Amino acid analysis, however, yields low

to normal values of tyrosine residues (Vyas et al., personal communication, February 1972) and it is expected that the high extinction coefficient is due to tryptophan which is destroyed by
acid hydrolysis. Indeed, examination of the continuous UV scan of
the 20 nm form of HBAg (Figure 4B) reveals a shoulder at 290 nm
suggesting that the HBAg proteins are rich in tryptophan residues.

The various forms of HBAg (ad) and HBAg (ay) purified by
the four-step procedure described above were solubilized and
analyzed by SDS-acrylamide gel electrophoresis under reducing
conditions.

The aqueous samples were concentrated to dryness by rotary
evaporation and solubilized by heating at 60°C for 10 minutes in
1% SDS, 6M urea and 1% 2-ME. The solubilized samples were electrophoresed on 10% SDS-urea-pH 7.6 gels at 5 ma/gel, fixed, stained
with Coomassie Brilliant Blue, destained and scanned at 550 nm on
the Gilford 2400 linear transport device. Analysis of the HBAg
(ad) 20 nm form (JMCs2R1Cs1) revealed two major polypeptides of
26,000 and 32,000 MW and three additional minor proteins with
molecular weights ranging from 40,000 to 95,000 (Figure 5A).

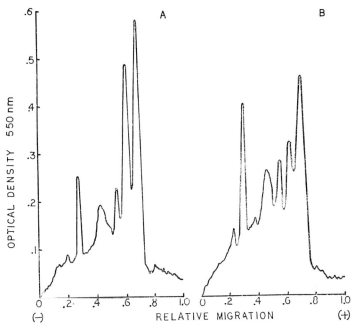

Figure 5. Proteins of the 20 nm form of HBAg (A) JMCs2R1Cs1 (ad)
subtype), (B) YtrCs2R1Cs1 (ay) subtype). Proteins were solubilized
by heating at 60°C for 10 minutes in 6M urea, 1% SDS, and 1% 2-ME
and electrophoresed on 10% SDS-urea-pH 7.6 acrylamide gels at 5 ma/
gel. Gels were stained with Coomassie Brilliant Blue and scanned
at 550 nm.

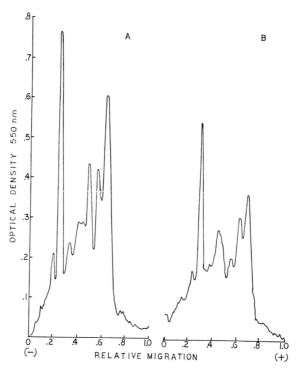

Figure 6. Proteins of filamentous forms of HBAg (ay). (A) short filaments of YtrCs2R1Cs1. (B) Large filaments of YtrCs2R1Cs1. Proteins solubilized and electrophoresed as described in Figure 5.

Electropherograms of the three forms of HBAg (ay) [20 nm forms (Figure 5B); short filaments (Figure 6A); long filament (Figure 6B)] reveal the same six polypeptides and an additional one with an estimated molecular weight of about 65,000. Except for the 65,000 MW minor component both preparations contain the same polypeptides but in different proportions (Table 3) as judged by staining affinity; alkylation of solubilized HBAg followed by electrophoresis does not alter the patterns. Recall that the JMCs2R1Cs1 material, at least, was immunochemically pure as evidenced by the lack of antibodies to normal serum proteins in hyperimmunized animals. The molecular weight estimates for proteins 4-7 are rough estimates and are used only for identification purposes for this presentation. We are presently obtaining better separations on 5% gels and more accurate estimates of the molecular weights of proteins 4-7 will be published shortly.

Comparision of the polypeptide patterns, of course, cannot be generalized to represent basic differences between the two subtypes; many more samples of each type must be analyzed. However, it is interesting that the same antigenic form can exist with different ratios of the various proteins, and would suggest that not all of the polypeptides are structural proteins coded

Table 3.   Proteins of HBAg

Protein	Estimated MW x 10^{-3}	HBAg (ad)*	HBAg (ay)**
1	26	Major	Major
2	32	Major	minor
3	(40)	minor	minor
4	(55)	minor	minor
5	(65)	-----	minor
6	(75)	minor	Major
7	(95)	minor	minor

*20 nm form of JMCs2R1Cs1
**20 nm form of Ytr Cs2R1Cs1

for by the viral genome. Millman et al. [316] have suggested that HBAg actually represents a complex of virus-specific antigens and normal serum proteins. This finding raises many possibilities as to the relationship between the circulating antigen and the pathologic manifestations of hepatitis.

The accumulated evidence would indicate that the predominant form (20 nm) of HBAg is not itself the virus of HBV, but rather an incomplete form containing virus-specific surface proteins. The virus itself may be present in much lower concentrations and is masked by the huge mass of incomplete material. The Dane particle would seem to fit many of the criteria for the virus and much effort is presently being expended to isolate this antigenic form from sera rich in Dane particles and finally establish the question of whether nucleic acids or reverse transcriptase activity are associated with HBAg.

Our knowledge of the physicochemical properties of HBAg has contributed to almost all phases of hepatitis research over the last few years. Although sophisticated biochemical studies are only now being applied, the results of these investigations should contribute greatly to our understanding of HBAg, its relationship to the virus of type B hepatitis, and the immunopathogenic mechanisms related to this disease.

As a final example of the worth of the biophysical approach, I would like to refer to several experiments done in collaboration with Drs. Carver and Seto at Johns Hopkins. Carver and Seto [83, 316] described the production of hemadsorption-negative areas (intrinsic interference) in WI-38 cells by sera containing HBAg and, presumably, HBV: A sample of MS-2 serum (Newell) obtained from Dr. Krugman was banded in a sucrose gradient and the resultant fractions assayed for HBAg by CF and "infectivity" by intrinsic interference (Figure 7). The antigen was well separated from the biological activity and, in fact, did not sediment under

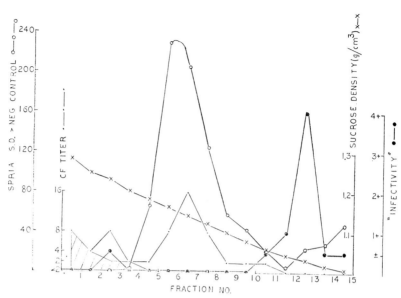

<u>Figure 7</u>.   Isopycnic banding of Newell serum on sucrose density
gradient using SW41 rotor (16 hrs. at 30,000 rpm and 5°C). Recovered fractions were assayed for sucrose density, CF activity,
HBAg by solid phase radioimmunoassay (SPRIA) and ability to induce
hemadsorption-negative areas in WI-38 cells ("infectivity").
Baseline for the SPRIA assay is 10 standard deviation's (SD) above
the negative antigen control; "infectivity" is only a rough attempt
to quantitate the biological assay, and the shaded area represents
anticomplementary activity.

these experimental conditions; subsequent experiments established
that failure of the biological activity to sediment was due to
its low buoyant density in sucrose.

    The results appeared to indicate no relationship between HBAg
and the production of hemadsorption-negative areas, however, when
the fractions were assayed by the more sensitive SPRIA technique
(courtesy of Dr. H. Alter) a small proportion of HBAg activity
was found in the low density region of the gradient in conjunction
with the biological activity described by Dr. Carver. Although
these experiments do not definitively establish the relationship
between HBV and the factor responsible to intrinsic interference
in Dr. Carver's system, the biophysical approach does contribute
to our understanding between the virus and future biological
systems.

    <u>Acknowledgments</u>. The author gratefully acknowledges the con-
tributions of his colleagues in the original data reported in this
manuscript: B. Gerwin, J. Shih, E. Hoffman, R. Faust and E. Ford
of the MAN Program; R. Purcell and D. Wong of the NIAID: H. Alter
and P. Holland, Clinical Center, NIH; M. Suggs of the NCDC, Atlanta; D. Carver of the Johns Hopkins Medical School.

The Rockville Laboratory of the MAN Program is supported by a collaborative program between the Division of Biology and Medicine, U.S. Atomic Energy Commission, and the National Institute of Allergy and Infectious Diseases.

29. Discussion
ISOLATION AND PHYSICOCHEMICAL CHARACTERISTICS OF HAA

Howard E. Bond

Electronucleonics Laboratories, Incorporated

Bethesda, Maryland

Dr. Gerin has raised some points pertaining to the immuno-logical, physical, and chemical characteristics of HBAg that I would like to enlarge upon to some extent based upon personal experiences.

We have separated the antigenic particles into their three morphologic types consisting of the nominal 22 nm sphere, fila-ments, and the 42 nm sphere [67], and we have prepared antisera against each type. Subsequently we have done the appropriate cross-absorption and reaction studies using the hemagglutination system to evaluate the results. Consistent with the reports from several laboratories, we find common antigenic determinants on all three morphologic forms. Also consistent with other reports, we find additional antigenic determinants peculiar to the 42 nm particle alone. We observe the outer coat of this particle to be structurally very delicate, and there is no way of knowing whether these are surface antigens or antigens of the inner core exposed during the red blood cell coating process. We cannot distinguish any differences whatsoever between the 20 nm particles and the filaments. Particularly, we cannot find ev-idence for an antigenic determinant common to the filament and 42 nm particle and absent from the 20 nm form. This is in con-trast to the evidence presented by Dr. Gerin and also possibly to that of Cross et al. [116], who were working with fecal anti-gen.

Dr. Gerin has referred to our studies on the determination of sedimentation coefficients in the analytical ultracentrifuge and to the fact that the predominant particle type that we find, approximately 23 nm, has a sedimentation velocity of 43.6 $s_{20,w}$. Interestingly, this value is exceedingly close to a theoretical value of 43.5 that we compute for the 22 nm form. We also find a similar correlation, an excellent correlation in fact, with other particles examined over a range of approximately 18 to 30 nm which we isolated by sedimentation velocity separations in the zonal ultracentrifuge. In addition, we find that the hydrated molecular weight of 3.5 million daltons computed for the 22 nm particle corresponds very closely to the actual anhydrous molecular weight determined in the Model E ultracentrifuge.

A result of these various determinations has been to give us confidence that the HBAg particle is relatively non-hydrated, or at least not excessively hydrated, and that the apparent hydrated particle weight of 5.8×10^{-18} grams per particle is a realistic value.

We have also compared particle counts with a number of analytical criteria and have reasonable assurance that our particle counting techniques are reliable.

A consequence of all this is that we can only account for less than about 20% of the particle's weight in terms of its apparent protein content as determined by nitrogen. Lipids are known to be present, and possibly some nucleic acid, but the quantities would be incompatible with physical data to account for the remaining mass. We do find a substantial anthrone reactivity in the particle, but as yet I cannot give quantitative data on this nor can I evaluate the significance of the reaction. However, the point is that there appears to be a substantial amount of the particle mass as yet unaccounted for that could have important significance relative to its immunological characteristics. Clearly this should be taken into consideration in future work.

A final point, the enigma of the high extinction coefficient, I believe will have to remain an enigma until further work is done. The 1% extinction at 280 nm relative to protein content is approximately six times that of serum albumin, and this is in spite of the fact that there is a low tyrosine content in the particle. It is quite possible that further amino acid analyses with alkaline hydrolysates will, in fact, disclose large quantities of tryptophan. I am somewhat pessimistic of this outcome, however, assuming we might have confidence in the amino acid analyses that have already been done. It would appear that most of the nitrogen has been accounted for.

30. ULTRASTRUCTURAL FEATURES OF AUSTRALIA ANTIGEN

A. J. Zuckerman

London School of Hygiene and Tropical Medicine

London, England

Viruses were among the first objects to be examined in the electron microscope over 30 years ago, yet little information was gained on the fine structure of viruses, except in the bacterio-phage field, until the advent in 1959 of the negative contrast technique for high resolution electron microscopy. Briefly, the principal advantages of negative staining are that the technique is relatively unaffected by impurities of small molecular size which merge with the background and conversely large sized impuri-ties are clearly discernible from virus particles. There is often very good preservation of biological material under test with min-imum distortion of structure. Furthermore, negative staining has yielded clear images revealing many detailed and intricate features of particular structures. Finally, only relatively small amounts of the material to be tested are required. The main disadvantage of this technique is that a high concentration of particle suspen-sion is usually required, often 10^9 to 10^{12} particles per ml, a condition which seems to be frequently satisfied in both patients and carriers of the serum hepatitis virus. An additional degree of sensitivity may, however, be obtained by the technique of immune electron microscopy, by looking for aggregates of antigen rather than individual particles by themselves.

Bayer, Blumberg and Werner [39] examined in the electron mi-croscope by the negative staining technique serum fractions rich in Australia antigen but containing no serum protein after rate zonal separation of whole serum on a 10%-30% (W/W) sucrose density gra-dient followed by electrophoresis in cellulose acetate. The orig-inal serum specimens containing Australia antigen were obtained from three different patients, one suffering from acute myelogenous leukemia, another with chronic reticuloendotheliosis and the third patient with Down's syndrome and chronic hepatitis. Negative staining with sodium silicotungstate revealed spherical particles 19-21 nm in diameter with surface knob-like "subunits" about 3 nm in diameter. In some fields spherical particles of approximately 15 nm in diameter were found. A central core of about 7 nm was observed in some of the particles whereas a few other particles appeared empty. Elongated particles varying in length from less than 50 nm to 230 nm were also noted. The particles were aggregated by the addition of specific rabbit antibody to Australia antigen. Such particles were not found in normal human sera nor in the sucrose gradient fractions not containing Australia antigen.

Almeida et al. [11] and Zuckerman [495] described the morphological features of virus-like particles visualised by electron microscopy in immune aggregates of serum containing Australia antigen obtained from a known long-term asymptomatic carrier of serum hepatitis and from two heroin addicts who contracted serum hepatitis after sharing syringes. The principal antigenic constituent was a rather pleomorphic roughly spherical particle measuring approximately 20 nm in diameter, but with a range of 16 nm to 25 nm. A notable feature was the presence of many tubular forms with a constant diameter close to 20 nm and often several hundred nm in length. The very marked morphological heterogeneity of the particles, which included many different shapes and forms, was a constant and striking feature. It was possible to resolve that the spherical particles were formed of subunits but it was not possible to interpret the surface structure. The tubular forms frequently displayed a regular transverse periodicity of approximately 3 nm on the surface. Many tubules displaying several right angles were also seen and this angularity appeared to be a unique feature of these structures. Bulbous or rounded swellings were frequently seen at either or both ends of the tubules. None of these particles or structures were found in normal human sera reacted with antisera to the Australia antigen.

Dane, Cameron and Briggs [123] described a third class of virus-like particles in the serum of 3 of 16 patients with Australia antigen-associated hepatitis. These particles measured about 42 nm in diameter and consisted of an inner body about 28 nm in diameter with a 2 nm shell and an outer coat about 7 nm in thickness. Several tadpole-like forms were found, with the tail resembling a typical tubular form in continuity with the outer coat of a large spheroidal particle. The large and small spherical particles and the tubules formed a mixed aggregate when reacted with antiserum to Australia antigen indicating that they all shared a common surface antigen. It was suggested that the double shelled 42 nm particles represent the virus of serum hepatitis whereas the small particles and the tubular forms of Australia antigen are non-infectious surplus virus-coat material.

   Cossart and Field [109] pointed out the striking morphological
resemblance between Australia antigen particles and the forms produced through the in vitro reassembly on polyanions of proteins
extracted from several groups of small RNA isometric plant viruses.
Zuckerman [496] extrapolated this situation further from the plant
virus kingdom and extended the covirus concept, whereby a combination of two or more morphological structures is required to produce infection, to human viral hepatitis. A logical corollary to
these observations was successfully applied by Almeida et al. [10]
on the premise that if the Australia antigen is reaggregated viral
protein then the parent virus could resemble cubical plant viruses,
the counterparts of which among the animal viruses are the picornaviruses. Examination by electron microscopy of liver homogenates
prepared from two patients who died of acute Australia antigen-
positive hepatitis revealed virus-like structures measuring 25-27
nm in diameter and displaying the morphology of many small entero-
viruses. It was proposed that these particles might represent the
serum hepatitis virus. However, another possibility, which has
been proposed by Almeida, Rubenstein and Stott [8] is that these
new particles might be the inner 28 nm bodies described by Dane
et al. and others and which are devoid of the outer shell and further that these particles may be the same intracellular particles
in liver biopsy material described by Nowoslawski et al. [364], by
Nelson, Barker and Danovitch [351] and others. More recently,
Almeida et al. [8], treated pellets of Australia antigen obtained
by centrifugation of whole serum with the detergent "Tween-80".
The large 42 nm spherical particles separated into an outer coat
of Australia antigen and an inner spherical component, 27 nm in
diameter, which resembled morphologically the rhinoviruses. Antibody present in the serum of patients after recovery from serum
hepatitis reacted with the inner component, but not with the outer
Australia antigen component, to yield immune aggregates resembling
those seen in homogenates of liver taken post-mortem from patients
with Australia antigen-associated hepatitis. An important observation is that antibody to the inner component was absent from
pre-hepatitis sera from the same convalescent patients. It was
suggested that antibody to Australia antigen develops in serum
hepatitis but that it is subsequently cleared from the serum with
clinical improvement, while a normal immune response is produced
in all patients to the internal component of the large 42 nm particles. The presence of this specific inner component antibody may
therefore be used to determine previous infection with the serum
hepatitis virus. The electron microscope may thus be used not only
for the study of the structure of Australia antigen and the serum
hepatitis virus but also for the investigation of Australia antigen-
antibody interactions.

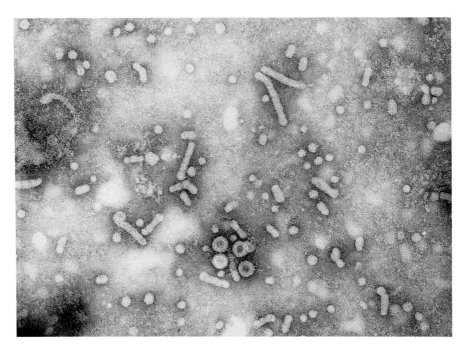

Figure 1. The general appearance of Australia antigen in serum without the addition of specific antibody (X 252,000).

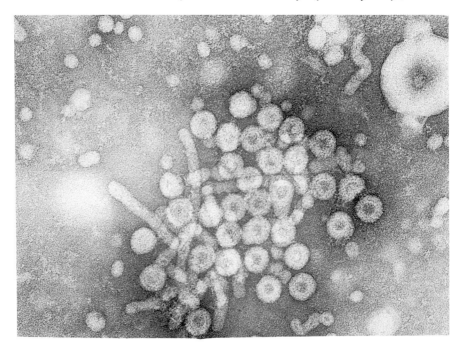

Figure 2. Australia antigen-antibody complex (X 252,000).

Acknowledgements. These studies are supported by generous grants from the World Health Organization, the Medical Research Council and with equipment and a grant from Pfizer Ltd, England.

31. Discussion

ULTRASTRUCTURAL FEATURES OF AUSTRALIA ANTIGEN

William T. Hall

Electro Nucleonics Laboratories, Incorporated

Bethesda, Maryland

I think all of us who have seen Dr. Zuckerman's figures and listened to his presentation today and followed his reports in the literature have come to envy the beautiful work produced by him and his colleagues. It is envied all the more by those trying to work on the Australia antigen with the electronmicroscope. I can do little more than support the morphological data already presented and comment very briefly on work in progress with Dr. Bond, Mr. Brandt and Mr. Strafford at Electro Nucleonics.

For some time now, Dr. Bond and I have been interested in centrifugally resolving the polymorphic Australia antigen (HBAg) into the three classes described by Dr. Zuckerman to provide material for investigating each class separately. We have already met with some degree of success [67] as this series of figures will indicate.

Figure 1 is a graphic representation of the results of the rate velocity separation in cesium chloride of HBAg-positive plasma from which most of the plasma proteins have been removed by two previous isopycnic bandings in a B-29 ultracentrifuge rotor. Three distinct peaks occur.

Figure 2 shows the appearance of the starting sample for the rate velocity run. The three types of particles already described are present: the small 18-30 nanometer particles, the Dane particles [123] and the filaments.

The center of the first and major (A, figure 1) peak is illustrated in Figure 3 and contains a fairly homogeneous complement of 22 nanometer particles. If one takes samples from successive fractions across this peak, a distribution of particle sizes is found such that the smaller ones (16-18 nanometers) occur closer to the center of the rotor and the larger ones more centrifugally.

The particles in Figure 4 come from the area between the first two peaks (B, Figure 1). These are the larger spherical particles and small filaments.

The larger filaments are concentrated in the second peak (C, Figure 1) and range in size from about 40 nanometers to several hundred nanometers, as shown in Figure 5. Some Dane particles also occur in this fraction.

A mixture (Figure 6) of filaments and Dane particles is found between the second and third peaks (D, Figure 1) and finally in Figure 7 we get the third peak (E, Figure 1), where we have, for the most part, isolated Dane particles. Since working with these 40-45 nanometer particles, it has been our experience that once isolated and allowed to sit around, the particles tend to break down rather quickly. Thus, we feel that we now have an opportunity to get purified cores of Dane particles by separating them from the rest of their coat material. This should provide an opportunity to further the work recently reported by Almeida, et al. [8].

Although most of the research on these fractions has thus far been biochemical and immunological, we have recently begun morphological studies on antibody-antigen complexes. Since we had pre-

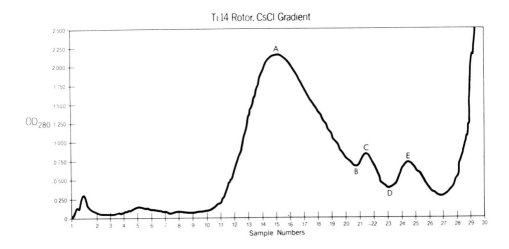

Figure 1. Graphic representation of results of rate velocity separation in cesium chloride of HBAg- positive plasma in a B-29 ultracentrifuge rotor.

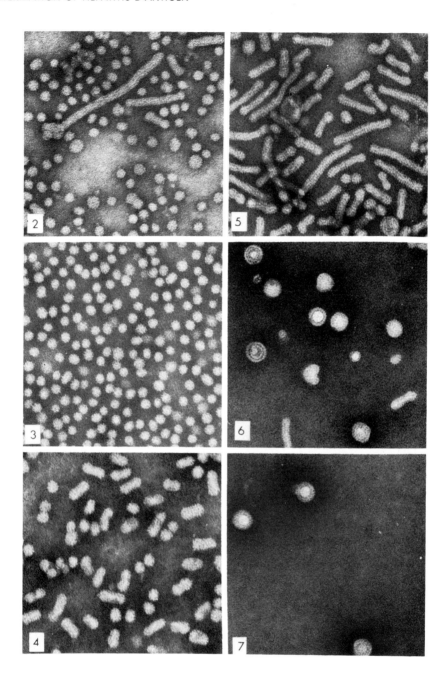

Figures 2-7. Electronmicrographs (x 150,000) of fractions from rate velocity separation 2) starting material 3) first, peak A, material 4) particles from area between peak A and B 5) second, peak B, material 6) mixture from area between B and C peaks 7) Dane particles, peak C.

viously made antibody to the various fractions, it seemed appropriate to look at the complexes formed by several anti-HBAg sera
against purified classes of the antigen. Our work is still somewhat preliminary, but I have included a series of lantern slides
to show the effect of reacting two-fold dilutions of goat antisera
to 20 nanometer particles with a purified sample of HBAg from peak
1. I was primarily interested in seeing if one could clearly distinguish between a genuine antibody-antigen complex and mere clumping. I tend to believe personally that some of the micrographs
shown previously by Dr. Zuckerman are examples of clumping. When
we let our material sit around, we get very heavy clumps. One of
the distinguishing characteristics of complexes would be the presence of the fine filamentous antibodies around the particles of
antigen. Excellent examples of this phenomenon have been shown by
both Dr. Gerin and Dr. Zuckerman in their presentations here today.
Since the antibody would have to be, at least in some dimension,
almost as large as the antigen, one would reasonably expect to find
antigen particles separated by these filaments. When a group of
particles is found in which the members of the group are quite
contiguous, I think it is hard to justify calling the aggregation
an antibody-antigen complex.

Figures 8-12 illustrate the effect of reacting a sample of
purified 22 nanometer particles of HBAg against several dilutions
(1:32, 1:64, 1:128, 1:256, 1:512) of goat anti-HBAg sera. The
steady diminution of aggregate with antibody dilution until, in
this example, at 1:512 the appearance of the antigen is as the
starting sample of antigen alone, strongly suggests that we are
looking at real complexes and not just clumps.

Figures 13 and 14 show two complexes at higher magnification.
Notice the filamentous material between the 22 nanometer particles
- and I think this is the important consideration. If we are
talking about complexes, then we have to find antigen and antibody.
And if both of them are present then we must have a spacing between
the particles of antigen.

Finally, since we had samples of isolated Dane particles, we
obtained from Dr. Shulman a convalescent serum and tried several
times to repeat the work of Dr. Almeida [8]. Thus far I must say
that we have not been very successful, although we have formed
complexes using an antibody made against a preparation of Dane
particles. We hope to continue further research on these particles.

Dr. Gordon: Dr. Zuckerman has called attention to the fact
that electron micrographs of the HBAg particle resemble the ultra-
structure of cowpea chlorotic mottle virus. This is an exciting
observation which deserves emphasis; because cowpea chlorotic
mottle virus is one of several plant virus (dubbed "coviruses" by

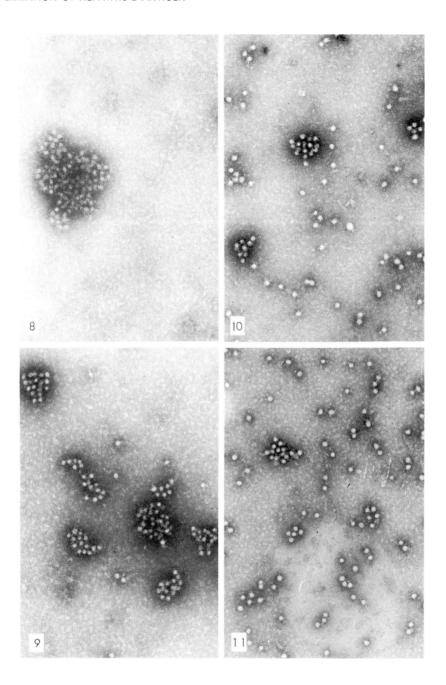

Figures 8-11. Electronmicrographs (x 75,000) showing effect of HBAg reacted with increasing dilutions of goat anti-HBAg. Antibody dilutions are: 8) 1:132 9) 1:64 10) 1:128 11) 1:256.

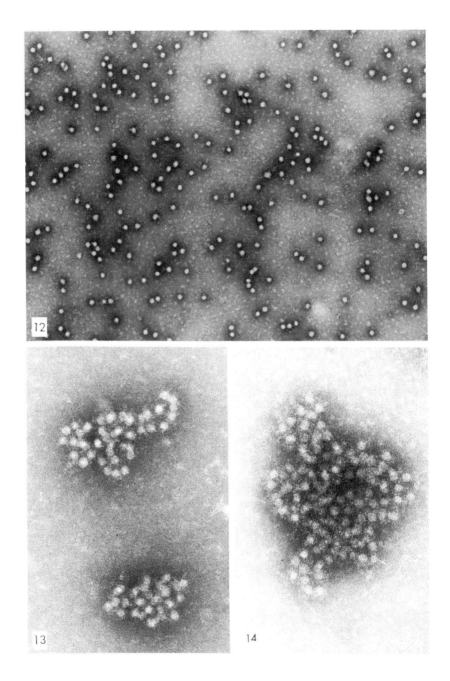

Figure 12. Electronmicrograph (x 75,000) of HBAg reacted with anti-HBAg, 1:512 dilution.

Figures 13-14. Complexes showing the filamentous material believed to be antibody which attaches to the antigen particles (x 150,000).

Fraenkel-Conrat) whose virions occur in two or more different sizes containing different amounts of RNA. Neither a single virion type nor a single RNA type is infectious; infectivity results only from coinfection with the combination of virions or RNA's. In short, the viral RNA genome appears to be distributed over two or more molecules, which are housed in two or more virion structures, and at least one essential function seems thus to be divided. As a historical note, Dr. Melnick, who is also here, pointed out the similarity between the particles he and his colleagues saw in electron micrographs of lymph node cultures inoculated with hepatitis B inocula, and cowpea chlorotic mottle virus [234].

32.   IMMUNOFLUORESCENCE AND IMMUNOELECTRONMICROSCOPY

I. Millman, S.N. Huang, V. Coyne, A. O'Connell,
A. Aronoff, H. Gault, and B.S. Blumberg
The Institute for Cancer Research, Philadelphia, Pa. and

McGill University, Montreal, Canada

Since the early publication of Coons et al. [104] the fluorescent antibody technique has mushroomed in popularity as a method
for detecting antigen-antibody reactions. Applications of the
fluorescent antibody technique in the diagnosis of communicable
diseases have been an invaluable aid to the diagnostic public
health laboratory. More recent uses of the technique have been
the detection in mammalian tissues of antigens and antibodies. It
is essentially here that the novice with only little experience in
diagnostic microbiology becomes disillusioned early. It is unfor-
tunate that this happens so often. One cause of this trouble is
that mammalian tissues are sticky and liver and tissues of the
hematopoietic system appear to be the worst. A recognition of this
fact was probably the reason that liver and bone marrow powders
were chosen for absorption of the coupled reagent to eliminate non-
specific fluorescence. While absorption helped to a degree, it was
no solution. To the diagnostic microbiologist it mattered little
whether background mammalian cells fluoresced brightly or dimly
since he could easily distinguish, by morphology alone, the brightly fluorescing microorganisms within a smear. An example is the
examination of vaginal smears for the detection of Neisseria gonor-
rhea. How does one determine, on the other hand, the presence of
soluble antibody on or within mammalian cells when these very cells
fluoresce non-specifically? How does one determine the presence of
Australia antigen within liver cells when the liver cell itself is
used for the absorption of non-specific fluorescence? The literature contains several articles and reviews on attempts to solve
this problem. I will not have time to go into these but, generally
speaking, they amount to the selection of different protein dye
ratios for coupling, variations in coupling procedure and counter-

staining or covering up of non-specific fluorescence with albumin-coupled dye of a different color.

It remained for an Australian investigator, Curtain [121], some 10 years ago to come up with a workable solution. He noted that electrophoresis patterns of fluorescent-antibody preparations showed a marked heterogeneity and that most of the non-specifically staining material could be isolated in the faster fractions which contained an excess of negatively-charged fluorescein groups. The coupling procedure, regardless of the ratio of antibody to fluorescein used, results in a heterogeneous mixture of molecules of gamma globulin from those with imperceptibly small quantities of dye to those that are saturated. By first passing the coupled globulin through "Sephadex" G-25 (Pharmacia, Inc.) to remove the unreacted dye and then through a DEAE-cellulose column, fractions could be separated with different 495/280 ratios indicating the separation of molecules with different quantities of coupled fluorescein. Of interest was the fact that the least coupled (fluorescent) material had the highest antibody activity (Figure 1).

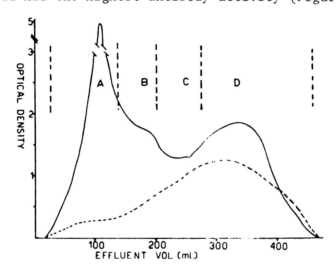

Fraction.....................	A	B	C	D
Antibody Titer	1,250	1,040	520	200
Relative brightness of non-specific fluorescence.	0.25	1.95	5.87	10

Antibody titers are reciprocal dilutions.

Figure 1. Chromatography of fluorescein-rabbit IgG on N,N-dimethyl-aminoethyl-cellulose. The solid line is the plot of optical density at 280 mμ, the broken line optical density at 490 mμ.

We, therefore, set about to make a fluorescent reagent, in which we would have confidence, to determine the location of Australia antigen in the body. We would make use of the method described by Curtain to isolate that reagent fraction which would be specific, and free of non-specific fluorescent activity. We strongly considered the possibility of using dissociated antibody from Australia antigen-antibody complexes for coupling with fluorescein but we abandoned the idea because of the extremely small yields that could be expected. Instead high-titered rabbit antisera was absorbed with normal human serum by the procedure described by Melartin [311]. The immune globulin (IgG) fraction was separated from 5.0 ml aliquots of absorbed rabbit antiserum by passage through a DEAE "Sephadex" column (100 x 2.5 cm) [424]. It has been shown that antibody to Australia antigen is in the IgG fraction of human and hyperimmunized rabbit sera [13]. The purity of the IgG pool was confirmed by immunoelectrophoresis and immunodiffusion. The IgG pool also produced a single precipitin line with sera which contained Australia antigen and no reaction with normal human sera which did not contain Australia antigen. The IgG pool was conjugated with fluorescein isothiocyante isomer I (Baltimore Biological Laboratories) by the method of Cherry et al. [92], and the conjugate was purified by a modification of the procedure of Curtain [121]. We found that little to no material was eluted from our column with 0.02 M potassium phosphate buffer pH 6.0. This difference from the results described by Curtain could have been due to either the labeling procedure we used or to the isomer I fluorescein isothiocyanate used. We therefore altered the buffer to include a small amount of NaCl. We found that any amount of NaCl up to 0.5 M did not alter the elution results. Five to six fluorescing bands could be seen migrating down the column with the aid of a Mineralight UVS 11 (UV Products, Inc., San Gabriel, Calif.) The fractions of each band were pooled, adjusted to pH 7.4 with 0.1 N NaOH, and concentrated by lyophilization to approximately 5-fold. Spectrophotometric 495/280 ratios were recorded for each fraction. In addition a 5.0 ml portion of each fraction was dialyzed in 0.01 M phosphate buffer pH 7.4 and concentrated 15-fold by lyophilization. These concentrates were used to determine immunoreactivity by immunodiffusion. As a rule the first 2 fractions proved best in having 495/280 ratios that were less than 1 and good precipitin activity. Figure 2 shows the appearance of a precipitin band made with fluorescein-coupled IgG and also unconjugated anti-Australia antigen. It will be noted that a continuous line of identity is produced when 2 negatives, 1 photographed with UV and the other with visible light, are superimposed. The conjugated anti-Australia antigen fractions were also shown to be unreactive with normal sera (those not containing Australia antigen).

Initially our fluorescent reagents were used to determine the presence of Australia antigen in a variety of materials including

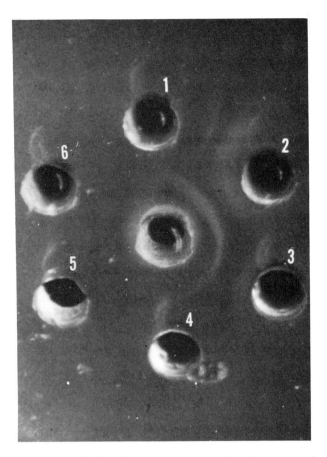

Figure 2. Micro-immunodiffusion pattern showing continuous line of identity between fluorescein isothiocyanate conjugated rabbit antiserum, well 2; unconjugated rabbit antiserum, well 3; and human serum containing Australia antigen, center well. Wells 1, 4, 5, and 6 contain normal rabbit sera. The thick band between well 2 and the center well fluoresces. Photo taken under reflected UV light superimposed over one taken with transmitted visible light.

liver, blood, jejunum loop, bone marrow, etc. With liver and jejunum loop we made the mistake of initially using impression smears, thinking that these would be better than cryostat slices which would require some manipulation of the tissue. Unfortunately, we seldom observed fluorescence in more than an occasional cell and much fluorescent debris surrounding cells. No fluorescence was seen with bone marrow cells or peripheral blood smears. Since we were also trying to grow liver cells in tissue culture from finely minced liver tissue we decided one day to stain a drop of the minced tissue. A drop minced in tissue culture fluid was placed on a slide, allowed to air dry (under a vertical laminar flow hood), acetone fixed (room temperature for 15 minutes) and stained with the fluo-

rescein-coupled reagent.   One of us (V.C.) shouted with surprise
when she first observed discrete fluorescing intranuclear granules
under the UV microscope.   It appeared at first that nucleoli were
the structures which fluoresced.   However, a number of cells with
intranuclear fluorescing granules could be shown to contain non-
fluorescing nucleoli which could be identified easily under phase
microscopy.   The numbers of fluorescent granules observed (from 1
to 12) also differed with different specimens.   The technique also
allowed us to prepare specimens immediately after needle (Menghini)
biopsy.   After fixation on slides the specimens could be stored for
months at -30°C.   Figure 3 (A and B) shows liver cells stained by
this technique under UV.

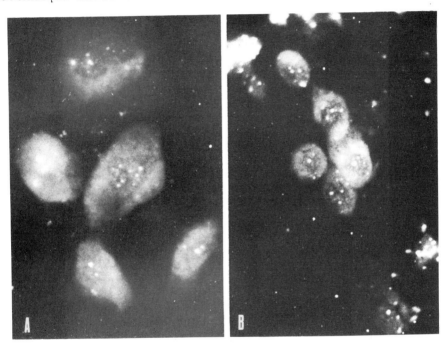

Figure 3.   (A) Fluorescent granules visible within nuclei of liver
cells of patient with infectious hepatitis;   X 3900.   (B) Same from
patient with post-transfusion hepatitis;   X 2600.

Liver cells, from patients with no Australia antigen in their blood,
as a rule appeared to have black nuclei and a faint blue-grey auto-
fluorescent cytoplasm.   Several tissues from one patient with Down's
syndrome, chronic anicteric hepatitis and acute myelogenous leukemia
were examined before and after death.   Practically all of these tissues contained fluorescing cell nuclei except for the spleen where
cytoplasmic fluorescence was seen.   Figure 4 shows testis tissue
from this patient.

Two of eight bone marrow smears of patients with acute and
chronic hepatitis showed fluorescence confined to the cytoplasm of

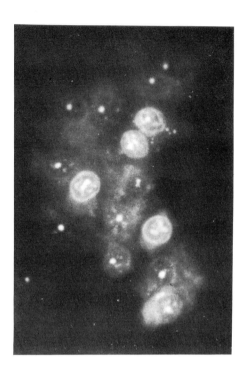

Figure 4. Testicular tissue from a patient with Down's syndrome,
chronic anicteric hepatitis, and acute myelogenous leukemia stained
with conjugated rabbit anti-Australia antigen antiserum; X 2700.

the cells. In both these cases only a few of the bone marrow cells
on the slide were involved. None of the other tissues studied,
including buffy coat smears, cells obtained from bile, duodonal
drainage and seminal fluid, showed fluorescence. In addition peripheral lymphocyte cultures in 6 patients with chronic hepatitis
and Australia antigen in their blood also were negative.

    Some 61 liver biopsies were examined by the mincing technique.
Figure 5 (A and B) shows 2 x 2 contingency-table analyses of the
results. There is a significant association between Australia antigen in the blood or histological hepatitis and fluorescence in
the nuclei. Those cases where cells were fluorescent and no Australia antigen was found in the blood might be attributed to the
lack of sensitivity of the immunodiffusion method which at that
time was the only test used to detect antigen in the blood. It is
significant that of the 15 patients in this category (Figure 5A)
6 had a histological diagnosis of viral hepatitis, 2 were alcohol-
ics and drug users, one was a patient with postnecrotic cirrhosis
and 2 were residents of an institution for the mentally retarded
and had been exposed repeatedly to patients with known hepatitis
and Australia antigen. Of the remaining four, two were patients
with malignancies involving the liver and had undergone surgery,

Chi Square and P Values

A. FLUORESCENCE VS. SERUM Au(1)

Fluorescence	Serum Au(1)		Total
	+	0	
+	26	15	41
0	0	20	20
Totals	26	35	61

Chi square = 19.58

p value ∠ 0.001

B. FLUORESCENCE VS. HEPATITIS (Histologic diagnosis)

Fluorescence	Hepatitis		Total
	+	0	
+	30	11	41
0	3	17	20
Totals	33	28	61

Chi square = 16.05

p value ∠ 0.001

Figure 5. (A) Comparison of immunofluorescence with presence of Australia antigen in patient's serum. (B) Comparison of immunofluorescence with pathologic diagnosis.

one had a biliary atresia and the other primary biliary cirrhosis.

At this point something should be said about variations of the technique as described here. We tried the indirect staining "sandwich" technique and after initial unsuccessful attempts resolved the difficulty. We discovered that the intranuclear fluorescent granules were not permanently fixed but easily dissolved in serum after prolonged contact. We determined this accidently when we tried an inhibition reaction with uncoupled antiserum. Fluorescence was quenched but negative (control) sera also inhibited or quenched the fluorescent reaction. By decreasing the time allowed for all of the individual steps in the indirect staining procedure, including the washing steps, we were able to see fluorescing particles in the nuclei. These same fluorescing particles appeared to "migrate" into the cytoplasm and eventually out of the cell completely, depending on the timing used for each step of the indirect procedure. Figure 6 (A and B) shows particles on the nuclear membrane and within the cytoplasm of 2 cells. We tried a variety of fixatives such as glutaraldehyde, formalin, phenol and alcohol in

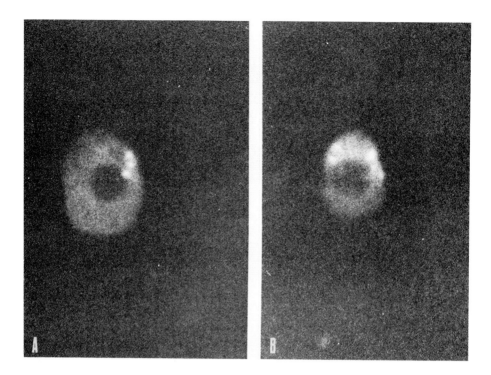

Figure 6. (A and B) Liver preparation from a patient with viral
hepatitis stained by the indirect method. Particles have been dis-
lodged from the nucleus and appear in the cytoplasm because of the
prolonged washing procedure; X 3900.

an attempt to permanently fix the granules within the nucleus.
None of the fixatives tried were effective. In fact, fixatives
other than acetone and alcohol appeared to destroy antigenic determinants since no fluorescent staining could be obtained after
fixation. A successful true inhibition test to determine specificity could be obtained only by absorbing the fluorescent reagent with Australia antigen. After absorption with Australia
antigen no fluorescent staining could be observed with coupled
antiserum. Controls (absorbed with normal sera) stained as expected.

Finally, it should be emphasized that 2 x 2 contingency tables
are important in evaluating a newly coupled reagent. Lack of association could mean the presence of anti-nuclear antibodies which
would give false positive reactions. Some 10 determinations may be
necessary to rule out this possibility.

Immunoelectronmicroscopy. Confirmation of our work with the
fluorescent-antibody technique came after 2 years when the Polish
workers Nowoslawski et al. [364] reported positive results with
liver sections of six patients with lymphoproliferative disorders

taken at necropsy. All six had Australia antigen in their serum
and fluorescence was seen in the nuclei of all six livers. Reports
from other investigators (unpublished) indicated that our data
either could not be confirmed or that fluorescence occurred in the
cytoplasm and not the nuclei of liver cells from patients with hepatitis. The issue was rather frustrating until the work of Ahmed
et al. [3] and Huang [223] appeared. These investigators used
electron microscopy to study liver biopsy tissue from a group of
renal transplant patients suffering from persistent Australia antigenemia and chronic active hepatitis. The nuclei of the hepatocytes
contained virus-like particles very much like that of Australia
antigen in 5 of 6 cases. No such particles were seen in the nuclei
of patients without Australia antigenemia. Although particles were
also seen in the cytoplasm of hepatocytes, they were far fewer in
number.

At this point in time I contacted Dr. Huang (McGill University,
Montreal) and we decided on a research plan of mutual interest. We
would attempt to identify as Australia antigen these particles observed under the electron microscope with the use of specific antisera coupled with ferritin.

Guinea-pig antisera to Australia antigen, either monovalent by
immunization with purified fractions of Australia antigen or absorbed with normal human sera, were fractionated by DEAE-cellulose
column chromatography [378]. The IgG fractions were coupled to
ferritin by the method of Hsu [222]. Some of the ferritin-coupled
fractions were further purified by starch block electrophoresis
[272]. The latter procedure separated unreacted ferritin and apo-
ferritin from the conjugate.

The specificities of the ferritin-coupled reagents were confirmed by immunoelectrophoresis and immunodiffusion analyses. By
immunodiffusion a single colored precipitin band resulted from reaction with Australia antigen. This colored band formed a line of
identity with that formed by other anti-Australia antigen antisera
and Australia antigen. By immunoelectrophoresis the conjugate
formed a broad precipitin band in the beta-and alpha-globulin region against anti-guinea pig IgG, anti-ferritin, and Australia
antigen. The reaction was strongest in the beta-globulin region*
when reacted against anti-IgG, in the alpha-globulin region when
reacted against ferritin, and in between when reacted against Australia antigen. The length of the precipitin band was somewhat
reduced when the conjugate was fractionated by starch block elec-

---

*Apparently the strongly-charged ferritin pulls IgG from the
normal gamma to beta position.

trophoresis. No reactions were observed with the ferritin reagents against normal sera by either immunodiffusion or immunoelectrophoresis.

The specificities of the reagents were also tested by reacting them with purified preparations of Australia antigen purchased from Electro Nucleonics, Inc., Bethesda, Md. The Australia antigen particles and the ferritin coupled antisera were prepared for electron microscopy by smearing a small drop of diluted material on carbonized formvar-coated copper grids. The grids were air dried, then rinsed briefly with distilled water and a drop of 3% phosphotungstic acid, aqueous solution, was added to the grids as the negative stain. Some grids were not stained with phosphotungstic acid but with osmium vapor in a closed chamber for one hour. One drop of diluted Australia antigen (1:8 dilution with 0.1 M phosphate cacodylate buffer, pH 7.4) was preincubated with varying amounts of ferritin-conjugated antiserum in glass capillary tubes for 30 minutes at room temperature. A small drop was spread on carbonized formvar-coated copper grids and air dried. Some of these preparations were osmificated in a closed chamber for one hour or negatively stained.

Needle biopsies were performed on 3 patients. Two had chronic active hepatitis and persistent Australia antigenemia. The third, a non-transplant patient without Australia antigenemia, served as a control. The biopsy material was divided into several pieces, each of which was handled differently: one piece was minced fresh, a second was frozen in liquid nitrogen and then thawed at room temperature, and a third was fixed for 20 minutes in cacodylate-buffered 3% glutaraldehyde, then rinsed in the buffer. Following these procedures the tissue fragments were incubated with ferritin-conjugated guinea-pig anti-Australia antigen antiserum for 45 minutes in a moist chamber at room temperature. After rinsing in 0.1 M phosphate buffer pH 7.4 the fragments were fixed in cacodylate-buffered glutaraldehyde for one hour. All preparations were then post-fixed in 1% osmium tetroxide for 1 hour and processed for embedding in Epon-812. The ultra-thin sections were mounted on uncoated copper grids and examined with or without uranyl acetate and lead citrate staining.

Several control experiments were included. In one, normal guinea-pig serum was substituted for the ferritin reagent; in a second, normal guinea-pig serum was added to the biopsy material before the addition of the ferritin reagent to determine whether there would be non-specific blocking of the ferritin reagent reaction; and in a third, tissue was frozen and thawed without addition of reagents before fixation. Biopsy material was also fixed in Bouin's for light-microscopy examination as well as minced in buffered saline and fixed in acetone for fluorescent

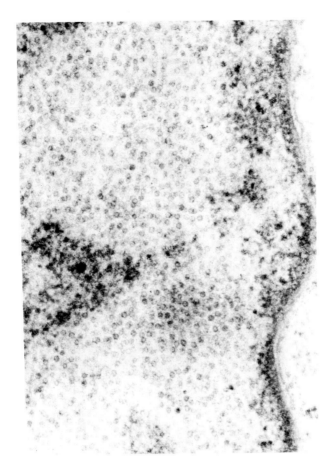

Figure 7.   A liver cell nucleus showing the presence of numerous spherical particles. The nuclear membrane is visible on the right. Glutaraldehyde fixed, not treated with antiserum. Uranyl acetate and lead citrate stain; X 74,000.

microscopy examination.

The light-microscopic findings of the liver biopsies showed features consistent with chronic active hepatitis. The immuno- fluorescent preparations from the chronic hepatitis cases showed apple green fluorescence in the form of specks and strands in the liver cell nuclei as well as granular and diffuse green fluores- cence in the cytoplasm. The control (negative for Australia anti- gen) showed no nuclear fluorescence but a weakly positive cyto- plasmic fluorescence. Regular electron microscopic preparations of liver biopsy material from the chronic hepatitis cases showed a large number of virus-like particles in the liver cell nuclei. A few particles were also evident in the cytoplasm (Figure 7).

The particles were uniform, spherical in shape, about 210-250 Å in size, and showed internal granular subunits. In spite of the

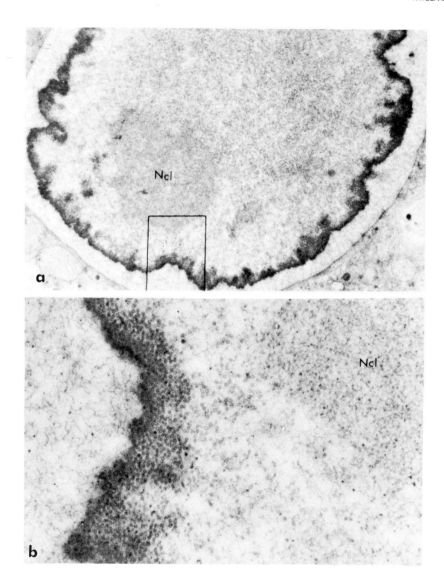

Figure 8.   (A and B) A liver cell nucleus showing densely stained
agglutinates of virus-like particles with formation of a coastline-
like precipitation pattern.   Smaller aggregates are seen to the
left of the nucleolus (Ncl).   Frozen and thawed tissues, treated
with ferritin coupled anti-Australia antigen antiserum.   Uranyl
acetate and lead citrate stain;   (A) X 12,000,   (B) X 56,700.

massive number the particles retained their discrete individuality
and were neither confluent nor agglutinated.   The control specimen
showed no particles as such in the liver cells.   Electron microscopic preparations of liver biopsies from chronic hepatitis cases
treated with ferritin reagents showed striking evidence of agglutination of the intranuclear and cytoplasmic virus-like particles

in fresh minced and frozen-thawed preparations. In nuclei containing massive numbers of particles, the large agglutinates often showed a deep osmiophilic boundary (Figures 8A, B) which resembled the precipitin line seen in agar gel diffusion. The specific ferritin label was seen intimately in association with clumps of particles within nuclei or at the periphery of intranuclear clumps of particles in osmium-fixed and stained preparations (Figure 9).

Figure 9. An aggregate showing heavy deposits of intranuclear virus-like particles. Frozen and thawed liver tissue, treated with ferritin coupled anti-Australia antigen antiserum. Osmium stain; X 114,800.

Tissues first fixed with glutaraldehyde and then treated with ferritin reagent showed no evidence of agglutination nor ferritin deposits. Control preparations treated with normal guinea-pig serum showed no agglutination of particles nor interference with the subsequently applied ferritin reagent. Control preparations frozen and thawed without reagent showed no effect on the particles. Liver cells prepared from the control patient (negative for Australia antigen) showed no particles or evidence of any specific reagent effect within the cells.

    Acknowledgements. Supported by U.S.P.H.S. grants CA-06551, CA-06927 and RR-05539 from the National Institutes of Health and by an appropriation from the Commonwealth of Pennsylvania.

33. Discussion
IMMUNOFLUORESCENCE AND IMMUNOELECTRONMICROSCOPY

G. N. Vyas

University of California, School of Medicine

San Francisco, California

Dr. Millman has presented a lucid, comprehensive and interesting paper on "Immunofluorescence and Immunoelectronmicroscopy". It illustrates the sterility of possessing conceptual skills without adequacy of technical skills in investigating this area. We set out to investigate whether subacute hepatic necrosis and the bridging between the triads of the liver resulted from an immunologic injury initiated by HBAg-anti-HBAg complexes binding complement. To test this concept, we decided to employ immunohistochemical methods using fluorescein-isothiocyanate (FITC)-labelled IgG from human anti-HBAg for demonstration of HBAg in liver and counterstaining with rhodamine-labelled IgG from rabbit anti-β_1c. Six specimens of liver biopsies obtained from patients with HBAg-positive hepatitis were examined by the immunofluorescence method. Only one biopsy was positive with FITC-labelled anti-HBAg and none of them were reactive with rhodamine-labelled anti-β_1c. In spite of the technical difficulties and frustrations involved in this laboratory procedure, once standardized, the positive results may have significance in laboratory diagnosis and prognosis. This approach may also shed more light on the immunologic mechanisms involved in tissue damage observed in viral hepatitis.

34. IN VITRO CORRELATION OF DELAYED HYPERSENSITIVITY TO HEPATITIS B ANTIGEN (HBAg) IN GUINEA PIGS

A. B. Ibrahim, S. Adelberg and G.N. Vyas

Department of Clinical Pathology and Laboratory Medicine
University of California School of Medicine
San Francisco, California

The humoral antibody response to hepatitis B antigen (HBAg) has been studied by several investigators since the initial discovery of Australia antigen by Blumberg, et al. [49]; specific antibodies to HBAg have been reported in man and in experimental animals such as goats, rabbits, guinea-pigs and chimpanzees [135, 398, 430, 432]. However, the development of delayed hypersensitivity (DH) to HBAg remained uninvestigated until recently when Irwin, et al. [229] showed its induction in guinea-pigs. Independently, our studies have demonstrated similar induction of DH to HBAg in guinea pigs. Our objectives were to study the in vitro correlates of DH in an animal model and extend the system to a study of the HBAg carrier state in man, particularly with reference to the carriers of ad and ay [283]. This report presents our data on the induction of DH to HBAg of ad and ay subtypes, its in vitro correlation with macrophage migration inhibition tests and the apparent cross reactivity between the two subtypes.

HBAg was isolated from the plasma of normal healthy carriers of ad or ay types by a combination of isopycnic banding and differential sedimentation velocities in cesium chloride gradients [67]. The first peak containing 20 nm particles, devoid of detectable human plasma proteins, was used as purified HBAg for all experimental work [478].

Adult albino guinea-pigs of the Hartley strain (Simonsen's Laboratories, Gilroy, California), weighing 600 - 700 grams were sensitized by injecting into each hind foot-pad 100 μg of either HBAg subtype, ad or ay, in Freund's complete adjuvant (FCA). Control guinea-pigs were either left uninoculated or were inoculated only with FCA. Ten days later all animals were skin-tested with an intradermal (ID) injection of 0.1 ml (100 μg) of purified HBAg subtype ad or ay. The animals were observed thereafter for both immediate and DH reactions over a 72-hour period. None of the animals showed any reactions immediately or at 6 - 8 hours after ID injection of purified HBAg. All animals sensitized with HBAg subtype ad or ay showed positive DH reactions at 24 hours characterized by erythema and induration upon ID injection of the respective antigens. In addition, animals sensitized with ad and skin tested with ay also exhibited DH reactions (Table 1). All skin reactions reached a maximal intensity by 24 hours and then subsided over the next 48 hours. Nonsensitized controls as well as animals sensitized with FCA alone failed to show DH reactions to either ad or ay. HBAg-sensitized animals did not give any reactions to ID injection of 1:16 dilutions of HBAg-negative human serum.

Sera were obtained from all animals before sensitization, prior to skin testing on the tenth day, and one week after skin testing. All sera were tested by hemagglutination assay for the detection of antibody to HBAg [477]. Ten-day sera from ad or ay sensitized guinea pigs exhibited low hemagglutination titers such as 1:8 to 1:16. However, the titers rose to 1:8,000 or higher approximately one week after the initial skin testing with the respective antigen (Table 2).

The capillary macrophage migration-inhibition technique of David, et al. [124] was applied to both peritoneal exudate and pulmonary alveolar macrophages. Alveolar macrophages were harvested by the pulmonary lavage technique of Myrvik, et al. [340]. Medium 199 with Earle's salt base (Grand Island Biological Company) containing normal guinea-pig serum (15%), 50 units of penicillin per ml, 50 μg streptomycin and 50 μg neomycin per ml was used [148]. Macrophage migration-inhibition tests were performed on guinea-pigs sensitized with HBAg type ad. A dose response study indicated inhibition of macrophage migration with HBAg in a dose of 6 - 100 μg. Therefore, 6.0 μg of purified ad was added to each test chamber containing ad sensitized cells. Peritoneal exudate as well as pulmonary alveolar macrophages from ad sensitized animals exhibited 80- 90% inhibition of migration in the presence of 6.0 μg ad but the migration was unaffected in its absence (Figure 1). Similar cells from nonsensitized animals migrated normally even in the presence of 100 μg ad (Figure 2).

Because all the animals sensitized with HBAg subtype ad or ay exhibited DH reactions to the respective antigens and since none of the control animals reacted to HBAg, it can be inferred that DH was induced in guinea-pigs against the HBAg. In addition, the HBAg-sensitized animals did not give any reactions to HBAg-negative human serum indicating that the DH induced to HBAg was specific.

Table 1.   24-Hour Skin Reactions of HBAg-Sensitized Guinea Pigs.

Guinea Pigs Sensitized With:	Guinea Pig Sensitized	Guinea Pigs Skin-Tested With: ad	ay
		[E/I]*	[E/I]*
HBAg Subtype ad	1	22/4	17/4
	2	17/5	15/5
	3	21/4	--
	4	21/4	--
	5	18/4	--
HBAg Subtype ay	1	--	20/6
	2	--	27/5
	3	--	22/5

*E = Erythema diameter in millimeters. I = Induration, thickness of skin in millimeters minus normal skin thickness (approximately 4.0 mm).

Table 2.   Hemagglutination Titers of HBAg Sensitized Guinea Pigs.

Guinea Pigs Sensitized With:	Guinea Pig Sensitized	Hemagglutination Titers Prior to Sensitization	Prior to Skin Test	A Week After Skin Test with ad or ay
HBAg Subtype ad	1	0	1:8	1:8,000
	2	0	1:8	1:10,000
	3	0	1:16	1:20,000
	4	0	1:16	1:10,000
	5	0	1:8	1:10,000
HBAg Subtype ay	1	0	1:8	1:8,000
	2	0	1:8	1:8,000
	3	0	1:16	1:8,000

These findings are in agreement with the recent observations of Irwin, et al. [229], who have also induced DH to purified HBAg in guinea-pigs. The cross reactions between the two subtypes is consistent with the fact that a is a common determinant [283]. It is noteworthy that a sharp rise in antibody titers following ID injection of HBAg to sensitized guinea-pigs may be useful in a prompt preparation of antisera within a period of three weeks.

Anergy has been reported in several infections such as tuberculosis [231], lepromatous leprosy [479], candidiasis [96], histoplasmosis [77] and coccidioidomycosis [437]. Conceivably the chronic carrier state to HBAg could be attributed to a state of

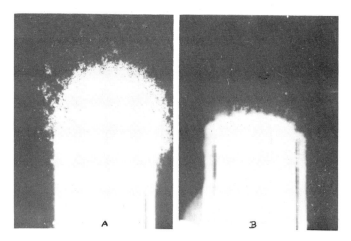

Figure 1. Peritoneal exudate cells from an HBAg-sensitized
guinea pig. A: without HBAg. B: with 0.6 μg HBAg.

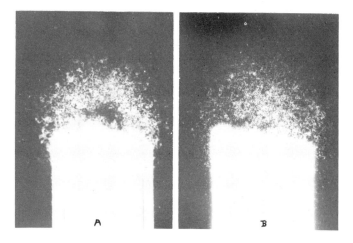

Figure 2. Peritoneal exudate cells from a normal guinea pig.
A: without HBAg. B: with 100 μg HBAg.

anergy. The exact mechanism of implicated anergy in these diseases is unknown at the present time. However, Ibrahim [227] has
reported successful induction of anergy to coccidioidin in sensitized guinea pigs without altering their DH to tuberculin. The
in vitro demonstration of the migration inhibition of macrophages
from the HBAg-sensitized animals confirms our in vivo observations
of DH to HBAg in guinea-pigs. Therefore, the concepts of DH and
anergy may well be extended to the HBAg carrier state in man.

        Acknowledgements. This research was supported in part by
Research Grant CC-00578 from the USPHS Center for Disease Control
and Contract 71-2355 from the National Blood Resource Branch of the
National Heart and Lung Institute. Communications regarding this
work should be addressed to Dr. Vyas.

HEPATITIS B ANTIGEN IN BLOOD DONORS

Chairman: H. A. Perkins

35. OCCURRENCE OF HBAg AND ANTIGENS IN EXCRETA AND SECRETIONS

N.R. Shulman, R.F. Lange, C.S. Knepp and C.R. Coleman

National Institute of Arthritis and Metabolic Diseases, Clinical Hematology Branch, National Institutes of Health Bethesda, Maryland

There is evidence from the epidemiology of hepatitis B reviewed by Dr. Krugman (see Section I) that this disease can be transmitted non-parenterally. The only direct experimental evidence bearing on the oral transmission of hepatitis B was Krugman's study [261] where infectious plasma, fed orally, transmitted this form of hepatitis. However, there is no other direct evidence that body fluids or excrement can transmit hepatitis B. In recent years a number of investigators have attempted to determine whether the antigen associated with hepatitis B (HBAg)*, which is present in infectious plasma, is also in materials such as saliva, stool and urine which are likely sources for transmission of a viral agent. While some investigators have reported finding HBAg in stools, urine, or bile, others have not been able to confirm these observations and our own attempts to measure HBAg in stools, urine, and saliva have been unsuccessful. However, during our attempts to demonstrate HBAg in stools from patients with hepatitis B (using sera from patients with acute hepatitis as a source of antibody) we discovered a new antigen system that appears unrelated to HBAg. First we will review information on the presence

---

*The nomenclature used in this paper is that recommended by the National Research Council Committee on Viral Hepatitis, as follows:
Diseases: Viral hepatitis, type A (infectious hepatitis)
            Viral hepatitis, type B (serum hepatitis)
Viruses: Hepatitis A Virus (HAV)
            Hepatitis B Virus (HBV)
Antigen: Hepatitis B antigen (HBAg) [Australia/SH/hepatitis
            associated antigen (HAA)]

Table 1. Stools in Hepatitis.

Author	Material Studied	Patients	Technique	Results
6 studies 1942-46 [152,153,193, 302, 345, 375]	Stool extract	Volunteers	Oral Administration	34 cases of hepatitis, 98 trials (most short incubation)
S. Krugman Virology '63 [267]	Stool extract	Volunteers	Oral administration	30 cases of hepatitis, 63 trials (most short incubation, 5 cases 60+ days, not proved to be hepatitis B)
N.R.Shulman Amer.J.Med. '70 [426]	20% stool extract	5 acute viral hepatitis; 5 chronic hepatitis	Agar gel diffusion, immunoelectrophoresis, complement fixation and hemagglutination	None of patients with HBAg in serum had HBAg in stool. 7 of 10 patients with hepatitis had new stool antigen
N.R.Shulman et al. '72	20% stool extract	30 patients with HBAg-positive hepatitis and other diseases. 57 normal individuals	Agar gel diffusion, immunoelectrophoresis, complement fixation, hemagglutination, and electronmicroscopy	None had HBAg. 22 of 30 patients with HBAg hepatitis and 43 of 57 normals had new stool antigen. No virus-like particles seen in precipitin lines by EM
I.E.Cossart & J.Vahrman BMJ Feb.'70 [111]	10% stool extract	4 patients with acute hepatitis. 3 had HBAg in serum	Agar gel diffusion	None had HBAg

Reference	Preparation	Subjects	Method	Findings
I.D.Gust et al. Lancet Apr.'71 [187]	Stool extract, unknown preparation	15 patients with acute HBAg-positive hepatitis	Agar gel diffusion & immunoelectro-phoresis	47 extracts collected within 2 weeks of jaundice all negative for HBAg and anti-HBAg
A.A.Ferris et al. Lancet, Aug.'70 [149]	20% stool extract	220 with viral hepatitis; 158 controls with other diseases	Agar gel diffusion and immunoelectron-microscopy; antibody made in rabbit against positive stool absorbed with normal stool extract	90 of 220 hepatitis cases positive for 18-25 nm and 35-40 nm virus-like particles different from HBAg. 5 controls positive for same particles by EM. Antigen present only during acute hepatitis or convalescence
G.F.Cross et al. Austr.J.Exp.Biol.Med.Sci. Jan.'71 [116]	Stool, unknown preparation	8 positive stools (criteria Ferris et al.) from acute hepatitis patients; 5 negative stools from non-hepatitis patients	Agar gel diffusion and immunoelectron-microscopy; antibody made in rabbit and guinea pig against positive stool absorbed with normal stool	In positives, 15-25 nm virus-like particles distinct from HBAg which aggregated with specific rabbit or guinea pig antibody (Anti F); 40-45 nm virus-like particles that cross react with anti-HBAg also noted. In negatives, very rare 15-25 nm and 40-45 nm particles that did not aggregate
P.J.Grob & H. Jemelka, Lancet Jan.'71 [183]	20-30gms of stool mixed with 3 ml Hanks solution	11 patients with acute HBAg-positive hepatitis	Agar gel diffusion and immunoelectro-phoresis	All positive for HBAg, 2 of 11 had anti-HBAg

of HBAg in various body fluids and excreta, and then describe
briefly the new stool antigen(s) and the antibodies that may arise
against it during acute hepatitis.

Table 1 summarizes the evidence for and against the presence
of HBAg in stools. The early studies from 1942 to 1946 indicated
that hepatitis could be transmitted by stool extracts but in almost all instances the hepatitis occurred after a short incubation
period, hence was probably hepatitis A rather than hepatitis B.
Krugman's similar studies in 1963 on administration of stool extracts to volunteers [267] resulted in 30 positive cases of short
incubation hepatitis (hepatitis A) and 5 cases that had an incubation period of over 60 days which Dr. Krugman has interpreted as
being secondary cases of hepatitis A from contact with the other
patients, (see Dr. Krugman's discussion).

The remaining studies in Table 1 concern attempts to detect
HBAg in stools by laboratory techniques rather than by human
transmission studies. In our initial studies using stool extracts [430] we did not find HBAg in stools of patients who had
high titer HBAg in their blood. The techniques employed were agar
gel diffusion (ID), counterimmunoelectrophoresis (CIE), complement-
fixation (CF), and hemagglutination (HA). Cossart and Vahrman [111]
and Gust et al. [187] were also unsuccessful in their attempts to
demonstrate HBAg in stool extracts of hepatitis patients by ID and
CIE.

Although Ferris and associates [149] were unable to identify
HBAg in stools, they reported finding an antibody in the serum of
a multi-transfused hemophiliac that formed a precipitate in ID
with stool extracts from 90 of 220 hepatitis patients tested but
with only 5 extracts of 158 controls. The antigen was immunologically distinct from HBAg and was present in the stools of
patients only during acute hepatitis or the immediate convalescence
period. In electronmicroscopy of the stool antigen precipitates
virus-like particles were seen; most were 20 nm in diameter but
some were 40 nm.

In further studies on the antigen reported by Ferris et al.,
Cross and co-workers [116], using the heterologous antibody made
in rabbits and guinea pigs, found that 8 stool extracts positive
for stool antigen by ID contained 20 nm particles that were aggregated only by anti-stool antibody, not by anti-HBAg. The stool
20 nm particles did not cross react with serum HBAg. However, they
also found some 40-45 nm particles in stool that did cross react
with 20 nm particles in HBAg-positive sera. Their conclusion was
that the 40-45 nm stool particles may share group specific antigens
with HBAg. In contrast to all others, Grob and Jemelka [183]
reported finding HBAg as well as anti-HBAg in stools of all 11

patients with hepatitis that they tested, a result which is still unconfirmed.

Normally 5 to 10 ml of blood is lost in the gastrointestinal tract each day; and when certain commonly used drugs are taken, such as aspirin, possibly 10-fold that amount may be lost. It is apparent that patients with HBAg in their blood do transfer some of that antigen to the gastrointestinal tract but using current methods HBAg cannot be readily identified in stools. The difficulty in finding HBAg in stools may be due simply to dilution or to denaturation of the antigen as it is exposed to strong acids, proteolytic enzymes and detergent action of bile salts as it passes through the gastrointestinal tract. In that respect it is of interest that Serpeau et al. [426] found that 2 patients with HBAg-positive hepatitis had HBAg in gall bladder bile obtained after administering cholecystokinin but did not have HBAg in duodenal bile and HBAg was found by Akdamar et al.[3] in the bile of one of 4 patients with HBAg-positive hepatitis (Table 2).

Table 3 lists studies on the transmission of hepatitis by urine and attempts to measure HBAg in urine. The 4 cases of hepatitis caused by administration of urine from patients with acute hepatitis to a total of 48 recipients in studies from 1944 through 1964 were short incubation hepatitis, probably hepatitis A. In our studies of patients with HBAg-positive hepatitis, we found no evidence of HBAg in the urine by a variety of techniques, even when urine was concentrated up to 100-fold. On the other hand, there have been two recent reports indicating success in measuring HBAg in urine. Blainey et al. [43] found 8 of 8 urine samples from patients with high blood levels of HBAg following renal transplantation were positive for HBAg by CF but only 1 of 7 was positive by ID or CIE. One might have expected more of the samples to be positive by CIE since CIE and CF have similar sensitivities in detecting HBAg [430]. Since hematuria is common after renal transplantation, it is not surprising that HBAg was found in urine of some patients. However, no determination of the amount of blood in the urine was made and no studies were done on the recovery of HBAg in mixtures of blood and urine. Apostolov et al. [22] found HBAg in urine in 12 of 48 patients with viral hepatitis, 8 of whom had HBAg in their blood, and 4 of whom did not. An additional 13 patients with HBAg-positive and 9 with HBAg-negative hepatitis did not have the antigen in their urine. In this study, 4 of 13 individuals who had chronic liver disease without HBAg in their blood, nevertheless had the antigen in their urine as did 2 of 7 normal controls. There is no explanation for finding HBAg in the urine of patients whose blood was negative for the antigen.

Table 4 summarizes the observations on attempts to transmit hepatitis via the nasopharyngeal route with nasopharyngeal washings

Table 2. Bile in Hepatitis

Author	Material Studied	No. of Patients	Techniques	Results
K.A. Akdamar Lancet May '71 [3]	Bile & gastric juice	4	Agar gel diffusion & immunoelectro-phoresis	1 patient positive for HBAg in bile but negative in gastric juice; 3 patients negative in bile & negative in gastric juice
D. Serpeau et al. Lancet Dec. '71 [426]	Bile obtained from duodenal drainage & bile obtained after cholecystokinin	2	Immunoelector-phoresis	Both positive for HBAg in gall bladder bile but negative in duodenal bile

Table 3. Urine in Hepatitis

Author	Material Studied	Patients	Techniques	Results
Five studies 1944-46 [153,193,302, 345,346]	Urine from patients with hepatitis	36 normal recipients	Oral administration	3 of 36 developed hepatitis, probably Hepatitis A
J.P. Giles et al. Virology '64 [161]	Urine from patients with hepatitis	12 retarded children	Oral administration of 5 ml	1 of 12 developed hepatitis, probably Hepatitis A
N.R. Shulman Am.J.Med. Nov. '71 [430]	Urine concentrated x 100	6 with HBAg (+) hepatitis	Agar gel diffusion, immunoelectrophoresis complement fixation and hemagglutination	None positive for HBAg
J.D. Blainey et al. Lancet April '71 [43]	5 samples unconcentrated; 3 samples concentrated x 25-60	7 HBAg (+) post renal transplant patients	Complement fixation immunoelectrophoresis agar gel diffusion	8 of 8 samples positive for HBAg by CF; 1 of 7 by immunoelectrophoresis; 1 of 7 by agar gel diffusion
K. Apostolov et al. Lancet June '71 [22]	Urine concentrated x 70-80	48 patients 7 controls	Agar gel diffusion, immunoelectrophoresis and complement fixation	8 positive for HBAg of 13 with HBAg (+) acute hepatitis; 0 of 9 with HBAg (-) hepatitis; 4 of 13 with HBAg (-) chronic liver disease, 4 of 13 with HBAg (+) chronic liver disease; 2 of 7 controls.

Table 4. Nasopharyngeal Secretions in Hepatitis

Author	Material	Test	Evidence of Hepatitis
J.D.S. Cameron Quart.J.Med. 1943 [79]	Nasopharyngeal washings from hepatitis patient	1 recipient injected	0/1
G.M. Findlay & N.H. Martin Lancet 1943 [152]	Nasopharyngeal washings from patients jaundiced following immunization for yellow fever	4 recipients via nasopharyngeal route	3/4
F.O. MacCallum & W.H. Bradley Lancet 1944 [261]	Nasopharyngeal washings from hepatitis patients	22 recipients via nasopharyngeal route	2/22- Elevated bilirubin only
W.P. Haven J.Exp.Med. 1946 [193]	Nasopharyngeal washings from hepatitis patients	3 recipients via nasopharyngeal route	0/3
J.R. Neefe & J. Stokes Jr. JAMA 1945 [153]	Nasopharyngeal washings from hepatitis patients	8 recipients via nasopharyngeal route	0/8
J.R. Neefe et al Amer.J.Med. 1946 [345]	Nasopharyngeal washings from hepatitis patients	4 recipients via nasopharyngeal route	0/4
N.R. Shulman Amer.J.Med. 1970 [430]	Saliva from 6 patients with HBAg (+) hepatitis	Agar gel diffusion, immunoelectrophoresis, complement fixation, and hemagglutination	None of 6 were positive for HBAg

from patients with acute hepatitis. Of 42 individuals subjected
to these transmission studies in the years 1943-46, five developed
hepatitis, and all of the cases were the short incubation type,
apparently hepatitis A. In one study of the saliva of 6 patients
with HBAg-positive hepatitis, the antigen was not found by in vitro
techniques [430].

Although direct tests for HBAg in excreta or secretions have
varied from negative to equivocal to positive in different laboratories, the epidemiological evidence, especially from the work
of Krugman et al. strongly indicates that the virus of hepatitis B
can be transmitted by ingestion of these materials. Since the
sensitivity of the biological transmission test is known to be
several orders of magnitude greater than any current in vitro test,
it must be assumed that body secretions, particularly those that
may contain even minute amounts of blood, may transmit hepatitis B
if ingested.

We will now describe newly recognized serum antibodies that
arise during acute hepatitis and react with antigens in the stool
that are distinct from HBAg. In our attempts to identify HBAg in
stools of patients with hepatitis we reacted stool extracts with
sera from patients convalescing from hepatitis and found that a
number of these sera formed a precipitin line with stool extracts
but the stool antigen was immunologically distinct from HBAg as
indicated by the crossing of precipitin lines in Figure 1. Antibodies

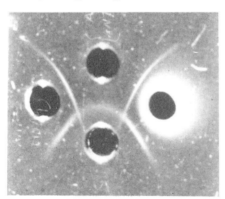

Figure 1. Agarose diffusion pattern. Stool extract from patient
with HBAg-positive acute hepatitis in lower well; stool-precipitating
antibody and anti-HBAg in upper well; and in left and right wells,
serum from two different patients with acute viral hepatitis containing high titer HBAg and stool-precipitating antibody but no
measurable anti-HBAg. The HBAg in the left and right wells reacted
with anti-HBAg in the upper well; the stool extract in the lower
well reacted with the stool-precipitating antibody in the lower
three wells. Lines of the HBAg precipitate and stool precipitate
cross without evidence of partial identity.

against the stool antigen appeared in patients shown in Table 5.

Table 5. Prevalence of serum antibodies to stool antigen

Patient Group	No. Tested	No. Positive	% Positive
HBAg positive, acute hepatitis	30	6	20
Multiply transfused patients with high titer anti-HBAg	25	6	24
Chronic liver disease, HBAg negative	66	2	3
Normal	151	0	0

the highest frequency being in patients with acute hepatitis, whether HBAg-positive or -negative, and in multiply-transfused patients. Some patients with chronic liver disease and an occasional patient with severe chronic bowel disease also developed similar antibodies. The antibodies characteristically were 7S gammaglobulin (Figure 2) which did not fix complement. Their reactions were of low avidity, forming reversible complexes that were

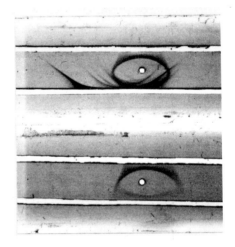

Figure 2. The top and third trough contain anti-Gamma g. The second and bottom trough contain anti-whole human serum. The first eluate from DEAE at low ionic strength is in the bottom well and all other serum proteins eluted at high ionic strength are in the top well. The antibody that precipitated stool antigen is in a fraction containing only Gamma g.

soluble in saline.

The stool antigen(s) appears distinct from substances that have been described as reacting with naturally occurring human antibodies (Tables 6 & 7). The antigen appears as frequently in normal stools

Table 6.   Characteristics of stool antigen.

Prevalence --------	In more than 75% of stools. Same prevalence in stools from normals and patients with hepatitis or other diseases. Not found in urine, bile, serum or extracts of liver, pancreas, stomach, or intestine.
Molecular Weight --	Varies from less than 60,000 to greater than 300,000 by Sephadex G-200.
Morphology --------	Immune complex precipitates showed no structure in electron microscopy. No virus-like particles were identified.
Stability --------	Immunologically stable after heating at 56° for 1 hr., boiling for 10 min., freezing or exposure to ether. Immunologically unstable after exposure to trypsin or sodium dodecyl sulfate, 1%.
Immunologic Characteristics ---	Forms distinct precipitin lines in agar gel diffusion or agarose counter immunoelectrophoresis; is immunologically distinct from HBAg and its subtypes AY or AD. Does not cross-react with any derivative of HBAg made by physicochemical treatment or with extracts of stool bacteria. Does not fix complement or coat red cells for hemagglutination tests.

as in stools of patients with hepatitis and is apparently in almost all stools if the extracts are sufficiently concentrated. The antigen is not found in urine, bile, serum or extracts of liver, pancreas, stomach, or various other organs including the intestinal tract. The molecular weight of the antigen varies from 60,000 to greater than 300,000. It appears to be a protein in that it is digestible by trypsin and degraded by detergents. Table 7 lists the immune precipitins formed with human sera that have been reported previously and appear to be distinct from the new stool antigen system.

Since the stool antigen(s) is recognized by an antibody that develops during acute hepatitis or occasionally severe bowel disease, it appears that during acute hepatitis (or severe bowel disease) a number of substances from the intestine, which are ordinarily filtered from the portal blood by Kupfer cells or parenchymal cells

Table 7.   Immune phenomena distinct from the stool antigen system

---

HBAg and related antigens [116,149,183]

Gram negative bacterial extract precipitins and hemagglutinins
(E. coli, Bacteroides, Pseudomonas, Serratia marscens, and
meningococci) [42,117,118,141]

Candida precipitins [406]

Dietary protein precipitins and hemagglutinins [147,465]

Lipoprotein precipitins

Ruminant serum protein (bovine thrombin) precipitins [18]

Tween 80 treated HBAg immunoelectronmicroscopic aggregates [8]

Polyribonucleotide - heat labile serum factor precipitins [341]

---

of the liver, are not effectively removed and gain excess to antibody tissue. Although not fully characterized as yet, these antigens could be bacterial or dietary in origin. HBAg-anti-HBAg
complexes have recently received much attention as possibly accounting for certain manifestations of hepatitis that might be caused
by immune complexes. It is well to be aware of other antigen systems, such as the one described herein, that could conceivably play
a role in immunologic manifestations of acute hepatitis and other
forms of liver disease.

36. Discussion

OCCURRENCE OF HBAg AND ANTIGENS IN EXCRETA AND SECRETIONS

Saul Krugman

Department of Pediatrics, New York University

School of Medicine, New York, New York

Dr. Shulman has summarized the studies concerned with the occurrence of hepatitis B antigen (HBAg) in urine and in stool. The detection of HBAg in urine has been observed by various investigators. The evidence for the presence of HBAg in stools is still controversial.

Objective data are available to support the observation that HBAg-positive blood is infectious. As yet, there are no objective data to support the hypothesis that HBAg-positive urine or stool are infectious. If these secretions were tinged with blood they undoubtedly would be infectious.

Dr. Shulman has referred to cases of viral hepatitis, type A (infectious hepatitis) which allegedly had an incubation period of 60 days or longer. The usual incubation period has been 25 to 50 days. The longer incubation periods were observed in individuals who were probably not infected during the first exposure; infection resulted from subsequent contact with one of the initial cases of infectious hepatitis.

37.   INCIDENCE OF HBAg IN BLOOD DONORS: AN OVERVIEW

Howard F. Taswell

Mayo Clinic and Mayo Foundation

Rochester, Minnesota

Soon after the association between Australia antigen and viral hepatitis became apparent [52], the Australia or SH antigen was detected in patients with serum hepatitis and post-transfusion hepatitis [367,384] and in some donors [169,367]. This important relationship to post-transfusion hepatitis has led to the screening of many donor populations for the presence of this antigen, in both retrospective and prospective studies. Many other studies have used blood donor populations as a normal healthy control group to study the relationship of Australia antigen to acute and chronic hepatitis and a variety of other hepatic and nonhepatic diseases. As with previous studies of many normal and diseased populations throughout the world, large variations in the incidence of Australia antigen -- or what came to be known as hepatitis-associated antigen (HAA) or, more recently, hepatitis B antigen (HBAg) -- were noted in various blood donor populations. These variations have been related to geographic and ethnic origins, socioeconomic status, age, sex, ABO blood group, and the sensitivity and specificity of the method of detection used.

Wide variation was found [461] in the incidence of HBAg in blood donors from Rochester (Minnesota), Denver, Chicago, Baltimore, Pittsburgh, and Boston. The incidence of HBAg was lowest in Rochester (0.06%) and highest in Chicago (1.47%). Excellent correlation was noted between the incidence of HBAg in the donor population and the incidence of overt hepatitis at each medical center studied when adjusted for the mean number of units transfused. The donor populations at each medical center were composed of varying percentages of voluntary and professional paid donors. In another study of more than 2.5 million volunteer Red Cross donors [134],

similar regional variations were noted throughout the United States.
The lowest incidence was in the north central region (0.06%) and
the highest was in the south eastern region (0.17%) and Puerto Rico
(0.34%). Many smaller studies [95,171,203,250,337] in individual
cities or areas of the United States report a similar range of
incidence of HBAg. Several studies throughout Europe and Great
Britain report higher incidences: Scotland, 0.13% [320]; Norway,
0.16% [439]; Denmark, 0.18% [31]; Germany, 0.20% [410]; Spain,
0.40% [185]; France, 0.40% [443]; and Yugoslavia, 4.0% [131]. An
incidence of 0.11%, which is comparable to that in the United States
and Great Britain, has been noted in Sydney, Australia [352]. However, throughout most of Southeast Asia, Japan, and Africa the
reported incidence of HBAg is much higher, ranging from 1 to 2% among
donors in Tokyo [367] to 4.2% among Chinese donors in Singapore
[434] and 6% in Nairobi, Kenya [27].

   Both genetic and environmental factors appear to be important
in determining the wide geographic variations seen in the incidence
of HBAg. Incidences of both post-transfusion hepatitis and HBAg have
been observed to vary with factors such as the socioeconomic status
of the donor, whether he is a volunteer or paid donor, whether he
is a paid donor known or unknown to the transfusionist, and whether
the donor is a prisoner or a known or suspected narcotic addict.
In a recent national study of post-transfusion hepatitis [178],
1.5% of more than 1,000 patients receiving an average of 7 units
of blood from volunteer donors developed overt hepatitis. In contrast, 5.3% of 625 patients receiving similar amounts of blood
from paid donors developed hepatitis. Previous studies [180,482]
have yielded similar results, suggesting an increased risk (5 to
15 times) of post-transfusion hepatitis following use of commercial
blood sources. In studies of donors in New York (94,95), Barcelona
[185], Tokyo [367], and Philadelphia [171], the incidence of HBAg
in commercial blood was found to be 2 to 15 times greater than that
in blood from volunteer donors (Table 1).

Table 1.   Incidence (%) of HBAg-positive blood donors

City	Paid	Volunteer
New York	1.2	0.09
Barcelona	1.0	0.4
Tokyo	2.2	1.2
Philadelphia	1.57	0.11

   Friends and relatives acting as replacement donors at an inner
city hospital serving a low-income population had an HBAg incidence
of 0.81% while the same type of donor at a neighboring hospital
serving a higher income group had an incidence of only 0.32% [171].

In several other studies, blood collected from prisoners or
from narcotic addicts has been found to have increased incidences
of HBAg, approximately 1.7 to 2% [250,337,352] and 2 to 5% [95,352,
362], respectively.

In virtually every report in which HBAg-positive donors were
studied with regard to their age and sex, the majority of HBAg-
positive donors were males in the younger age groups, as has been
true in many studies of other normal population groups [178,300,
461] and of patients with acute hepatitis [197,235]. Among HBAg-
positive donors in New York City [95], the large majority were
males under age 30. In a study in Sydney, Australia [352], 86% of
HBAg-positive donors were male while only 64% of the 56,140 donors
tested were male; 62% of the positives were 18 to 26 years old
while only 30% of all donors were in that age group. In Tokyo,
the ratio of male to female HBAg-positive donors was 6:1; 2.32%
of all male donors and 1.14% of all female donors were found to
be HBAg-positive [366]. In Paris, 80% of HBAg-positive donors were
male but only 60% of all donors were male. In contrast, 57% of
anti-HBAg is seen in female donors while only 40% of all donors
are female [443]. A similarly high incidence of anti-HBAg was
found in Danish female donors, 0.58%, in contrast to 0.18% in
male donors. The ratio of HBAg was reversed, with 0.08% in females
and 0.21% in males. Those donors who were HBAg-positive were
primarily between ages 18 and 29 years [31].

No relationship has been found between HBAg and the ABO or Rh
blood groups [443,457].

A wide variety of methods -- including agar gel diffusion (AGD)
counterelectrophoresis (CEP), complement fixation (CF), hemagglutination-inhibition (HAI), and radioimmunoassay (RIA) -- have been
described for the detection of HBAg. These methods vary in their
sensitivity in terms of their ability to detect in vitro dilutions
of known antigens and, to varying degrees, to detect increased
numbers of HBAg-positive donors. In a study in Tokyo [366] using
an AGD method, approximately 1% of volunteer donors were HBAg-
positive; however, with a more sensitive immune adherence agglutination method, approximately 2% were positive. In a study in
Yugoslavia [131], 2.3% of donors were positive by AGD and 4.08%
by CEP. Although an increased percentage of HBAg-positive donors
may be detected by more sensitive methods, the clinical importance
of these weakly positive donors in causing post-transfusion hepatitis has not yet been well established. In a study, by AGD, of
the serum of 92 donors implicated by the occurrence of hepatitis
in 103 transfusion recipients, 32% of the expected number of hepatitis carriers were found to be HBAg-positive [461]. When these
sera were retested by RIA, nine previously negative (by AGD and
CEP) donors were found to be HBAg-positive [459]. A study, by RIA

of 300 donor serum samples from Chicago and Rochester collected
for a previous study [461] revealed 7 of 150 donors in Chicago
and 4 of 150 donors in Rochester who were positive by RIA and
previously negative by AGD (and CEP). It will be important to
establish clear criteria for an HBAg-positive result by RIA, which
is significantly related to the infectivity of the donor and to
clinical or subclinical hepatitis and the hepatitis carrier state.

Variations in the specificity of antisera and in antigen
subtypes [243,283,290] which have been reported in several donor
populations may also account for variations in reported incidence
of HBAg and may be clinically and epidemiologically significant.

The ultimate purpose of screening blood donor populations,
determining the HBAg incidence in population subgroups, and avoiding
transfusion of HBAg-positive blood is, of course, to decrease the
incidence of post-transfusion hepatitis. That this in fact has
been accomplished, or to what degree, has not yet been firmly established. Until this has become evident, all HBAg-positive blood
should be detected by the most sensitive and practical methods,
donor populations with the lowest incidence of HBAg should be used
when possible, and donor populations should be increased by encouraging a greater percentage of voluntary blood donation.

INCIDENCE OF HBAg IN BLOOD DONORS

Paul V. Holland

Clinical Center Blood Bank, N.I.H.,

Bethesda, Maryland

I would certainly agree with Dr. Taswell that there is a variable frequency of hepatitis B antigen (HBAg) carriers among blood donor populations. The incidence found is dependent on a number of factors, especially the test method employed and the commercial or non-commercial status of the blood donor.

I would like to emphasize two points. First, screening of blood donors for HBAg, by even the most sensitive techniques currently available, will not affect the incidence of hepatitis A (infectious hepatitis) transmitted by blood. And, second, even using a radioimmunoassay test (RIA) for HBAg, all HBAg carriers cannot be currently detected and hence not all hepatitis B transmitted by transfusion can be prevented. I will illustrate these two points by summarizing the results of a recent study by Dr. Alter of our group [14].

For some time now we have been using only volunteer blood which has been screened by a counterelectrophoresis technique. Our incidence of posttransfusion hepatitis (PTH) is considerably lower now than ever before but not insignificant. Among our open-heart surgery patients, who received an average of 16 units of blood, we still found that 7% developed PTH, of which 2% were icteric. Let us examine in detail those patients who developed PTH after receiving blood from volunteers which did not contain HBAg detected by CEP (Table 1).

Nine patients developed PTH with one patient, J.K., apparently experiencing two bouts. Using the radioimmunoassay for HBAg and this same assay for antibody to HBAg, as well as the hemagglutination

Table 1.   Serologic Analysis of 10 Episodes of Posttransfusion
Hepatitis.

Recipient	Incubation Period (Days)	Recipient HBAg	Recipient Seroconversion Anti-HBAg	Donors' HBAg
N.A.	25	No	No	No
J.C.	28	No	No	No
M.K.	39	No	No	No
J.K.*	14	No	No	No
J.K.*	89	Yes	Yes	No
J.S.	95	Yes	Yes	No
M.W.	105	Yes	Yes	No
V.F.	75	Yes	Yes	Yes
A.T.	89	Yes	Yes	Incomplete
J.G.	106	Yes	No**	Incomplete

*Same patient with two distinct episodes of posttransfusion
hepatitis
**Became chronic carrier of HBAg

test, the original donor sera and the serial patient sera were
carefully restudied.

As you can see from the upper half of the table, these episodes of PTH were of relatively short incubation and entirely
unrelated to HBAg. This included J.K.'s first episode of hepatitis.
We believe these cases were undoubtedly due to hepatitis A and
could not have been prevented by available tests on the donor
bloods.

In the group of the lower half of the table, all patients had
a longer incubation period, all had HBAg at the time of their
hepatitis, and all but one seroconverted, that is, developed anti-
HBAg after recovery. One became a chronic carrier of HBAg and did
not produce antibody. All of the donors to four of these patients
were available for retesting by complement fixation and radioimmunoassay. In only one donor to one of these patients were we
able to detect HBAg. His blood had HBAg detectable by both RIA
and CF, but missed by CEP. All of the donors to three patients
who developed clearcut HBAg-positive PTH did not have detectable
HBAg by even the most sensitive test available, the RIA.

We, therefore, need to develop a means of detecting donors
with the hepatitis A virus, plus, even more sensitive techniques
for HBAg detection.

39. CARRIER BLOOD DONORS

Thomas C. Chalmers

National Institutes of Health, Department of Health,

Education, and Welfare, Bethesda, Maryland

The title of this paper is really what is referred to in the publishing business as a "running head". The true title should be "Elimination of the Carrier Blood Donor". I believe that we have it within our power at the present time to accomplish this with over 90% efficiency. It is the purpose of this paper to review the steps required to attain this goal. It can be accomplished by continuing or intensifying procedures that are well known and already carried out to varying degrees: screening of donors, elimination of high risk populations from the donor-pool, and identification and reporting of all chronic carriers not picked up by the other two procedures. Although it is probable that post-transfusion hepatitis could be virtually eliminated by applying all of the measures we now have available, the cost will be high, both in money and strain on the blood collection and delivery systems. However, 30,000 attacks of hepatitis and 2 to 3,000 deaths a year are also expensive; it is likely that cost-benefit analyses will come out in favor of prevention.

SCREENING OF INDIVIDUAL DONORS

Testing for hepatitis B antigen is now required of all federally licensed blood banks and by some state health departments. Eventually no blood will be administered that has not been tested. Other screening procedures, such as an adequate physical examination and a transaminase test, may be necessary to eliminate all patients with active hepatitis.

Testing for HB antigen. It has been estimated from data

gathered during the transition period between the discovery of the
hepatitis B antigen and routine testing that application of the
latter would result in a reduction of hepatitis incidence of
approximately 25% [16,167,211]. Actual reductions have been larger
than this [425] but undoubtedly reflect the screening out of commercial and other high risk donors [16]. Two groups of patients
will probably never be screened adequately by antigen tests currently on the horizon.

The studies of Barker [36] and Murray [339] indicate that HBAg
can be transmitted parenterally to produce symptomatic hepatitis
in concentrations of infected plasma of 10^{-4} and to produce antigenemia in concentrations of 10^{-7}. The original plasma had titers
of 1 to 10, by the complement fixation technique, and it is not
expected that any test likely to be developed will detect antigen
in dilutions of that serum greater than 10^{-2} or 10^{-3}. So some
cases of hepatitis B are bound to continue to occur after application of the most sensitive, practical tests.

There is now evidence appearing to document what was previously only suspected--that at least some post-transfusion hepatitis
is the result of the transmission of short incubation period virus
A, for which no test is available. Experimental transmission data
gathered by Neefe et al. [345] and by Paul et al. [375] during
World War II clearly showed that virus A could be transmitted
parenterally, albeit much less consistently than virus B. However,
two types of epidemiologic data have suggested that virus A was not
a common cause of post-transfusion hepatitis. The distribution
of incubation periods in large series of post-transfusion hepatitis
is not bimodal as it should be if two agents of distinctly different
incubation periods were involved [180]. Furthermore, one might
expect that post-transfusion disease caused by virus A might be
prevented by the same gamma globulin preparations that prevent
oral transmission of acute infectious hepatitis. However, four
recent controlled trials of gamma globulin have not revealed any
lengthening of the mean incubation period among the gamma globulin
patients when compared with controls [177,213,241,322], as might
be expected if the short incubation period disease was being prevented. Since the advent of routine testing for HBAg, three groups
of investigators [16,179,330] (Table 1) have confirmed the World
War II data by demonstrating that patients with HBAg-negative
post-transfusion hepatitis have significantly shorter incubation
periods than HBAg-positive cases. Although there is a great deal
of overlap in all series, these data suggest that from one-third
to one-half of the residual cases may be virus A disease or, more
correctly, caused by a virus not identifiable by any known hepatitis B antibody. Information as to the exact proportion will
have to await careful studies of sero-conversion, which should be
much more accurate because of the increased sensitivity of available methods of measuring antibody.

Table 1.   Post-transfusion hepatitis incubation periods

Author	HBAg-			HBAg+		
	#	Mean	S.E.	#	Mean	S.E.
Grady	23	71	6.6	28	92	6.5*
Mosley	26	49	4.0	13	83	11.9***
Alter	4	26	5.1	7	93	4.0***

t- test
* P <.05   *** P <.001

It is possible that virus A is more commonly transmitted from patients with acute disease rather than from carriers. Infected sera employed in the World War II experiments came from patients sick with acute virus A disease, whereas the B serum often came from carriers. Similarly, Krugman has demonstrated disappearance of virus A (MS-1) from the serum early in the course of the disease [266]. The prevention of virus A hepatitis is a two-fold problem: Development in the future of a test for virus A, and successful screening at present for asymptomatic acute hepatitis.

Tests for active hepatitis. There are conflicting data in the literature on the value of screening all blood for the signs of active hepatitis [88,315]. There is no doubt that bloods with high transaminase values are more likely to contain a virus than those with normal values. For instance, the rate of HB antigenemia is much higher in patients with chronic hepatitis or non-alcoholic cirrhosis than in the normal population. Whether this is an indication that the virus is causing the disease or that the disease causes the antigen to be measurable and transmissible is not pertinent here. The important point is that the two are sufficiently associated to proscribe donation of blood by all patients with acute and chronic hepatitis. Singleton [435] found that 8 of 25 donors found to be HBAg-positive had active hepatitis. In the survey of active health care personnel described below, 9 of 1189 were HBAg-positive; 3 of the 9 had acute hepatitis; one, chronic; and one had a transient antigenemia. Three of 11 with an SGPT >50 and negative HBAg probably had asymptomatic acute hepatitis for a total rate of 5 per 1,000.

Reluctance to employ transaminase tests as a routine screen has its genesis in the lack of demonstrated specificity and the possibility that too many bloods would have to be discarded. However, it is entirely possible that transaminase tests will be more predictive once HBAg-positive donors without active hepatitis have been eliminated. Adequate data on this will be available if follow-up of transfused patients becomes routine, as advocated below. A cutoff of three standard deviations above the normal mean will only eliminate approximately 1% of donors. The availability of automated procedures minimizes the cost per test.

Adequate physical examination. Blood banks have not carried out adequate physical examinations of prospective donors because it is impractical to have each donor examined by a physician. However, the advent of physician's assistants is teaching the medical profession that any trained person can do an adequate physical examination. A blood bank technician can learn to recognize jaundice, spider angiomata, ascites, and hepatosplenomegaly. It might be impractical to examine the abdomen of volunteer donors, but this could be required of commercial blood banks.

Tests for drug addiction. If America is never able to convert to an all volunteer blood collection system and payment for donation continues, the elimination of heroin addicts from the donor pool will be of paramount importance. There is about to be available in kit form a simple radioimmunoassay method of detecting minute amounts of morphine and its derivations in serum--possibly effective 48 to 72 hours after the last injection [444]. This could be required of all commercial blood banks.

HIGH RISK POPULATIONS

It is certain that some infective donors will slip through all available and feasible screening procedures, and this emphasizes the importance of considering the elimination of whole populations of donors who might have a higher than acceptable rate of sub-measurable antigenemia. There are now enough epidemiologic data based on transmission and screening studies to indicate that certain populations may be identified as having a higher infectivity rate than others. It is reasonable to assume that those that have a higher rate of HBAg will also have a higher rate of sub-measurable quantities of the antigen [36,339] and will therefore entail a greater risk, even though they are screened by routine testing procedures. Proof of this assumption is now available in the case of commercial blood [16,211] and should be forthcoming for other populations in future epidemiologic studies. Until the data are available, it is likely that elimination of whole high risk populations from donating blood will reduce the incidence of post-transfusion hepatitis beyond that attained by screening, but in each case such a move must be weighed against the resulting loss of donors.

Commercially supplied blood. Allen [5] and Kunin [271] first demonstrated in 1959, by retrospective studies, that blood purchased from commercial blood banks resulted in a higher hepatitis rate than that collected from volunteers. This has been confirmed by prospective studies carried out by Walsh et al. [482] and by Grady et al. [178] (Table 2) (Figure 1). Grady was able to calculate differential rates for those hospitals that used only volunteer blood (.21%), higher rates for those that purchased blood

Table 2. Rates of hepatitis in volunteer vs. commercial blood

Author	Percent Commercial Blood	Total Units of Blood	Total Cases of Hepatitis	Cases/ 1000 Units	Ratio of Rates Comm./Vol. Blood
Allen, 1959 [5]	0	14,549	5	0.3	
	40	56,543	184	3.3	11.0
Kunin, 1959 [271]	0	243,481	110	0.5	
	29	9,869	28	2.8	5.6
Walsh, 1970 [482]	2	496	0	---	
	95	1,449	42	28.0	+30
Goldfield 1970 [173]	0	297,949	153	0.5	
	100	155,280	267	1.7	3.4
Grady, 1972 [178]	0	7,557	16	2.1	
	100	3,062	33	10.7	5.1

in the hospitals in which it was administered (.52%), and highest (1.07%) among those hospitals that used some blood from commercial banks. The data establish without a doubt the fact that, on the average, purchased blood is more infectious than that donated by volunteers. Alter [16] has demonstrated that the post-transfusion hepatitis rate can be reduced by as much as 60% by the elimination of commercial blood, i.e., that employing only volunteer blood is twice as effective as screening alone.

The higher infectivity rate of purchased blood may be the result of poorer sanitary customs among people who need to sell their blood for cash, but there are abundant data indicating that narcotic addiction is the principal cause of the high HBAg-positive rate among people who sell their blood. Cohen and Dougherty [98] first demonstrated the striking increase of the rate of hepatitis among recipients of blood from known narcotic addicts. Since then, studies of populations of addicts have demonstrated HB antigenemia rates of 1.1 to 4.2% (Table 3).

Health care personnel as a potential source of HBAg-positive blood. Because of the established higher rate of viral hepatitis among hospital employees [78,442], a study was undertaken to determine whether they also had a higher rate of chronic HB antigenemia,

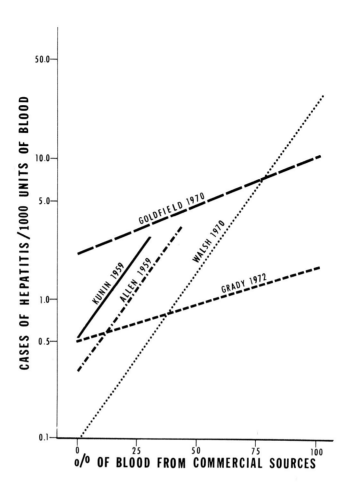

Figure 1.

Table 3.   Frequency of HBAg among "asymptomatic" natcotic addicts

	Total	Positive	Percent
Albany	180	2	1.1
Australia	104	4	3.8
New York	340	5	1.5
Philadelphia	215	9	4.2
Totals	839	20	2.4

and might thus represent an increased hazard as blood donors and
as health care delivery workers. N.I.H. Clinical Center employees
who are either physicians, nurses, or laboratory technicians were
requested to donate 30 cc of blood and at that time a questionnaire
was filled out with regard to their past history. Pertinent details recorded were: Their exact occupation, the locale in which
they grew up and lived with regard to the population density, and
whether or not they had ever had viral hepatitis or been exposed
to someone who had, had pricked themselves with a needle that had

been in a patient who had had hepatitis, had received a blood
transfusion, or had lived outside of the United States for more
than two months. Controls were matched with regard to broad
categories of age, sex, and GS rating--the salary level of the
employee. The latter was thought to be important because of the
possibility that the less educated had grown up and lived under
more crowded conditions and might have a higher rate of antigenemia
as a result of that. Thus an attempt was made to control all
variables except that of exposure to patients with acute viral
hepatitis that might have been antigen positive, or to their blood
or other excreta.

One deficiency of the study needs to be emphasized. Since
the blood-letting was only on a voluntary basis, one might expect
a systematic trend in each of the groups: Those in the high
risk group who thought they might be or knew they were antigen
positive might not volunteer for fear that knowledge of the information would impair their opportunities to work; conversely, those
in the low risk group who thought they might be antigen positive
might be inclined to volunteer in order to find out. Thus, the
bias in the study was toward minimizing the difference between the
two groups.

Preliminary data presented in Table 4 indicate that after the

Table 4. Health care personnel survey

	High Risk	Low Risk
Total	1189	1376
Previous hepatitis	8%	4%
Previous blood transfusion	9%	13%
Previous needle pricking	62%	1%
Blood donation (last 2 yrs.)	32%	35%
HBAg-positive	9	5
Acute hepatitis	3	0
Transient HBAg	1	0
Chronic hepatitis	1	0
HBAg carrier	4	5
Previous transfusions	0	4
SGPT over 50	15	16
With HBAg-positive	4	0

elimination of health care workers with acute hepatitis and the
controls who have been transfused there is only a slight difference
in the rate of chronic antigenemia. Unfortunately, the rate found

among health care workers is low enough to require a study involving
many times as many as those in this survey to establish an accurate
rate. However, health care workers are a population with a mildly
increased risk of transmitting hepatitis, which is in part the result of the coincidental occurrence of asymptomatic acute hepatitis.

Previously transfused normals. In the course of the health
care personnel survey, it was found that four out of the five
volunteers with HB antigenemia in the low risk control group had
previously received a transfusion. When this group was supplemented
by 40 more volunteers who had been transfused in the past, and the
tests re-run by the slightly more sensitive solid phase radioimmunoassay procedure, it was found that 6 of 322 transfused employees
were positive (1.9%), compared with none in 291 matched controls
selected by computer from among the 2,279 volunteers who had not
been transfused. These data suggest that the rate among previously
transfused normals may be almost as high as that among narcotic
addicts. If the findings are confirmed, a serious problem will be
presented to blood banks, since between 8 and 15% of normal adults
who ordinarily give blood have received a transfusion in the past.

A past history of acute hepatitis. This has been a traditional
reason for excluding normals from donating blood and has resulted
in the rejection of approximately 5% of the people who would ordinarily donate. There has never been any epidemiologic evidence
that they are more infectious than people who do not know that they
ever had viral hepatitis. Although 5 to 10% of patients with acute
HBAg-positive hepatitis have persistent antigenemia for an unknown
period of time, the Health Care Personnel Survey reviewed above
shows no relation of antigenemia to a history of hepatitis (Table
5), but the numbers are small. Further data of this kind are needed.

Table 5. Health care personnel survey

	History of previous hepatitis			
	YES (6.2%)		NO	
	Number	Percent	Number	Percent
Total cases	155		2410	
HBAg-positive	1	0.6	13	0.5
SGPT over 50	3	1.9	28	1.2

Geographic and socioeconomic factors. The data in Dodd's
paper [134] presented at this Symposium suggest that HBAg-positive
rates among volunteer blood donors are much higher in the southern
parts of the United States than in the north. Rates vary from
0.2/1,000 in Iowa to 3.4 in Puerto Rico. There are also data suggesting that inhabitants of ghetto areas have a higher rate than
those in the suburbs [93]. If commercial blood banks are to
continue in operation they should locate in the north central areas
of the country.

IDENTIFICATION OF CHRONICALLY INFECTED DONORS WHO SLIP
THROUGH ALL AVAILABLE SCREENS

It is impossible to estimate accurately what proportion of
infective donors who would slip through all available screens have
acute hepatitis, a transient antigenemia without disease, or are
chronic carriers of the antigen in too low concentrations to be
identified in the laboratory. It is entirely possible that the
majority would fall into the last category, and for this reason an
accurate system for detecting and reporting all cases of post-
transfusion hepatitis to the relevant health department and blood
bank becomes crucially important, and the ultimate step in eradi-
cating the disease and learning more about its epidemiology in the
process.

Identification and reporting of all possible cases. Available
data [180] indicate that a search of hospital records uncovers one-
third as many cases of recognized hepatitis with jaundice as are
found by a prospective followup. That number can be multiplied by
a factor of 3 or more [178] by the measurement of blood transaminase
every two weeks following transfusion. Obviously, the last maneuver
is not possible except in specific research situations. However,
it could and should be made a responsibility of blood banks to obtain information from all living recipients of their blood to the
effect that they have or have not had something that might be diagnosed as viral hepatitis in the six month period after transfusion.
This could be accomplished both by tightening up reporting procedures within hospitals and by conducting a routine followup by
means of a postcard sent both to the patient and his doctor.

At present the operators of blood banks could be considered
to be worrying about post-transfusion hepatitis one-tenth as much
as they should because they usually hear of less than 10% of the
hepatitis cases caused by their blood. In Boston during one 2-year
period [253], 103 cases of acute hepatitis were seen in six teaching hospitals. Twelve were reported to the local health department.
There were 24 patients with post-transfusion hepatitis and one was
reported. It is not known how many were reported directly to the
blood banks involved but it probably was a small percentage of the
total cases. Among seven hospitals in New Orleans [279], the percentage of cases of serum hepatitis reported to the health department varied from 0 to 54%, averaging 34%.

There are a number of examples in the literature of blood
donors who have been associated with more than one recipient of
their blood [198,460]. An effective reporting system could have
prevented many of those cases.

The Veterans Administration, in its latest Manual of Operations, requires that all hospitals have a transfusion committee which reviews all cases diagnosed as definite or possible viral hepatitis and makes sure that those which might in any way be related to blood transfusion are reported to the responsible blood banks.

Exclusion of implicated donors. Successful exclusion of implicated donors will have ramifications throughout the whole blood collection and delivery system. Two important steps in the proper direction have already been made. The Red Cross is now compiling a list of voluntary donors with chronically positive HB antigen tests. The Veterans Administration, for several years, has been requiring in its contracts for purchased blood that the name, address, and social security number of the donors be maintained by the collecting agency. It is not clear that the link between the compiling of names and social security numbers of the donors, the reporting of cases of post-transfusion hepatitis, and the exclusion of implicated donors from future donations has yet been closed, but the V.A. is moving in that direction.

The problem is complicated by the fact that many patients receive multiple pints of blood. There is no question about excluding donors of a single, double, or even triple transfusion of a patient who develops hepatitis, but beyond that the problem becomes one of weighing the risk of hepatitis versus the loss of too many potentially useful donors. This problem is the same as exists in deciding which populations of donors should be excluded on the chance that they have sub-measurable amounts of hepatitis B antigen. To some extent, the degree of exclusion will depend on the efficiency of the blood collecting system. In the voluntary sphere, the keeping of a list of implicated donors has suggestions of invasion of privacy and might result in less of an inclination to donate on the part of well-intentioned citizens. In the collection of blood under commercial auspices, it might be possible for documented HBAg-positive donors to give a false social security number or borrow someone else's blood donating identity card. This could be prevented in part by making out a check only to the person identified on the card, but it is also possible that, if commercial collection of blood is to continue, a system of identification by fingerprinting could be added. All of these maneuvers will add to the cost of blood transfusions, but the prevention of hepatitis will save at least as much money as will be spend on extra precautions.

A COST-BENEFIT ANALYSIS OF ELIMINATING THE CARRIER BLOOD DONOR

It has been estimated that there are 30,000 cases of post-transfusion hepatitis in the country each year and 3,000 deaths, resulting from the administration of about 6 million units of

blood to 2 million people.   If we assume an average hospitalization
charge of $100 per day for 30 days each, the total cost of hospi-
talization alone is 90 million dollars per year, not to mention
time lost from work and the cost of death.   So, hospitalization for
post-transfusion hepatitis adds a mean cost of approximately $15
per unit of blood administered and $45 for each patient transfused.
Data dependent on varying rates of hepatitis are presented in Table
6.   Screening for HBAg will probably cost $1 per unit, and SGPT

Table 6.   Cost-benefit analysis of the prevention of post-transfusion hepatitis.

Type of Blood Collection System*	Expected Hepatitis Rate/1000 Units**	Cost of Hepatitis per 1000 Units***	Cost per Unit
Some commercial donors	10	$30,000	$30
Some paid donors	5	15,000	15
All volunteer donors	2	6,000	6
Maximum screening	1	3,000	3

* As defined by Grady et al. [178]
** Rates from intensive followup study [178], completed before
   testing for HBAg was routine
*** Cost of hospitalization alone estimated as 30 days x $100 per
    day.   Costs of disability, occasional chronic illness, and
    death not included.

another $1.   That leaves plenty of money to be spent on recruiting
volunteer donors, followup of recipients, reporting of cases, and
maintaining lists of infected donors.   The principle of applying
the cost of treating a disease to its prevention is an important
one that is eminently applicable to blood banking.

     Finally, would the supply of blood be dried up by too rigid
screening and exclusion of possibly infective donors?   At present
only 3% of the eligible donors in this country give their blood an
average of 2 to 3 times a year.   Doubling that number would more
than take care of any decreases resulting from screening and reporting.   Furthermore, commercial blood would be perfectly safe if
it were collected from the north-central, rural areas of the United
States, from adequately screened and tested donors whose blood is
followed carefully in recipients.

SUMMARY AND CONCLUSIONS

     The exact degree to which the incidence of post-transfusion
hepatitis can now be reduced can only be predicted when more data
are available on residual hepatitis from blood that has been

screened for HB antigen.   It seems likely, however, that further
screening for anicteric acute hepatitis by serum enzyme determination and detection of chronic carriers by universal reporting and
exclusion of suspected infective donors could practically eliminate
the disease.   This could be done for less than a third of the
present cost of hospitalizing patients with post-transfusion
hepatitis.

40. HEPATITIS-ASSOCIATED ANTIGEN IN BLOOD FRACTIONS

Milton M. Mozen, Duane D. Schroeder and Victor J. Cabasso

Biochemical and Microbiological Research Departments,

Cutter Laboratories, Inc., Berkeley, California

Introduction. The technical advances of recent years in blood component isolation and in large scale plasma fractionation have resulted in greatly increased usage of blood fractions. Although many therapeutically useful components are available, the risk of transmitting serum hepatitis remains a serious deterrent toward fulfilling all potential applications. As a result, the administration of some fractions can only be justified under circumstances where their expected benefits outweight the hepatitis risk.

The emergence and significance of the hepatitis-associated antigen have amply been reported by others. It is now clearly accepted that the presence of HBAg in donor blood sharply increases the risk of hepatitis B in the recipient. Extending these findings to blood fractions has not been as rewarding, since no meaningful test is available yet which can be applied prior to the administration of fractions. The distribution of HBAg in blood fractions is described below, with comment on the quantitative and qualitative relationships between HBAg in fractions and their infectivity.

Hepatitis related to components. Just prior to and during World War II, from the time pooled human plasma was transfused into battle casualties and human sera were administered for prophylaxis, the icterogenic potential of these biological fluids was clearly recognized. Subsequent experience allowed a classification of blood derivatives to be made in terms of the risk of transmission of viral hepatitis. In 1966, attributing to whole blood an average risk, Mosley and Dull [334] classified human blood products and protein derivatives then in use according to whether they produced a similar incidence of viral hepatitis, a higher incidence, or

none.   Derivatives of plasma or serum pools such as pooled plasma,
fibrinogen and antihemophilic globulin, were recognized as high
risk products.   Whole blood and other single unit derivatives were
assigned an average risk, whereas pooled plasma stored 6 months
at 31.6°C, and the protein fractions albumin, plasma protein
fraction and immune serum globulins were recognized as safe derivatives.   Since that time, however, Redeker and collaborators [404]
have shown that hepatitis infectivity persisted in pooled plasma
stored 6 months at 30-32°C.   The safety of albumin and plasma protein fraction is attributed to pasteurization at 60° for 10 hours
during their manufacture, and immune serum globulins are generally
accepted as non-icterogenic as a result of the manufacturing process used.   Consequently, even minor deviations from standard
isolation procedures are not possible without first establishing
that the immune globulin so derived will not transmit serum hepatitis; a task which experimentally presents great difficulty.

HBAg in fractions.   With the discovery of the hepatitis
associated antigen (HBAg) by Blumberg [99] and the proliferation
of methods for its detection and quantitation, it became possible
to test various blood fractions for the presence of HBAg and to
determine if there existed some quantitative correlation between
HBAg content of a fraction and its propensity to transmit serum
hepatitis.

Of the many schemes which have emerged for the fractionation
of human plasma to yield protein fractions of therapeutic usefulness,
the cold alcohol procedures developed by Cohn and his collaborators
[99,370], namely methods 6 and 9, have been most widely adapted
for industrial scale fractionation.   In the U.S. these methods
are used exclusively with only slight modifications, whereas elsewhere more extensive alterations have taken place.   The operational
details of Cohn Methods 6 and 9 as currently employed are charted
in Figures 1 and 2.   The successful application of these processes
depends on strict control at each fractionation step of the important variables: alcohol concentration, pH, temperature, protein
concentration and ionic strength.   Cryoprecipitate fraction serves
as a starting material for the preparation of antihemophilic factor concentrates used therapeutically in the treatment of classical
hemophilia [204].   Fibrinogen, another of the coagulation factors,
is purified from Fraction I.   Albumin, which is isolated in greater
than 95% purity, is found in the form of Fraction V.   In our laboratories Supernatant I is adsorbed with DEAE-Sephadex from which
the Factor IX Complex, containing also coagulation Factors II, VII
and X, is subsequently eluted.   This product was specifically
developed for the treatment of hemophilia B or Christmas disease
[209].   Fraction (II + III) is the source for the preparation of
gamma globulin by Oncley's Method 9 [370] shown in Figure 2.   Fraction III containing a myriad of proteins among which are plasminogen,

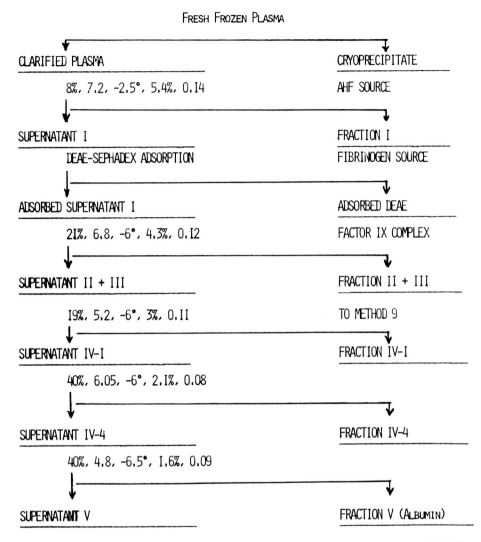

Figure 1. Cold ethanol fractionation of plasma. Method 6 of Cohn [99].

prothrombin and the isoagglutinins, may be further subfractionated after its removal from Fraction II. The latter fraction is employed in the production of immune globulin products without further purification.

To determine the distribution of HBAg in these various plasma fractions, several groups of investigators have applied fractionation procedures to HBAg-positive plasma pools [20,41,210,421,502]. We have carried out such studies in our laboratories [421] and the

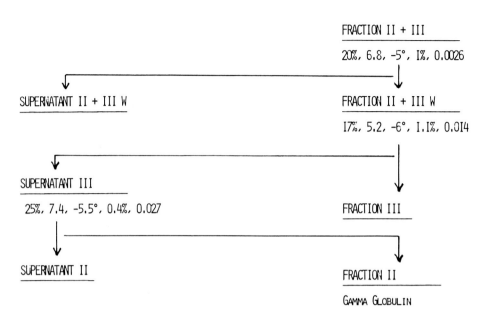

Figure 2. Fractionation of Fr. II+III. Method 9 of Oncley et al [370].

data from two fractionations are summarized in Figure 3. The HBAg
content of the various fractions was determined by gel diffusion
measurements. From the results of titration, arbitrary total units
are calculated for each fraction, and compared to the starting
plasma to establish the relative concentrations in each fraction.
The data show that HBAg is distributed throughout most fractions
and that the total amount varies substantially in the different
fractions. The highest content of HBAg is seen in Fractions IV-1,
IV-4 and III, and when the latter is subfractionated into III-1
and III-2,3, essentially all of the HBAg is found in III-1, the
isoagglutinins. These observations are consistent with earlier
reports that preparations from these fractions which were used in
human therapy have been implicated with the transmission of hepatitis B. Porter et al. [381] in 1953 confirmed in human volunteers
the infectivity of a specific batch of thrombin which had been prepared by the activation of prothrombin isolated from Cohn Fraction
III. Fortunately, the thrombin material and serums from the recipients had been successfully preserved until the time, some 17 years
later, when they could be examined for HBAg. Thus Barker et al.
[36] found that the thrombin sample did indeed contain HBAg in a
titer of 1:10 by CF, and virus-like particles were seen by electron
microscopy in an HBAg concentrate of the material. These studies
must be considered as the most direct demonstration that a plasma
fraction which has transmitted serum hepatitis contained measurable
HBAg.

FRACTION	HAA (UNIT/FRACTION)			
	FRACTION I		FRACTION II	
PLASMA	400,000		400,000	
CRYOPRECIPITATE	5,000		1,250	2,000
FRACTION I	2,750		2,500	
SUPERNATANT I	490,000	367,000	224,000	
FACTOR IX COMPLEX	66		10	
ADSORBED SUPERNATANT I	477,000	358,000	222,000	
FRACTION II + III	33,000		NEGATIVE	7,700
FRACTION IV-1	56,000		87,600	
FRACTION IV-4	22,000	27,000	34,000	
SUPERNATANT V	NEGATIVE		NEGATIVE	
FRACTION V	20,000	23,000	NEGATIVE	
FRACTION III	36,400			
FRACTION III-1			28,800	
FRACTION III-2,3			200	
FRACTION II	NEGATIVE		NEGATIVE	

Figure 3. Distribution of HBAg in Cohn fractions. Data of authors [421].

Hepatitis B was also reported following the injection of Fraction IV. Hsia, Kennell, and Gellis [220] recorded serum hepatitis in 4 of 16 patients following treatment with Fraction IV prepared from pooled postpartum plasma, and concluded "the risk of hemologous serum hepatitis from Fraction IV of pooled plasma seems particularly great".

Perhaps one of the unexpected results derived from these data is the relatively low level of HBAg found in Fraction I, from which fibrinogen is obtained, since fibrinogen has long been incriminated as a carrier of hepatitis virus. Phillips [379], for example,

reported that the incidence of hepatitis from fibrinogen administration over a 10 year period in one medical institution was 14.1 percent among patients infused. Furthermore, Pennell [376] showed
that when plasma was seeded with measurable viruses and then
fractionated, the viruses were found predominately in Fractions I
and (II + III), with very little being present in Fraction IV.
When the crude Fraction I of our study [421] was subsequently processed to Fibrinogen U.S.P., the level of HBAg was further reduced
by some 80%, the balance being accounted for in the wash solution.
The obvious conclusion from these observations is that plasma
fractions are associated with a serious risk of hepatitis, albeit
they carry only a minor part of the total HBAg in the starting
plasma. This suggestion is also strongly supported by the fact
that almost negligible levels of HBAg are found in Factor IX complex, yet this complex has been associated with the transmission
of hepatitis [66,199,245]. This point will be further discussed
later on.

The one observation which fits into the pattern anticipated
from experience is the complete absence of HBAg from Fraction II,
the immune serum globulin fraction. This is consistent with the
long established non-infectivity of immune serum globulin products.
The antigen may have been totally removed by the fractionation
process or, more probably, antibody present in this fraction may
have masked its presence by complexing with it. We were unable
to detect HBAg antibody in this fraction by agar gel diffusion and
antigen neutralization assays.

The finding of HBAg in the albumin from one fractionation
supports the belief that albumin fails to transmit hepatitis as a
result of heat treatment rather than as a result of HBAg being
fractionated from it. When a sample of this albumin was heated
at 60°C for 10 hours in the presence of the usual stabilizers,
the HBAg precipitin reaction was neither destroyed nor diminished
[421].

The distribution of HBAg in fractions recovered from HBAg-
containing plasma was also reported by Berg et al. [41] and Zuckerman et al. [502], and excerpts of their data are shown in Figure 4.
In the Zuckerman study, presence of HBAg was determined by both
electron microscopy and immunodiffusion, whereas Berg employed
radial immunodiffusion for a more quantitative measurement of the
antigen. Fraction IV was found by Berg also to be a principal
repository for HBAg, with some 85% of the original being recovered
in it. HBAg in albumin was also relatively low: it was undetected
by Zuckerman, and found to be less than 1% of the total by Berg.
Neither group recovered HBAg from the washed fibrinogen product.
The chief discrepancy between these data and those of Schroeder
and Mozen just discussed resides in finding HBAg in Fraction II.

DISTRIBUTION of HAA in COHN FRACTIONS

| FRACTION | ZUCKERMAN Et AL. (9) | | BERG Et AL. (8) |
	IMMUNO-DIFFUSION	ELECTRON MICROSCOPY	PERCENT HAA of STARTING PLASMA
PLASMA	+	+	100
FRACTION I (After Wash)	- .	-	0.2
SUPERNATANT I	+	+	100
SUPERNATANT II	-	-	< 0.42
FRACTION III	+	+	1.7
FRACTION II	-	-	0.11
FRACTION IVa	-	+	86
FRACTION IVb	-	-	3.06
FRACTION V	-	-	.91
SUPERNATANT V	-	-	< .43

Figure 4.

One explanation might be that the fractionation carried out by Kabi
in Stockholm utilizes somewhat different modifications of the Cohn
procedures than those employed in our laboratories. Nonetheless,
there is no evidence that immune serum globulin products prepared
by either adaptation transmit hepatitis. In light of this, Berg
postulates that factors such as partial inactivation by the manufacturing procedure or neutralization by antibody may also be
operative.

     In a similar study by Holland, Alter, Purcell and Sgouris
[210] HBAg was found in all fractions except in Fraction II. They
also failed to detect HBAg activity in Fraction II even when it
was concentrated 20 times and tested by a most sensitive test, the
radioimmunoassay.

     Another study in which HBAg-containing plasma was fractionated
was reported in Heidelberg by Andrassy and Ritz [20] who studied,
in particular, fibrinogen and other coagulation factor concentrates.
HBAg was detected in a number of fibrinogen concentrates as well
as in cryoprecipitate, but it was not found in the PPSB (Factor IX
Complex) fraction prepared from a $BaSO_4$ eluate. This latter result
is not in agreement with data reported by Soulier [440] who cited

evidence that HBAg was in fact found in PPSB preparations. Since it is well established that blood which contains HBAg carries a considerably greater risk of transmitting hepatitis than HBAg-negative blood, it is often asked if there might be merit in routinely testing plasma products for the presence of HBAg.

The evidence just presented strongly suggests that routine testing could not be trusted to identify product lots which carry greater risk of inducing hepatitis: a safe fraction like ISG was found in one study to contain HBAg, whereas fractions known to be icterogenic, e.g. Factor IX Complex and fibrinogen, had barely detectable levels of HBAg. The quantity of HBAg in the latter two fractions was about 10,000 times lower than that in the starting contaminated plasma. If we assume that a normal plasma pool might contain 1% contaminated plasma, the dilution of HBAg in these fractions from this pool would be about 10^{-6}, a dilution several orders of magnitude below the detection limits of presently available methods. These products might be expected not to transmit hepatitis since Barker and associates [36] have shown that inoculation of human volunteers with infectious plasma diluted 10^{-5} to 10^{-7} produced no definite clinical hepatitis, whereas 7 of 15 of these volunteers became positive for HBAg. Despite this favorable arithmetic, antihemophilic and fibrinogen products do at times transmit hepatitis, and little hope exists at present to reduce the frequency of transmission by routinely screening these products for HBAg.

In spite of these discouraging facts, we have repeatedly attempted to find HBAg in Factor IX Complex fractionated from plasma pools from unscreened donors, but had no success [422]. A number of lots which had been implicated in transmitting hepatitis were found uniformly negative for HBAg. Further detection efforts were made by highly concentrating any HBAg which might have been present, with equally negative results. For example, in earlier studies [422] the elution volume was determined in which HBAg emerged when plasma was fractionated by gel filtration on Bio-Gel A-5m. A typical profile of such a separation is shown in Figure 5, wherein the region where HBAg was detectable is cross-hatched. Consequently, an identical gel filtration separation was carried out with Factor IX Complex and the eluate in the HBAg region was pooled, concentrated and tested. Although this procedure should have led to approximately 100 fold concentration of any HBAg, none was detected. Samples of Factor IX Complex were concentrated about 10 fold and freed of about 90% of their protein by chromatography, and assayed for HBAg by the radioimmunoassay. No HBAg could be detected.*

---

*We are indebted to Dr. R.H. Purcell, NIAID, National Institutes of Health, Bethesda, Maryland, for testing these samples by the RIA.

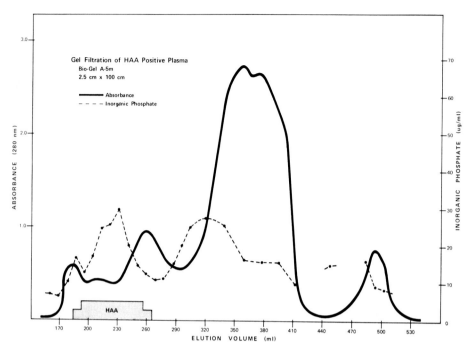

Figure 5.

From the findings reported in this review it is clear that the distribution of HBAg in various plasma fractions cannot always serve to predict the likelihood that a particular fraction will transmit the virus of hepatitis B. The failure to detect HBAg in a pooled plasma product can in no way be construed as evidence that it is safe from the hepatitis hazard. For the present, we must still be guided by the body of clinical experience as to which fractions are safe. All other fractions must be regarded as posing a definite hepatitis risk. Hopefully, today's plasma products which are derived solely from HBAg-negative donors may prove to have a reduced risk of transmitting hepatitis. However, experience on this point is still much too limited. With the short-comings of present screening procedures, and the large donor input to plasma pools, optimism should be guarded. It would seem that for the time being, eliminating the hepatitis hazard from a particular fraction resides more in the successful treatment of the fraction by procedures which might inactivate the virus of hepatitis B, than in the hope of fractionating the virus away.

Acknowledgment. The experienced and expert technical assistance of J.C. Smiley in plasma fractionation and Rita Nieman for assays is gratefully acknowledged.

41. THE EPIDEMIOLOGY OF HEPATITIS B VIRUS INFECTION IN BLOOD DONORS

Wolf Szmuness, Alfred M. Prince, Betsy Brotman and
Robert L. Hirsch
New York Blood Center

New York, N.Y.

The present report describes preliminary observations concerning the epidemiology of hepatitis B infections among volunteer blood donors of the greater New York metropolitan area. For comparison, data concerning the distribution of hepatitis B antibody (anti-HBAg) in a sample of paid donors from two commercial blood banks are also presented.

MATERIALS AND METHODS

From May 1970 to April 1971, there were 208,000 volunteer blood donors to The Greater New York Blood Program. Routine screening for hepatitis B antigen (HBAg) was carried out by the immunoelectroosmophoresis (IEOP) assay [388] in the Clinical Services Laboratories of The Greater New York Blood Program. All sera found to be positive by IEOP were retested adjacent to reference HBAg by agar gel diffusion (AGD) [384]. Only those sera showing clear-cut reactions of identity were considered positive. Approximately 50% of the sera containing HBAg were retested by the hemagglutination inhibition (HAI) assay [394, 477]. Volunteer blood donors from prisons were not included in this survey.

All specimens in which HBAg was detected were also tested for transaminase (SGPT) activity by the kinetic spectrophotometric method [492]. The interval between bleeding and separation of serum from clots was less than 24 hours. Serum was held from one to ten days at 4°C prior to SGPT determination. Previous studies have revealed that SGPT levels as determined by the kinetic spectrophotometric assay are unaffected by these delays (Prince, A.M., unpublished observations).

   2,002 blood specimens were screened for anti-HBAg using the
hemagglutination (HA) assay [394, 477]. 1,030 of these specimens
were obtained from volunteer blood donors: the first 700 were
collected systematically from donors who donated blood during
the first three months of 1971; the remaining 330 specimens were
obtained preferentially from females and blacks because of race-
sex predilections in the general donor population. 972 specimens
were obtained from consecutive paid donors at two commercial blood
banks: 500 specimens from New York City and 472 from Detroit,
Michigan.

   The following information concerning the tested donors was
collected and analyzed: for the 208,000 volunteer donors who
donated blood during the study period, data concerning sex, age,
residence, time and number of prior donations were available from
the computer files of The Greater New York Blood Program; in
addition, data concerning place of birth, ethnic group, religion,
education and family size was obtained from the sample of 1,030
volunteer blood donors selected for anti-HBAg determination. Since
the first 700 volunteer blood donors tested for anti-HBAg were a
random systematic sample drawn from a large donor population, this
sample was considered to be reasonably representative of the general
donor population of The Greater New York Blood Program (control
sample). Only data concerning sex, race and age were available for
the sample of paid donors screened for anti-HBAg. A personal
interview was carried out with most of the donors found to carry
HBAg. A total of 226 HBAg carriers were interviewed. These inter-
views were carried out in order to obtain more detailed data concerning possible exposure to hepatitis B infection.

RESULTS

   Duration of Antigenemia. HBAg was detected in the serum of
319 of the 208,000 volunteer blood donors tested, a frequency of
1.5 per 1,000 donors.

   210 of these carriers were followed with serial blood specimens
(2 to 4) drawn 4 to 20 months after the donation in which HBAg was
detected; of these, 197 (94%) again revealed the presence of HBAg.
This would suggest that nearly all New York City volunteer donors
in whom HBAg is detected by routine screening are chronic HBAg
carriers.

   Liver Disease in Carriers. 77% of all chronic carriers had
normal (<30 Karmen units) SGPT levels; in 11% the values ranged
between 30 and 60 units, and in 12% they were 60 units or higher.

Effect of Age and Sex on Frequency of HB Antigenemia. The HBAg carrier state in volunteer blood donors was found to be associated with both age and sex. In all five age classes, the antigen was detected more frequently in male donors than in female donors (Table 1). The overall crude prevalence rate was 1.70 per 1,000 male donors and 1.08 per 1,000 female donors. In both sexes, the highest prevalence was observed in the 20 to 29 year age group. In donors under 20 years and over 30 years, HBAg was detected two to three times less frequently. The prevalence of HBAg was found to decrease with advancing age (Figure 1).

EFFECT OF RACE AND ETHNIC ORIGIN ON FREQUENCY OF HB ANTIGENEMIA

The proportion of blacks among HBAg carriers was 3.3 times as high as expected on the basis of the ethnic distribution of the control sample (Table 2). The number of carriers of oriental origin (Chinese, Japanese, Philippine, etc.) was also higher than expected. On the other hand, Jews were significantly under-represented: they constituted 21% of all white donors but only 4.7% of the detected HBAg carriers. The age-sex composition of blacks, non-Jews and Jews in the control sample did not differ significantly and, therefore, could not have affected the ratios.

Exposure History in HB Antigen Carriers. Only a minority of the carriers interviewed gave a past history of overt viral hepatitis (3%), blood transfusion (4%), major surgery (6%), contact with a known case of hepatitis (28%) or shared-needle injections (4%). No differences in the frequency of such potential sources of exposure were found between blacks and nonblacks.

Distribution of HB Antibody Detectable by Passive Hemag-glutination Assay. 6.7% of the 1,030 volunteer blood donors showed detectable levels (>1:4) of anti-HBAg in the hemagglutination assay. The prevalence of antibody was found to be significantly higher among blacks than nonblacks; anti-HBAg was detected in 11% of blacks tested in comparision to 5.8% of nonblacks tested (Table 3).

Antibody distribution did, however, differ from antigen distribution with respect to certain other characteristics: in both blacks and whites the prevalence rates for anti-HBAg were the same, or even slightly lower, for males and for females; among whites, Jews showed the presence of anti-HBAg with the same frequency as non-Jews; the frequency of detectable antibody increased with advancing age, being lowest in donors under 30 years of age and highest in those 50 years or older (Figure 2); prevalence of anti-HBAg was found to be unrelated to education or family size.

Table 1. Sex-Age Specific Prevalence Rates of HB Antigen Among Volunteer Blood Donors.

Age Group	Males			Females			Both		
	Total No. of Donors (Thousands)	No. of Donors with HBAg	Rate per 1,000 Donors	Total No. of Donors (Thousands)	No. of Donors with HBAg	Rate per 1,000 Donors	Total No. of Donors (Thousands)	No. of Donors with HBAg	Rate per 1,000 Donors
<20	8.2	10	1.21	5.7	3	0.52	13.9	13	0.93
20-29	48.3	119	2.46	20.1	34	1.69	68.4	153	2.23
30-39	39.1	66	1.68	10.2	10	0.98	49.3	76	1.54
40-49	34.1	45	1.37	12.2	11	0.90	46.3	56	1.20
>50	21.1	17	0.80	9.1	4	0.43	30.2	21	0.69
Total	150.8	257	1.70* 1.69**	57.3	62	1.08* 1.30**	208.1	319	1.53

*crude rate: $\chi^2 = 3.86$, p<.05
**rate adjusted for age differences: $\chi^2 = 2.12$, p>.05

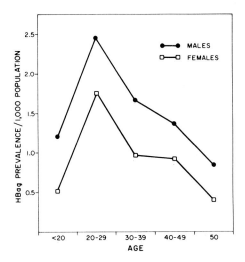

Figure 1. Prevalence of HBAg among male and female volunteer blood
donors in relation to age.

Table 2. Distribution of 226 HB Antigen Carriers According to
Ethnic Group.

Ethnic Group	Percent in Control Sample	Number of Carriers Observed	Number of Carriers Expected	Observed/Expected
Whites:	84	126	190	0.66
non-Jews	79	120	103	1.16
Jews	21	6	26	0.23
Blacks	10	77	23	3.34
Orientals	6	23	13	1.76
Total	100	226	226	1.00

The composition of the paid donor populations with respect
to age, sex and race, as well as the prevalence of anti-HBAg was
practically the same in donors from both blood banks screened; the
results are, therefore, presented for the entire sample of paid
donors. Taken together, anti-HBAg was detected in 20% of the paid
donors tested, or three times as frequently as in the sample of
volunteer blood donors (Table 3). The difference between paid and
volunteer donors was still significant when the rates were corrected
for age distribution. Among paid donors, blacks were found to
carry antibody more frequently than whites, though this difference
was smaller than among volunteer blood donors. The age distribution
of donors with detectable anti-HBAg among paid donors was also somewhat different than in the sample of volunteer blood donors. In
paid donors over 50 years old, the prevalence of detectable anti-
HBAg decreased and approached that found in volunteer donors (Figure 2). These data must be considered to be preliminary since

Table 3. Distribution of anti-HBAg Detectable by Passive Hemagglutination in Volunteer and Paid Blood Donors.

Group	# Tested	# with anti-HBAg (HA$\geq$1:4)	% with anti-HBAg
Volunteer Blood Donors - Total	1,030	69	6.7*
Whites and Orientals	857	50	5.8**
Blacks	173	19	11.0**
Males	508	32	6.3
Females	522	37	7.1
Paid Blood Donors - Total	972	194	20.0*
Whites and Orientals	438	72	16.4***
Blacks	534	122	22.8***
Males	963	192	-
Females	9	2	-

$*\chi^2 = 77$, p<.001
$**\chi^2 = 6.12$, p<.02
$***\chi^2 = 6.38$, p<.02

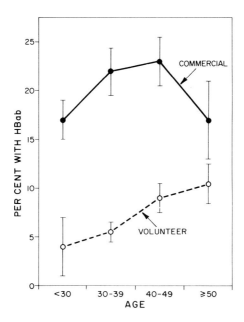

Figure 2. Age specific prevalence rates ($\pm$1 SE) of anti-HBAg
among volunteer and commercial blood donors.

both numerators and denominators in certain of the age classes
were rather small. The sex ratio could not be analyzed since only
a negligible portion of paid donors (1%) were females.

DISCUSSION

Mechanism(s) Responsible for Variations in HBAg/anti-HBAg
Prevalence in Different Populations. The data presented indicate
that prevalence of both HBAg and anti-HBAg is associated with
certain variables, e.g., sex, age and ethnic group. The association with age and ethnic group was still found to be valid
when adjusted for the remaining two variables. An excess prevalence of HBAg among male donors and young adults has been reported by other workers [31, 38, 251, 366], and by Chalmers and
Taswell at this Symposium. No entirely convincing explanation
for these findings can be given at the present time. The simplest
explanation for these observed differences would be drug addiction
since illicit drug use is known to be more prevalent among young
adult males and blacks. Although drug addiction certainly
contributes to the transmission of the HB virus, it seems unlikely
that this factor alone is responsible for the excess prevalence
in the three high-risk groups which we have identified. Only 4%
of all HBAg carriers and 7% of male carriers ages 20 to 29 years
admitted drug usage. A high HBAg prevalence in young males has
also been observed in institutionalized mentally retarded patients
and in some African populations [60, 454, 455] where shared needle
exposure could, at least in most cases, be entirely excluded. An
excess HBAg prevalence in young adult males has also been recently
reported from Israel [38] and some eastern European countries
[240] where, to our knowledge, drug addiction is less of an important social problem than it is in this country. It therefore
seems likely that in addition to drug addiction other factor(s)
are involved.

One of the factors which determines the development and
persistence of antigenemia is age at first exposure to infection.
Studies carried out in institutionalized mentally retarded patients revealed that the probability of becoming a chronic carrier,
as well as the persistence of antigenemia, is significantly higher
in individuals who have been exposed at an early age and, independently, in males [454, 455]. From these observations it might
therefore be assumed that young adult males acquire the infection
earlier in life.

Similar difficulties are encountered in attempting to explain the relatively high prevalence of HBAg and anti-HBAg among
black volunteer and paid blood donors. The excess prevalence
among blacks cannot be attributed to a genetically determined

susceptibility since no such differences in the prevalence of HBAg or anti-HBAg were observed between white and black residents in institutions for the mentally retarded [455, 458]. The high prevalence of HBAg in African populations also does not appear to be related to genetic factors since a similar high prevalence has been described among Indians from Peru [383], Chinese [60], Japanese [366], Greeks [188] and Jews from Arab countries [38].

It would appear more likely that excess prevalence of HBAg and anti-HBAg among blacks, as well as among paid donors, both white and black, is related to socio-economic factors [95]. The substandard social and environmental conditions under which a part of these populations live may in some way favor and sustain the circulation and dissemination of hepatitis B virus(s).

A striking finding of this survey was that a very small proportion of Jews were found to be chronic HBAg carriers. The number of Jews among white carriers was four times lower than expected. On the other hand, the prevalence of anti-HBAg among Jews was exactly the same as among whites of other religions. This would suggest that Jews were exposed to HB infection to the same extent as non-Jews. The low HBAg prevalence among Jews also seems unrelated to genetic determinants since in hyperendemic conditions such as institutions for the mentally retarded they were found to be chronic carriers with exactly the same frequency as non-Jews (27% for each) (Szmuness, unpublished data). An alternate explanation could be that some ethnic differences in socio-economic, cultural, behavioral or nutritional patterns are responsible for the discrepancy in the prevalence of HBAg between Jews and non-Jews. It should be noted that we cannot entirely exclude the possibility that the sample of HBAg carriers surveyed for religion was self-selected or otherwise biased. In any case, it appears that this question merits further exploration.

Self-Limitation of the HB Antigen Carrier State. There is renewed indication from these data that, as has been previously observed in studies in institutions for the mentally retarded [454, 455], the carrier state is self-limited. The repeated observation that HBAg prevalence declines with advancing age (after a peak incidence around the age group 20 to 29 years) and that anti-HBAg prevalence increases with advancing age appears to support the theory that the HBAg carrier state is not life long.

Acknowledgements. We are grateful to the personnel of the Clinical Services Laboratories of the Greater New York Blood Program for carrying out IEOP testing of donor blood under the supervision of Mr. D. Steele. We wish particularly to acknowledge Ms. M.E. Sullivan, Mr. S.A. Cohen, Ms. E. De Kosko, Ms. A. Zajac, and Ms. Claire Baumann, R.N., of the Virus Laboratory, The New York Blood

Center, for their conscientious assistance in gathering epidemiological data, and Ms. B. Clinkscale, Ms. E. Echenroth, Ms. A.M.
Moffatt, and Mr. D. Joss for technical assistance. We are indebted
to Mr. M. Seldeen and Mr. T. Lee for assistance in obtaining specimens from paid blood donors.

These studies were aided by Grant #HE-09011 and AI-09516 from
the National Institutes of Health, Contract #70-2236 from the
National Heart and Lung Institute, and Grants in Aid from the
Kresge Foundation and from the Strasburger Foundation. Dr. Prince
is a Career Scientist of the Health Research Council of the City
of New York under Contract #I-533.

42. Discussion
HBAg IN BLOOD DONORS

G. F. Grady

Commonwealth of Massachusetts, Department of Public

Health, Boston, Massachusetts

The hepatitis-associated antigen is unique in every sense--
its serendipitous discovery, the unprecedented amount of viral
capsular material shed into the blood, and the relatively small
loss of available blood occasioned by the screening out of antigen-
containing infective units. Since there has never been a test
system quite like this, there is no real basis for judging whether
we have been perspicacious or slow in implementation. But the
resultant new attention to the supply of safe blood, and the
bringing together of persons of many disciplines to help solve the
problem, may be the most lasting byproduct of the recognition of
the antigen-hepatitis association.

This meeting should not be concluded without some mention of
other developments such as autologous transfusions and washed-
frozen blood. Although there is no single study of washed-frozen
blood which is unassailable, the combined results of trials are all
very encouraging. Presumably the washing step is effective in
reducing or eliminating the hepatitis virus, and the frozen storage
helps stabilize the supply of the blood. I am told that the
Massachusetts General Hospital is now wash-freezing over 40% of
its bloods.

Dr. Chalmers has persuasively given a cost-benefit analysis of
the hepatitis burden and has stressed that even imperfect tests
such as the widely used counterelectrophoresis technique can
identify high risk populations of donors even if many infective
individuals slip through. While supporting his analyses and plea
for preventive measures, I wonder whether it is reasonable to vest
primary responsibility for policy in the blood bank. If the blood
bank is of exceptional quality such as the Irwin Memorial Blood

Bank in San Francisco, this might be reasonable. However, in my experience, most hospitals have been successful in improving the quantity and quality of their blood sources only insofar as it was of concern to the local prime figure in the clinical teaching and bedside care hierarchy. For example, if the Chief of Surgery of an outstanding surgical service thinks it is important to have low risk blood, it is usually provided by one means or another. If hepatitis risk is considered a relatively minor problem that has to compete and take its place among thousands of other problems, then improvements are unlikely in spite of technological advances. It is simply a question of leadership. So I think the antigen story, even if it per se did little to eliminate hepatitis, by focusing our attention on the problems and the question of who is accepting responsibility, has already been invaluable.

43.   OPEN DISCUSSION: HBAg IN BLOOD DONORS

R. H. Purcell

National Institutes of Allergy and Infectious Diseases
N.I.H.
Bethesda, Maryland

The very elegant physicochemical, electron microscopic and seroanalytical studies that we have heard about this morning and yesterday all point to the conclusion that what we call Australia antigen, or hepatitis-associated antigen, or hepatitis B antigen, is a very complex set of structures. Therefore, I think it is important to define what we mean by Australia antigen.

I prefer the original concept of the antigen as an antigenic specificity rather than an entity. There is only one antigenic specificity that seems to be consistently present on the various morphological forms which we tend to group together as Australia antigen. I believe that this one antigen specificity, the "a" specificity of Le Bouvier [283] should be the sine qua non of hepatitis-associated antigen.

I think it is exciting that Drs. Bond and Hall have found a specificity unique to the Dane particle [123], and it remains to be seen whether this has any relationship to the various subtype systems that have been described, perhaps most particularly the X antigen mentioned by Dr. Le Bouvier, which appears to be present at times and not at other times. This may be related to the concentration of Dane particles present in any given preparation.

Equally exciting are the studies of Almeida, alluded to by Dr. Zuckerman. Almeida demonstrated, in the liver of patients dying with HBAg-positive hepatitis, aggregates of virus-like particles [10]. These particles were morphologically indistinguishable from the virions of known small viruses (the picornaviruses) but were easily distinguished from aggregates resembling Australia

antigen which were also present in the preparation. The two kinds
of particles were found in separate aggregates; that is, they were
not co-precipitated by endogenous antibody which appeared to be
present in the patient's serum. Almeida interpreted this to mean
that the two kinds of particles did not share antigenic specificities. More recently, Almeida has treated HBAg-positive serum
rich in Dane particles with a nonionic detergent, Tween 80, and
demonstrated disruption of the Dane particle with release of an
internal component morphologically indistinguishable from the
virus-like particles she had found previously in livers from
hepatitis patients [8]. When she treated these disrupted preparations with appropriate antisera she found that antibody obtained from "hyperimmunized" individuals such as hemophiliacs
reacted with both Australia antigen (and the external coat of
Dane particles) and with the internal component. However, when
she reacted the Tween 80-treated preparations with convalescent
serum from persons convalescing from HBAg-positive hepatitis but
who lacked demonstrable antibody to HBAg, she found that these
convalescent sera had antibodies reactive with the internal component of the Dane particle but not with HBAg or the outer coat
of the Dane particle. She interpreted this to mean that the
immune response to hepatitis B may consist of the development of
antibody to the internal core component of the Dane particle as
well as, and independently of, the development of antibody to
HBAg. Dr. Almeida employed the negative staining technique for
the demonstration of virus-like particles and Australia antigen
and could not therefore localize these entitites in the liver cell.
However, others, using the thin sectioning technique, have demonstrated clusters of intranuclear virus-like particles in liver
cells obtained from patients with HBAg-positive hepatitis. These
have been shown most elegantly by Huang [223]. It is not yet clear
whether these intranuclear particles are identical with the
particles observed by Almeida but, if allowance is made for the
differences in technique employed by Almeida and Huang, the particles observed by these two workers resemble each other in size
and morphology. Huang also found the virus-like particles in the
cytoplasm of liver cells, but less frequently than in the nucleus.
Some of the intracytoplasmic particles were found to be enveloped
with an outer coat. Huang suggested that these may be analogous
to the Dane particles found in serum. He also demonstrated a
poorly resolved material in the cytoplasm that appeared to consist
of spherical and tubular structures. He suggested that these might
be the spherical and tubular forms of Australia antigen. On the
basis of these studies by Almeida, Huang and others, some new
concepts concerning infection of liver cells by hepatitis B virus
are beginning to emerge. Thus, as diagrammed in Figure 1, it
appears that hepatitis B virus nucleocapside may be synthesized in
the nucleus of the liver cell. This nucleocapside may then be
transferred to the cytoplasm where the viral coat protein is synthesized. The nucleocapside appears to be enveloped by viral coat

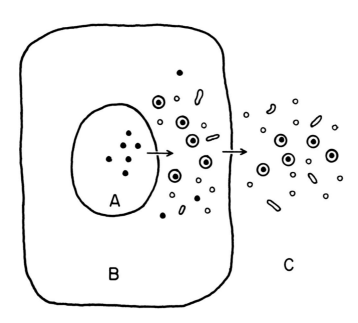

Figure 1. A hypothesis for the synthesis of hepatitis B virus.
Nucleocapsid is synthesized in liver cell nucleus (A) and enveloped with an outer coat in the cytoplasm, where viral coat protein is synthesized in excess (B). Enveloped nucleocapsids and
excess viral coat protein are released from the cell into the
circulation (C) and are recognized as Dane particles and spherical
and filamentous forms of Australia antigen respectively. Additional
work must be done to determine if this or an alternate interpretation of existing data is valid.

protein before being released from the cell. Viral coat protein
appears to be synthesized in marked excess in the cytoplasm of
infected cells. This excess viral coat protein, also released
from the cell, becomes the spherical and tubular forms which we
call Australia antigen. Additional studies are necessary before
we will know whether these hypotheses are correct, but they provide some exciting new ways to look at hepatitis B infection.

     If the concept of virus synthesis outlined above is proven
to be correct, one must ask what is being detected by the
various immunofluorescence studies described at this meeting,
as well as in the literature. Immunofluorescent staining of the
nucleus [318], cytoplasm [102, 140] and both nucleus and cytoplasm [364] has been observed by various groups. All have interpreted this fluorescence as representing specific staining of
Australia antigen. However, none of the groups reporting immunofluorescent staining of Australia antigen in liver cells have
adequately defined the specificity of their reagents in terms of
their reactivity with highly purified HBAg or with internal components of the Dane particle. If the hypothesis for the systhesis

of hepatitis B virus described above proves valid, then it is likely
that those individuals reporting intranuclear immunofluorescence
are not staining Australia antigen per se but the immunologically
distinct internal core component. The studies to answer these
questions of specificity are currently in progress in other laboratories.

These caveats concerning interpretation of immunofluorescence
results apply equally to the results of immunoelectron microscopy
with ferritin-labeled antibody described this morning by Dr. Millman. Until it can be proven that the reagents used in Dr. Millman's study are devoid of antibody to the internal components of
the Dane particle it seems premature to interpret the results as
proving that the intranuclear virus-like particles are indeed
Australia antigen.

Dr. Shulman gave a very excellent summary of the search for
Australia antigen in secretions and excretions of persons with
HBAg-positive hepatitis. As he indicated, the results of these
studies are still equivocal. However, I think his discussion does
serve to introduce the question of, "What is the origin of the
Australia antigen that we find in the blood donor who comes into
the blood bank with no history of hepatitis or drug usage or
transfusion?"

It is difficult to believe that all of this Australia antigen
originates from transfused blood or from a hypodermic needle. It
seems obvious, therefore, that another mechanism must be considered for the source of all this antigen. Among those mechanisms
suggested by various individuals have been fecal-oral and urinary-
oral spread, the razor or toothbrush shared by the husband and wife,
the barber's razor, and sexual intimacy, as well as arthopod vectors.

There are some serological data which might help to shed light
on the ecology of hepatitis B. We have surveyed a number of human
populations for antibody to Australia antigen, using a very sensitive radioimmunoprecipitation technique developed in our laboratory [277]. (W.C. Reeves, et al., C. Cherubin et al., manu-
scripts in preparation.) As seen in Figure 2, antibody to HBAg
appears to be acquired primarily after childhood, a pattern in
good agreement with most published surveys for age-specific ac-
quisition of HBAg in various populations. These studies have been
carried out now in a number of populations, both primative and
civilized. Thus, antibody appears to be acquired, not in infancy,
as is found with polio and a number of other viruses spread by the
fecal-oral route, but in late childhood and adulthood. Although
the frequency of antibody varies from population to population
and the exact age at which the frequency begins to increase varies
somewhat, this same general pattern is found in various parts of

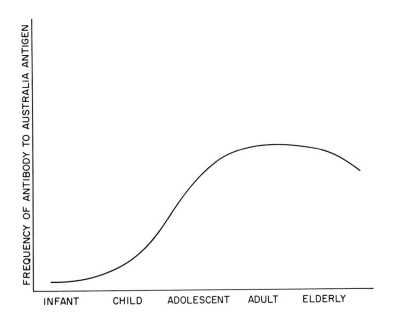

Figure 2. Relationship between age and frequency of antibody to Australia antigen as measured by radioimmunoprecipitation. This pattern, with slight variation, has been found in several human populations of diverse geographic, cultural and socioeconomic background.

the world and various societies.

These data do not provide support for most of the various postulated ways that Australia antigen may be transmitted, other than, perhaps, through the route of sexual intimacy, but I think further studies must be carried out before any firm conclusions can be drawn.

Finally, the plasma fractionation studies which Dr. Mozen described this morning were extremely interesting. I think it is going to be even more interesting to repeat these studies with antibodies directed against the core component of the Dane particles. Such studies may provide more important information on the potential infectivity of plasma fractions.

I agree with Dr. Mozen and Dr. Holland and others that there probably is no lower limit for Australia antigen, beneath which detectable antigen is not associated with infectivity for hepatitis B. I think that, like most other biological phenomena, there is going to be a bell-shaped curve of antigen levels and there are going to be certain materials which are clearly infectious for hepatitis B in which HBAg cannot be detected by any means. This does not mean that there are not levels of detection beneath which the tests become non-specific, but this is another problem.

Dr. Shulman: I wonder if there could be other ways of preventing hepatitis. From the comment that Dr. Holland made, I would expect that maybe gamma globulin is in vogue again, in view of the fact that there is an implication that one-third of the patients who get post-transfusion hepatitis after multiple transfusions may be getting hepatitis A. Could we hear a comment on that?

Dr. Paul Holland: I think it is very true, Dr. Shulman, that many patients are getting infectious hepatitis by blood, and after Dr. Ward's talk this afternoon, I plan to elaborate on the possible hazards of gamma globulin to these people.

From the Floor: A brief question. What about dental work as a mode of transmission, which was talked about in the past and has not been mentioned here?

Dr. R. H. Purcell: I am told that many dentists do not adequately sterilize their equipment, particularly their drill bits, between patients, presumably because heat sterilization is believed to damage them. These instruments frequently penetrate the gums or tooth pulp and opportunities for parenteral spread of hepatitis B would appear to exist.

From the Floor: As a microbiologist working for the Dental School here, I think I can answer the last question to the extent that the majority of dentists in the United States are not sterilizing their instruments.

Dr. M. Goldfield: I won't ask for equal time. There is a great deal of data related to dental-associated hepatitis. It is far too extensive to discuss extemporaneously.

There is a great deal of transmission in a dentist's chair and we have a lot of information epidemiologically on this.

There is a great risk of acquiring Australia antigen by dentists and by dental technicians, and particularly in low-income areas, or, for example, in a dental clinic handling patients who are drug abusers. It is not related to the use of a needle, so far as we know. It is related to almost any procedure involving some degree of manipulation, even cleaning of teeth, for example.

Although we reported some of this to the Society for Epidemiological Research last year, it will be subsequently published this year. If you are interested in details, I will be glad to give this to you.

SECTION V

POST-TRANSFUSION HEPATITIS

Chairman: J. M. Stengle

44. TRANSFUSION OF BLOOD CONTAINING ANTI-HBAg

D. J. Gocke and J. M. Panick

Department of Medicine, College of Physicians & Surgeons
Columbia University
New York, N.Y.

Transfusion of blood containing Australia antigen (HBAg) is frequently associated with development of hepatitis in the recipient [36, 166, 167, 367]. However, the safety of transfusing blood containing antibody to HBAg remains uncertain. The possibility that such blood may harbor infectious virus has given rise to the concern that transfusion of antibody-containing blood should also be prohibited. The rationale for this would be based on the possibility that the virus remains infectious despite being bound to antibody, as has been shown to be possible with some model systems [363], or that the anti-HBAg antibody may be directed against a non-structural component of the virus. Although objective evidence of either of these possibilities in the HBAg system is lacking, the implications are considerable since large scale screening of blood donors for anti-HBAg would require techniques for rapid, sensitive detection of antibody which presently exceed the capability of most blood banks, and would result in the elimination of significant numbers of potential blood donors.

This report describes prospective observations on a group of blood transfusion recipients followed at the Columbia-Presbyterian Medical Center in New York City. The donor blood transfused was screened for both HBAg antigen and antibody. The correlation between the presence of HBAg in the donor blood and the development of hepatitis in these recipients has been reported previously [168, 169]. This report describes observations in recipients of blood containing antibody to HBAg.

Patients and Methods. Patients in this study were transfused at the Columbia-Presbyterian Medical Center in New York City from December 1968 to January 1971. During this period all donor blood

entering the Blood Bank was tested for HBAg and anti-HBAg. The
recipients of all HBAg-positive blood were identified and followed,
and observations in this group have been reported [168, 169]. From
November 1968 to June 1970 all donor specimens were routinely
screened for anti-HBAg by the relatively insensitive two-dimensional immunodiffusion technique (ID); 32 of 30,200 donors had
detectable anti-HBAg by this method. In June 1970 routine screening
of donor blood for HBAg by the counterelectrophoretic method [168]
developed in this laboratory was instituted and routine screening
for anti-HBAg was discontinued. However, a second group of recipients of blood containing anti-HBAg detectable only by the more
sensitive hemagglutination (HA) technique [477] was followed
during the period March 1971 to February 1972. Two control series
composed of recipients of blood negative for anti-HBAg by ID and HA
were formed by following the recipient of every 10th unit of negative blood in the same manner as the positive recipients. There
were no differences in age, sex, race, or medical diagnosis between the various recipient groups. The average number of transfusions was the same in the positive and negative recipients.

The protocol for prospective followup consisted of observation of the recipients for signs and symptoms of hepatitis
every 1-2 weeks for a period of six months following transfusion.
Serum glutamic oxaloacetic transaminase (SGOT) and HBAg were
determined regardless of whether the patient was symptomatic.
In most instances, patients were seen and tests done at the
Columbia-Presbyterian Medical Center. Occasionally, followup was
accomplished with the aid of outside physicians and laboratories
with specimens sent to this laboratory for Australia antigen
testing. Hepatitis was defined in this study as an SGOT elevation
of greater than 100 I.U. on two consecutive occasions without other
evident cause. Icteric hepatitis was characterized by clinically
detectable jaundice and a serum bilirubin in excess of 4 mg%.

Results. Table 1 summarized observations on recipients of
blood containing antibody to Australia antigen. The study consists of two series of patients. One group received transfusions
of donor blood containing sufficient quantities of antibody to be
detected by immunodiffusion techniques. The second group consisted of recipients of donor blood containing small amounts of
antibody requiring the more sensitive hemagglutination technique
for detection. Comparable control groups consisting of recipients of transfusions negative for both Australia antigen and
antibody were followed during the same respective periods in time.
Hepatitis was observed in all groups. In those who received high
titer anti-HBAg (detected by ID) six cases of hepatitis occurred
in the 22 recipients who survived and were adequately followed for
six months after transfusion. In the recipients of low titer
anti-HBAg (detectable only by HA) two cases of hepatitis were seen

Table 1.   Summary of Recipients of Blood Transfusions Containing
Anti-HBAg

| | Anti-HBAg Titer of Blood Infused | | | |
	Pos. by ID	Neg. by ID	Pos. by HA	Neg. by HA
No. of Recipients	31	210	23	17
Survivors - 6 mo.	22	124	15	12
Hepatitis	4	23	2	2
Hepatitis with Anti-HBAg	2	0	0	0
Hepatitis with HBAg	0	3	0	0
HBAg	0	0	0	0
Anti-HBAg	0	2	0	1
Well	15	96	13	9

in 10 surviving recipients. None of the recipients who developed hepatitis following an antibody-containing transfusion
developed HBAg during the acute illness, nor was HBAg antigenemia
alone observed. Of these eight cases of hepatitis in anti-HBAg
recipients, three were jaundiced and the remainder were mild anicteric illnesses.

In the control patients followed during the same time period
as the high titer anti-HBAg recipients, 26 of 124 individuals
successfully followed developed hepatitis.   Three of these
illnesses in the control group were associated with the presence
of Australia antigen during the acute phase and probably represent
cases of weak HBAg-positive units which were missed by the less
sensitive ID techniques employed for screening at that time.   In
the control series followed with the low titer anti-HBAg recipients
2 of 12 recipients developed hepatitis. Comparison of these results by the Chi square method failed to reveal statistical
differences between the groups.

Discussion. The observations described here do not support
the idea that transfusion of blood containing antibody to the
Australia antigen is hazardous. While hepatitis is observed in
recipients of antibody-containing blood, the frequency with
which this is encountered is comparable to that seen in control
recipients who receive donor blood negative for anti-HBAg (and
HBAg). These observations constitute an in vivo assay for infectivity which, in the absence of tissue culture methods, is
the only presently available way of approaching the question of
the safety of antibody-containing blood, and is likely to be
more sensitive and meaningful than serological methods as well.

These findings provide no factual basis for prohibiting the
transfusion of donor blood containing anti-HBAg. A considerable
investment of time and effort would be required to develop simple,

sensitive, rapid methods for antibody detection on a large scale. Presently, the best methods for anti-HBAg detection are the hemagglutination and radioimmunoassay procedures, neither of which can easily be applied at the level of routine blood banking at the present time. In addition, if all donors with detectable hemagglutinating antibody titers were rejected, a significant segment (10-30%) of the donor population would be lost as a source of blood and the already acute shortage of donor blood in many areas would be worsened. Thus, any recommendation that donor blood be screened for anti-HBAg before transfusion should be deferred pending confirmation or refutation of these findings. Screening of blood donors to search for good sources of human anti-HBAg antibody can be done retrospectively and should be considered as a matter separate from the safety of the transfusion.

45. Discussion
TRANSFUSION OF BLOOD CONTAINING ANTI-HBAg

Vincent Caggiano

Sacramento Medical Foundation Blood Bank

Sacramento, California

Doctor Gocke has focused his attention on a very real and practical problem facing many blood banks today--namely--what to do with the donor who is found to have anti-HBAg.

At present, there are no regulations or guidelines, perhaps wisely so, from the American Association of Blood Banks for anti-HBAg testing of donor blood. Similarly, in California, no such regulations exist.

Most blood banks would exclude the use of donor blood reactive for anti-HBAg since, by inference, it would imply prior history of hepatitis, though the infectivity of such antibody (or blood) remains in doubt. Our own experience at the Sacramento Foundation Blood Bank, which is a completely volunteer donor bank, is quite small. Since July 1970, we have been testing for HBAg, initially by immunodiffusion and later by counter electrophoresis. We have tested for anti-HBAg exclusively by immunodiffusion in agar since January 1971. In our hands, we have found the immunodiffusion method to be more sensitive than counter electrophoresis for the detection of antibody. Thus far, of 60,270 donors tested, 80 have been found positive for the HBAg, an incidence of 0.13%. Seventy of the 80 donors were males, whereas only 10 were female donors. Female donors comprise 22% of our donor population. Of 47,628 donors tested for anti-HBAg, only 29 reactive sera were found (an incidence of 0.06%), no doubt representing only high titer anti-HBAg, due to the limitation of the method employed. Thirteen of these 29 donors were females, however, in agreement with the finding of others of a higher incidence of anti-HBAg in females. The blood from 23 of these

anti-HBAg positive donors was not used for transfusion purposes.
Since anti-HBAg testing was done by immunodiffusion and required
a minimum of 24 hours, in 6 instances, donor blood, subsequently
found to contain anti-HBAg, had been transfused to 6 individual
recipients. One recipient died postoperatively for reasons unrelated to transfusion, within 24 hours of receiving blood containing anti-HBAg. Five of the recipients were followed by their
physicians for up to six months without any clinical or chemical
evidence of hepatitis. HBAg and anti-HBAg were not detected in
any of their sera. Thus, in our small and uncontrolled series
of transfusions of blood reactive for anti-HBAg, we have not experienced any post-transfusion hepatitis.

Doctor Gocke's studies and our own experience certainly are
by no means conclusive. Further prospective studies are needed to
evaluate the role of donor blood containing anti-HBAg.

46. GAMMA GLOBULIN IN POST-TRANSFUSION HEPATITIS

Robert Ward, Ricardo Katz and Julio Rodriguez

University of Southern California School of Medicine
Los Angeles, California; University of Chile, El Salvador, Chile

The fact that gamma globulin is capable of preventing or
modifying infectious hepatitis (IH) or hepatitis A was established
more than a quarter of a century ago, and has been confirmed time
and time again. The same unqualified statement cannot be made for
serum hepatitis (post-transfusion hepatitis, or hepatitis B).

Evidence has been presented both for and against gamma globulin
preventing post-transfusion hepatitis. On the side of prevention,
Grossman, Steward & Stokes in 1945 [184] were the first to report
the effect of γ-globulin given to alternate battle casualty patients
who had been transfused with whole blood or plasma. Two doses of
10 ml each were injected intramuscularly, the first at the time
of admission (the interval between transfusion and injection of
γ-G was not stated) and the second, one month later. A significant
difference in the incidence of icteric hepatitis was seen in the
gamma globulin group (5 cases, 1.3%) as compared with the control
group (34 cases, 8.9%).

Two decades later Mirick and his co-workers [322] reported
the salutary effect of gamma globulin given in 2 doses of 10 ml
each, the first within a week after transfusion and the second
dose 1 month later. Seven of 656 treated patients acquired
icteric hepatitis as compared with 26 of 655 controls. The difference was significant at the 0.01 level.

Csapo, et al. [119] gave large doses of 10% γ-globulin (8 ml/
kg of body weight) to 182 premature infants and no γ-globulin to
205 infants. Both groups were transfused. In the group given
transfusions and γ-globulin only 1 case of hepatitis occurred; in

325

the group receiving transfusions but <u>no</u> γ-globulin, 15 acquired
hepatitis--a difference which is highly significant.

On the other hand, a considerable body of evidence has accumulated indicating failure of gamma globulin to prevent hepatitis. As long ago as 1947, Duncan, <u>et al</u>. [138] published a paper
indicating that a single dose of 10 ml gamma globulin given intramuscularly to more than 2 thousand battle casualty patients who
had received blood or plasma transfusions failed to reduce the
incidence of hepatitis. However, the authors failed to point
out that 20 of their 26 patients receiving gamma globulin received their gamma globulin between 30 and 130 days <u>after</u> they got
their last blood or plasma transfusions. One could <u>hardly</u> expect
gamma globulin to have an effect under these circumstances.

In 1966, Holland, <u>et al</u>. [213] gave gamma globulin in 2 doses
of 10 ml each--one was given shortly before open heart surgery and
the other 1 month later; there was no significant difference in
the incidence of hepatitis in the gamma globulin group as compared with the controls. A total of 17 patients acquired hepatitis with jaundice--11 in the treated group and 6 in the controls.
The authors do point out that the 167 patients were exposed to a
total of 4,085 units of blood (or an average of about 24 units per
person) and that 79 per cent of the blood came from commerical
sources. Gamma globulin failed to reduce the incidence of hepatitis in this experiment, but it may have been a pretty stiff
assignment.

A cooperative, prospective, controlled study [382] of over
5,000 cardiovascular surgery patients was carried out at 14
university hospital centers. It showed that hepatitis was not
prevented or modified by 10 ml of γ-globulin given during the
1st, 4th and 7th post-operative weeks.

It seems clear that in the last 2 studies described, there
is no evidence of protection against hepatitis afforded by 2 or
3 doses of γ-globulin given to patients receiving an average
of 24 and 7.5 units of blood, respectively.

In any event, even if it were accepted that 2 or 3 doses of
γ-globulin were effective in reducing the incidence of post-
transfusion jaundice, the problem must be examined from a
practical point of view. To inject each transfused patient with
20 to 30 ml of 16% γ-globulin would require 40,000 to 60,000
liters annually, assuming 2,000,000 patients transfused. The
total current production of γ-globulin in the U.S.A. is estimated
at 6,000 to 10,000 liters per annum.

On the other hand, if an average of about 3 units of blood
were given to approximately 2 million persons and if 10 ml of 6%

gamma globulin were added to each unit of blood, the total requirement might be about 60,000 liters of 6% modified γ-globulin; this is the equivalent of 22,200 liters of 16% gamma globulin. Current facilities are not able to cope with this amount, although 18,000 liters or 81% might be achieved.

Therefore, in view of this discrepancy between supply and potential demand, we have been working on the second approach: The working hypothesis or question asked by the present study is whether or not practicable amounts of gamma globulin modified for intravenous use and added directly to each unit of blood before transfusion will neutralize hepatitis viruses in vitro before they pass the portal of entry, and thus prevent or modify the disease.

With Dr. Ricardo Katz and his group in Santiago, Chile, we have tested this hypothesis in a controlled study [241]. Since ordinary γ-globulin may give rise to severe reactions when given intravenously, we used γ-globulin modified by the Swiss method [32]. Briefly, this method involves (1) Adjusting a 10% solution of gamma globulin to pH 4 by addition of 1N HCL. (2) Incubation at 37°C for 24 hours with added pepsin 1:10,000. (3) Neutralization with 1N NaOH, and diluting to 6% solution. The final product is filtered through Seitz sterilizing pads, and tested for sterility, toxins, pyrogens, antibody titers to polio virus and measles virus, and for anticomplementary activity. The latter has proven to be the key test for safety of γ-globulin for intravenous use.

Subjects were female patients over 19 years of age, admitted to various medical and surgical services of the Hospital del Salvador.

Ten ml of modified γ-globulin 6% solution was added to each unit of blood required by a patient whose hospital record number ended in an even digit. The γ-globulin was added to blood an average of 60-70 hours before transfusion. Patients with an odd last digit received blood alone, and served as controls. A third group consisted of patients admitted to the same hospital wards at the same time who received neither blood transfusion nor γ-globulin: These were considered as environmental controls.

After discharge from the hospital, all patients in the study were examined at home or in the Out-Patient Department, and liver function tests were performed at the time of the first transfusion and at 20 to 30 day intervals for 150 to 180 days.

The source of blood was the patient's family or friends. No professional donors were used.

During the 5-1/2 years (April 1965 to October 1970) of this trial, a total of 6,126 patients completed the study. The

Table 1. Post-Transfusion Hepatitis: γ-Globulin Modified for Intravenous Use Added to Blood Before Transfusion.

	γ-globulin in Transfusion	Transfusion Only	Neither γ-G nor Transfusion	Total
Total Patients	1970	2019	2137	6126
Icteric Hepatitis	5*	18*	1	24
Anicteric "	22	16*	6	44

*p .01

distribution was as follows: Group A (γ-globulin added to blood) 1,970 patients; Group B (blood only) 2,019 patients; and Group C (no blood) 2,137 patients (Table 1).

Hepatitis with jaundice was confirmed in 24 patients--5 in Group A, 18 in Group B, and 1 in Group C. The difference between Groups A and B is significant at the 0.01 level. Hepatitis without jaundice was observed in 44 patients--22 in Group A, 16 in Group B, and 6 in Group C (environmental controls). The difference between the incidence of anicteric hepatitis in Groups A and B is not significant.

The attack rates of hepatitis with jaundice per 1,000 cases also showed a difference when compared according to the number of units of blood received (Table 2). It is clear that the attack rates differed very little between Groups A and B in those patients receiving 1, 6 and 7 units of blood. By contrast, a striking difference is seen in recipients of 2 to 6 units, inclusively: One patient in Group A and 16 patients in Group B acquired hepatitis with jaundice. This is highly significant (p,0.001).

Another measure of the difference between Groups A and B was the severity of hepatitis (Table 3). All 6 of the severe cases occurred in the control Group B--2 with coma which ended fatally, 3 with pre-coma (cloudy sensorium, prothrombin complex concentration of 40% or less), and 1 with prolonged illness, i.e., persistence of jaundice for more than 90 days with eventual recovery. The difference between 6 severe cases in the control group and no severe cases in the γ-globulin group is significant at the 0.04 level.

The incubation period is important because post-transfusion hepatitis may include cases of viral hepatitis type A, (short incubation period hepatitis) as well as viral hepatitis type B, (long incubation period hepatitis). In five patients (22%) in the present study, the incubation period was less than 40 days (Table 4); in 14 patients it was 49 days or longer, and in 4 patients the

Table 2. Post-Transfusion Hepatitis: Distribution of Icteric Cases According to Number of Units of Blood.

Blood Units	Group A (γ-Globulin)			Group B (Controls)		
	No. of Patients Transfused	Icteric Hepatitis #Cases	Rate/1000	No. of Patients Transfused	Icteric Hepatitis #Cases	Rate/1000
1	1070	3	2.8	1024	1	0.98
2	504	0	0	517	8	15.5
3	178	0	0	190	2	10.5
4	93	0	0	105	2	19.0
5	47	0	0	62	3	48.3
6	18	1	55.5	28	1	35.7
7	17	1	58.8	26	1	38.4
8-24	43	0	0	67	0	0
Totals	1970	5	2.5	2019	18	8.9

(Group B rows 2–6, p.001)

Table 3. Post-Transfusion Hepatitis: Distribution of Icteric Cases According to Severity.

Group	Total No. of Patients	Mild	Average	Prolonged	Pre-Coma	Fatal Coma
γ-Globulin	1970	3	2	0	0	0
No γ-Globulin	2019	8	4	1	3	2

(No γ-Globulin Prolonged/Pre-Coma/Fatal Coma, p0.04)

Table 4. Patients with Icteric Hepatitis: Distribution According to Incubation Period.

Incubation Period	γ-globulin	Controls	Total
<40 days	1	4	5
49 " or >	3	11	14
Multiple Tx. some < some >40 days	1	3	4

incubation periods were multiple and straddled 40 days. In addition, it should be noted that in a patient in Group A whose incubation period was 29 days--just right for hepatitis A--γ-globulin added to the 1 unit of blood she received failed to prevent hepatitis.

Hepatitis-associated antigen (HBAg) and antibody (anti-HBAg) were sought by both immunodiffusion and complement fixation tests. The serum of 5 patients was positive for antigen by both tests with complement fixation titers of 1:512 (2 patients), 1:256 (2 patients)

and 1 with 1:64. As you might expect, all 5 of these antigen-
positive patients had long incubation periods--68, 81, 84, 93
and 75-89 days. No antigen was found in 39 anicteric patients. No
anti-HBAg was found in these patients or in any others in this
study.

In conclusion, the addition of modified γ-globulin to blood
before transfusuion resulted in a significant reduction in the
incidence of post-transfusion jaundice in this study.

47. Discussion
GAMMA GLOBULIN IN POST-TRANSFUSION HEPATITIS

Paul V. Holland

National Institutes of Health, Clinical Center Blood

Bank, Bethesda, Maryland

I had the opportunity to review Dr. Ward's manuscript ahead of time; to quote H. G. Wells, "No passion in the world, no love or hate, is equal to the passion to change someone else's draft..."

As Dr. Ward has pointed out, the evidence for the ability of immune serum globulin (ISG) to modify infectious hepatitis (IH or hepatitis A) has been consistent and overwhelming. However, the evidence for its modification of post-transfusion hepatitis (PTH) is conflicting.

Table 1 is a summary of all of the published studies to date which bear on the effectiveness of ISG in post-transfusion hepatitis. All included a control group for comparison. I have deliberately placed studies which were similar in design next to each other, and I have split two of the studies because they contain divergent treatment schedules and results. The dose is the total ISG in grams given singly or more than once as noted. In the third column is the time of administration of the ISG in relation to the transfusion. In the last column is the conclusion of the authors of each study relative to the significant reduction, P less than 0.05, of icteric, post-transfusion hepatitis.

In the first two studies, gamma globulin modified for intravenous use was added to each unit of blood prior to transfusion. As you have heard today, Drs. Ward, Katz and Rodriguez found a significant reduction in the incidence of icteric hepatitis. In a similar but smaller study, Creutzfeldt et al. did not find a statistically significant reduction of icteric PTH [115].

Table 1.   Immune serum Globulin (ISG) and the modification of post-transfusion hepatitis (PTH).

Study	Dose (gm)	ISG re Transfusions	↓Icteric PTH
Katz [241]	0.6/unit	in blood	YES
Creutzfeldt [115]	0.5/unit	in blood	NO
Csapo [119]	1.3/Kg	pre or with	YES
Ekbloom [143]	1.7	with	NO
Holland [213]	1.6 x 2	pre & post	NO
Mirick II [322]	1.6 x 2	pre & post	NO
Mirick III & I [322]	1.6 x 3 or 2	pre &/or post & post	YES
Torii Ia & II [464]	2.4 x 2 or 3	with or post & post	YES
Torii Ib [464]	1.6 x 2	post & post	NO
Grady & NTS [382]	1.6 x 3	post, post & post	NO
Grossman [184]	1.6 x 2	late post & post	YES
Duncan [138]	1.6	late post	NO

In the next two studies, ISG was given as a single dose before or on the day of transfusion. Csapo et al. in Hungary found that a single, massive dose of ISG given several days before, or on the day of, transfusion in neonates, reduced the resultant incidence of icteric PTH [119]. Ekbloom et al. found no such effect in adults with a more usual dose [143].

Our group [213], and Mirick et al. [322] with their schedule II, found that two doses of ISG, one given at or before transfusion and another one month later, were ineffective. But, when Mirick's group gave the ISG in the same dose to the same type of patient but one week after transfusion, and again one month later, or gave a pre-transfusion injection as well, a significant reduction in icteric hepatitis resulted [322]. Torii et al. in Japan found that a slightly larger dose, given at similar times was effective; but the same dose and timing as used in Mirick's schedule I was not effective [464].

Grossman, Stewart and Stokes were the first to find that ISG reduced the incidence of icteric hepatitis in transfused casualties of World War II [184]. They gave two doses of ISG; the first injection was as late as four months after overseas transfusion and the second, one month after this. With an identical patient group

treated with just one dose of ISG, Duncan et al. could not dupli-
cate these results [138]. They did, however, note, as did Stokes
et al. [445] in a subsequent study, that the incubation period in
the ISG group was significantly prolonged; so much so that the
study of Grossman et al. [184] may not have followed all of the
patients in the ISG group long enough to get a true hepatitis frequency. Finally, Grady and the National Transfusion Study (NTS)
found no reduction of icteric hepatitis in a large transfusion
series combining the doses and schedules of ISG found effective by
Grossman et al. [184] and Mirick et al. [322]. A large, cooperative VA ISG-PTH study is currently underway to again assess this
problem.

In addition to the aforementioned differences, these studies
utilized different lots of gamma globulin, with undoubtedly varying antibody titers, on diverse types of transfused patients. I
submit, however, that there is little agreement between the results
of apparently similar, controlled studies.

While ISG may not be overwhelmingly effective for PTH, let us
assume that it does modify the disease to some extent by making some
icteric cases anicteric and some anicteric cases milder or inapparent.
Is this desirable? The milder or inapparent disease might become
more chronic or might result in a silent hepatitis carrier state with,
eventually, chronic hepatitis, cirrhosis or even, perhaps, hepatoma
in the recipient. Barker and Murray [34] have shown in volunteers,
for instance, that decreasing the dose of HBAg-containing, icterogenic serum resulted in a higher proportion of minimal or inapparent
disease and more persistent carriers with residual hepatic dysfunction. Long term followup should, therefore, be performed on the
transfused patients in the aforementioned studies to see if there
is an increased, long term incidence of hepatic disease in those who
received concurrent ISG versus the controls. If this is so, then
the short term benefit of ISG given at the time of transfusion may
be outweighed by later sequelae. Until such studies are done, I
believe that reducing unnecessary blood transfusions, eliminating
commercial donors, establishing hepatitis carrier registries, and
screening for HBAg are more proven and practical measures to reduce
PTH.

48. HEPATITIS B IMMUNE GLOBULIN

A.M. Prince, W. Szmuness, B. Brotman, H. Ikram, A. Lippin,
M. Stryker, C. Ehrich, and N.C.D.C. Finlayson.
The New York Blood Center and New York Hospital, Cornell
Medical Center
New York, New York

The present discussion will review current knowledge concerning
passive immunization against hepatitis B infections. We shall summarize current knowledge of the efficacy of γ-globulin preparations
containing defined and elevated concentrations of hepatitis B antibody, hereinafter termed hepatitis B immune globulin (HBIG), in
prevention or modification of hepatitis B infections. In addition
we will present new data concerning availability, preparation, characterization, and safety of HBIG preparations.

While it is clear that γ-globulin preparations may prevent or
modify infections due to hepatitis virus A [157,195,257,265,446,447,
484,485], there is no agreement concerning the efficacy of γ-globulin
preparations in prevention or modification of infections due to
hepatitis virus type B. Grossman, Stewart and Stokes [184], and
Mirick et al. [322] have presented data suggesting that conventional
γ-globulin may reduce the incidence of post-transfusion hepatitis.
On the other hand, Holland et al. found no evidence of such protection in a carefully controlled study [213]. More recently a
large cooperative study designed to evaluate the possible effect of
three 10cc doses of conventional γ-globulin in prevention of post-
transfusion hepatitis suggested that this regimen was entirely without value in prevention or modification of this disease [382].

Katz et al. have reported on the effects of adding suitably
modified globulin directly to transfused blood as a possible prophylactic method [241]. The results of this work have been reviewed
in detail by Dr. Ward in this Symposium.

The rapidly growing body of knowledge concerned with hepatitis

335

B infections (serum hepatitis) which has resulted from work with what is now termed the hepatitis B antigen [44,384,390,393] has made possible a variety of new approaches to this problem [394]. In particular, the availability of sensitive assays for hepatitis B antibody (anti-HBAg) [477] resulted in the demonstration of marked variations in anti-HBAg activity of different preparations of conventional γ-globulin and also made possible the preparation of γ-globulin having greatly enhanced anti-HBAg content [394]. These new findings may help to explain the discordant results obtained by different workers in the past.

The realization that a major proportion of sporadic cases of hepatitis in adults who deny past exposure to blood or blood products are due to hepatitis B infection [384,390], and the availability of appropriate assays, has made it possible to ask whether conventional γ-globulin might protect against contact type (low dose) hepatitis B infections. Indeed, evidence has been reported [164,396] suggesting that a preparation of conventional γ-globulin thought to have an unusually high content of hepatitis B antibody did confer significant protection against icteric cases of hepatitis B infection among US Army personnel in Korea.

Recently Krugman, Giles, and Hammond, reported the results of an evaluation of hyper-immune hepatitis B immune globulin [394] in prevention or modification of hepatitis B infections when given four hours following a simulated "needle stick" type exposure [263]. Of 10 subjects who were exposed in this manner, only 4 developed hepatitis as compared to an attack rate expected on the basis of previous studies to be in excess of 90%. Five of the 6 subjects who did not develop hepatitis showed evidence of passive/active immunity.

Independently, Soulier and his colleagues at the National Transfusion Centre in Paris, have prepared hepatitis B immune globulin, and have administered it to 27 subjects, 19 of whom had received a transfusion later found to contain hepatitis B antigen, and 8 of whom had been accidentally exposed (needle sticks) to HBAg-containing blood [441]. HBIG was administered between 3 hrs and 7 days after exposure. None of the 27 recipients developed jaundice. Eighteen of the above subjects have been followed with serial blood samples; significant transaminase elevations were found in only 2 of these cases. Hepatitis B antigen was not detected in any of these 18 cases. Soulier concluded that passive immunization appeared to be both effective and innocuous. Indeed serological data suggested the occurrence of passive/active immunization, as was also suggested by Krugman. It was therefore suggested that passive immunization with HBIG would be long lasting. Soulier concluded that the major problem in passive immunization might be finding adequate supplies of hepatitis B immune plasma (HBIP).

Recently Soulier has summarized his additional experience between July 1971 and January 1972 (personal communication). Four lots of HBIG have been prepared from nine to twenty liter plasma pools. The resultant yields of 16.5% γ-globulin varied from 150 - 360 ml. The preparations of HBIG varied in anti-HBAg titer from 1:8 to 1:12 by AGD and from 1:3,000 to 1:10,000 by radioimmunoassay. HBAg was not detected in any of the final preparations by radio-immunoassay, or by electron microscopy. The above material has been administered to 85 subjects, 38 of whom were inadvertently transfused with HBAg-containing blood and 47 of whom were accidently exposed (needle sticks). The dose employed was 0.16 ml/kg for those exposed by transfusion, and 0.08 ml/kg for those accidently exposed. HBIG was again injected between 3 hrs and 7 days after exposure (mean 2-4 days). Only 2 cases of clinically evident hepatitis were observed in the above 85 HBIG recipients. Transaminase elevations were seen in three cases and hepatitis B antigen in only one case (who also developed clinical hepatitis).

The studies of Soulier and Krugman are indeed encouraging. However, it must be pointed out that neither study was adequately controlled, or "double blind" in nature.

These recent developments offer renewed hope that effective prevention or modification of hepatitis B infections may be possible; however, presently available data on this question are by no means conclusive. Extensive, well controlled, double blind evaluations are required before the safety and efficacy of hepatitis B immune globulin can be considered adequately evaluated for clinical use.

In the remainder of this paper we will summarize data which we have recently obtained which bear on the possible application of hepatitis B immune globulin for immunoprophylaxis, or immunotherapy. In addition to standard methods for detection of HBAg and anti-HBAg [384,388] we have relied heavily on a modification of the passive hemagglutination method first described by Vyas and Shulman [477]; our procedures have been detailed previously in this volume (p.147).

Passive Transfer of anti-HBAg. In our initial report [394] we described the administration of HBIG to children enrolled in a controlled double blind study designed to evaluate the possible protective action of HBIG against contact infections in institutions for the mentally retarded. The high attack rate of newly-admitted children to three institutions in which we have carried out epidemiologic studies [454,455] offered the possibility of an evaluation of efficacy of HBIG. Subject to informed consent, alternate newly-admitted children received either conventional γ-globulin, or HBIG (0.01 ml/lb) and then were followed with monthly blood samples. Repeat injections of γ-globulin were given at intervals of four months. Although it is too early to draw conclusions regarding efficacy from these studies, it has been possible to document passive transfer of

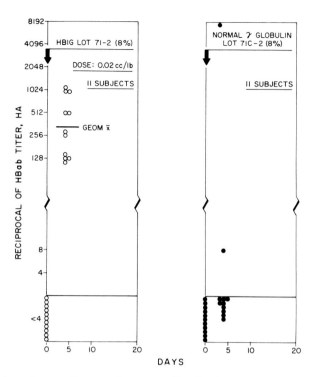

Figure 1.   Induction of passive antibody by HBIG.

antibody and its persistence in detectable quantities for 2-3 months [394].

      In an extension of the above study which is currently under way in collaboration with Dr. Morris Goodman at the Plymouth State School, Detroit, Michigan, we have obtained follow-up blood samples three to five days after administration of HBIG and conventional γ-globulin. As shown in Figure 1, children who received HBIG developed passive antibody titers varying between 1:128 to 1:1024 three to five days after injection of HBIG. This demonstrates the very considerable levels of passive antibody which can be induced by this method.

      Subtype antibody composition of HBIG. The characterization of subtype antigens associated with the HBAg particles by LeBouvier and others, which has been reviewed by Dr. LeBouvier at this symposium, raises important questions concerning the nature of the antigenic specificity which might be involved in neutralization of HB virus. We have therefore investigated the subtype hemagglutinating antibody composition of HBIG. We have taken advantage of the fact that the passive hemagglutination inhibition technique can be made subtype specific by utilizing two to four units of absorbed mono-specific (anti-d and anti-y) antiserum in the inhibition test. Quantitative precipitin curves are then carried out with antigen of defined subtype specificity, e.g., types adx, ayx, and ad(x⁻). Supernatant fluids from the quantitative precipitin curve mixtures (held 2 hours at 37°C and then six days at 4°C) were as-

sayed for specific antigenic subtypes and for antibodies reactive
with red cells coated with antigen of defined subtypes, as shown
in Figure 2.   The results of nine such graphs summarizing estimates

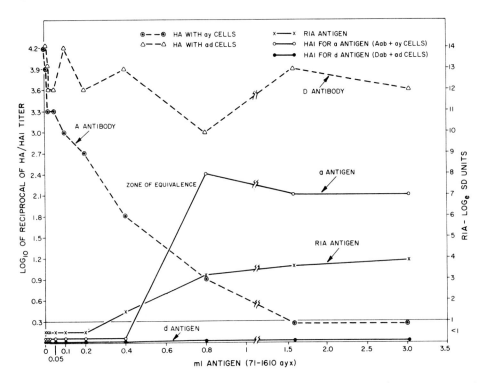

Figure 2.   Precipitin curve: AD antiserum (50μl) (NIH guinea pig
V801-502-558) with varying quantities of <u>ayx</u> antigen (71-1610).
All volumes were made up to 5.0 ml.

of subtype antibody content of (1) a well-characterized serum of AD
type, (2) serum from the wife of a carrier of <u>ayx</u> type antigen
which we had previously found to be AY type by agar gel diffusion
analysis, and (3) Hepatitis B Immune Globulin are summarized in
Table 1.   It may be seen that HBIG contains antibody against all

Table 1.   Subtype antibody characterization.

Subtype of Antibody	HA UNITS/ML	(% of A)	
	NIH Guinea Pig (AD)	71-3392 (AY)	HBIG 71-2
A	1,600,000	800,000	1,600,000
D	400,000 (25%)	<200 (0.01%)	400,000 (25%)
Y	<400 (<0.1%)	200,000 (25%)	6,300 (0.4%)
"X"	<6,400 (<3%)	<200 (<0.01%)	9,000 (0.6%)

of the defined subtype specificities; however, the antibody against
the common <u>a</u> antigen predominates.   This type of analysis permits
comparison of different hyper-immune globulin preparations and offers an approach to elucidation of the role of subtype antibodies

in protection.

Availability of HBIG.   Should HBIG prove safe and efficacious, the major problem will be the provision of adequate supplies for widespread clinical use.   The magnitude of this problem will depend on definition of antibody titer and dosage required for effective use.   As discussed in more detail below it is quite possible that hyper-immune HBIG contains considerably more antibody than is required for protection against certain types of challenge or exposure.

We have investigated the anti-HBAg titers of γ-globulin preparations from a variety of sources (Figure 3).   Highest titers

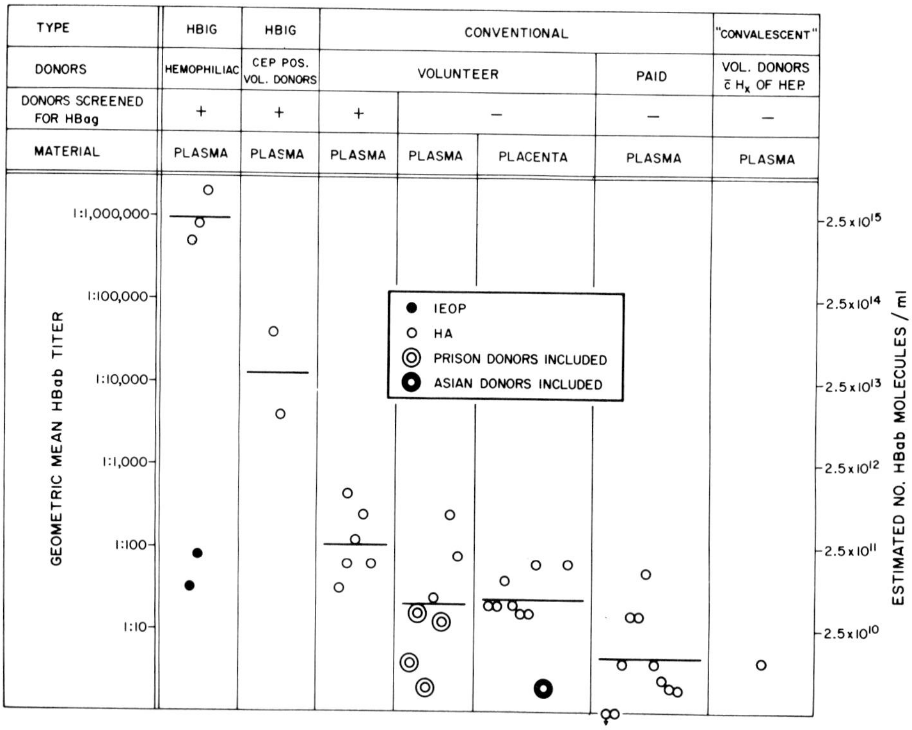

TYPE	HBIG	HBIG	CONVENTIONAL				"CONVALESCENT"
DONORS	HEMOPHILIAC	CEP POS. VOL. DONORS	VOLUNTEER			PAID	VOL. DONORS c̄ Hx OF HEP.
DONORS SCREENED FOR HBag	+	+	+	−	−	−	
MATERIAL	PLASMA	PLASMA	PLASMA	PLASMA	PLACENTA	PLASMA	PLASMA

Figure 3.   Anti-HBAg levels in γ-globulin preparations from different sources.

were observed in HBIG prepared from the plasma of patients with hemophilia.   Plasma from blood donors having antibody detectable by agar gel diffusion or counter electrophoresis methods also contained high titers of antibody; however, when measured by the hemagglutination technique, these were on the average 100 fold lower than those in hemophiliac plasma.   When agar gel diffusion was employed for evaluation, the difference was only 3-10 fold.

Conventional γ-globulin was found to vary widely in antibody content.   Paradoxically, highest antibody titers were found in plasma pooled from volunteer donors, especially donors who have been prescreened for HBAg and/or come from regions of the world in which the HBAg carrier state is relatively infrequent. This un-expected finding suggests that the anti-HBAg yield obtainable from pooled plasma or placental γ—globulin varies inversely with the quantity of HBAg in the starting pool. It appears likely that HBAg forms complexes with anti-HBAg, which reduces the quantity of the latter available for assay.

Production of HBIG. We have prepared three batches of HBIG. The first (lot 71-1) was derived from a 5 liter pool of plasma from a single hemophiliac donor. The second and third batches (lots 71-2, and 72-1) were prepared from 50 and 76 liter pools of plasma from 10-15 different donors with hemophilia.

Tables 2, 3, and 4 summarize recovery calculations from the fractionation of lot 72-1. In terms of protein recovery (Table 2)

Table 2. Recovery of proteins in large scale fractionation of HBIG

Fraction [1]	TOTAL PROTEIN			γ-GLOBULIN		
	Total (Gms)	% OF TOTAL	TOTAL (Gms)	% OF TOTAL PROTEINS	SPECIFIC ACTIVITY [2]	YIELD [3] (%)
Original Plasma	4058	100.0	584	14.4	0.14	100
II Super-natant	2376	58.6	<23	<0.5	<0.01	<3.9
II A Super-natant	176	4.3	<1.7	<0.1	<0.1	<0.3
III E Pre-cipitate	663	16.3	50	1.2	0.07	8.6
IV Super-natant	<4	<0.1	<0.5	<0.1	-	<0.1
γ Globulin	425	10.5	425	10.5	1.0	72.8

[1] Method of Nitschmann, Kistler and Lergier
[2] Gm γ-globulin/ Gm total protein in fraction
[3] Percent of γ-globulin in starting material

results are comparable to those obtained in our laboratory in routine fractionation of conventional γ-globulin. Recoveries of anti-HBAg are summarized in Table 3. Only 30% of the anti-HBAg was detected in the final product.

Table 4 summarizes the overall yield of this fractionation and emphasizes the large quantity of hyperimmune plasma required for production of one vial of HBIG.

Chimpanzee γ-globulin? The use of chimpanzee plasma as an

Table 3. Recovery of HB antigen and antibody in large scale fractionation of HBIG

| FRACTION | FREE HB ANTIBODY* | | | |
	RECIPROCAL OF HA TITER/ml	TOTAL UNITS	SPECIFIC ACTIVITY**	YIELD (%)
Original Plasma	2.4×10^5	7.1×10^{11}	1.7×10^8	100.0
II Supernatant	2.4×10^3	8.5×10^9	3.5×10^6	1.2
IIA Supernatant	1.3×10^3	2.1×10^9	1.2×10^7	0.3
IIIE Precipitate	1.3×10^5	1.1×10^{11}	1.7×10^8	16.1
IV Supernatant	$<2 \times 10^2$	$<5.9 \times 10^8$	-	<0.1
γ Globulin (4%)	5.0×10^5	2.1×10^{11}	5.0×10^8	30.2

* Bound forms of HB antigen and antibody not measured
**Antibody units/gm protein

Table 4. HBIG: Summary of yield: Lot no. 72-2

1 liter HB immune plasma (HBIP)	= 5.6 Gm γ-globulin
	= 7 x 5cc vials 16% γ-globulin

1 5cc vial 16% γ-globulin contains globulin from 143cc HBIP

alternate source for HBIG is under consideration in our laboratory. Precipitating quantities of hepatitis B antibody have been observed in unimmunized chimpanzees [385] and have been induced by immunization [291] in these animals. Immunization with highly purified antigen results in the appearance of monospecific high-titer antibody within two weeks after a booster injection of purified antigen suspended in Freund's adjuvant (Figure 4). The results presented are typical of those observed in 20 chimpanzees whom we have immunized during the past year; thus large volumes of hyperimmune plasma can be obtained by plasmapheresis. If γ-globulin of chimpanzee origin can be shown to be no more immunogenic in man than pooled γ-globulin of human origin, as would be expected, chimpanzee γ-globulin could represent a logical source for protective antibody for human use.

Is HBIG infectious? It is generally accepted that conventional γ-globulin prepared by the Cohn ethanol fractionation method is not infectious following administration to man. We have followed 50 recipients of conventional immune serum globulin, who had been treated following possible exposure to a case of fulminant hepatitis, with serial biweekly blood samples for 6 months. Transaminase elevations were observed in only one case, and HB antigen was observed in none of these cases (Prince, A.M., and Christenson, W.N., unpublished data).

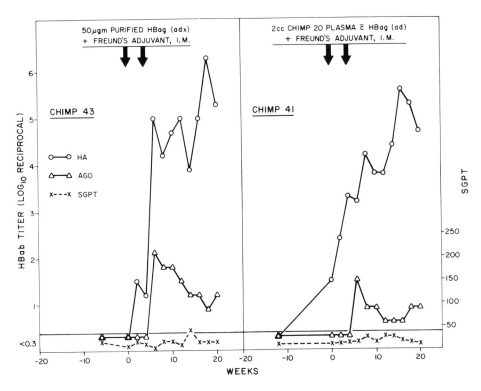

Figure 4.   Immunization of chimpanzees with HBAg.

Table 5 summarizes follow-up results on 17 subjects who received HBIG (lot 71-1) and who were then followed for four to fifteen months with monthly blood samples.   These subjects were par-
ticipants in a trial to determine the prophylactic efficacy of HBIG
in prevention or modification of infections among newly-admitted
residents to institutions for the mentally retarded [394].   Among
these 17 subjects only 2 showed transaminase (SGPT) elevations
above 30 Karmen units, neither case exceeding 50.   Three cases
showed mild anti-HBAg titer rises: one of these occurred in a
child who had detectable anti-HBAg prior to the first injection of
HBIG and could represent a booster response to the small amount of
HBAg present in the γ-globulin preparation.   One child developed
HBAg, detectable only in a single blood specimen taken four weeks
after a second injection of HBIG.   The transaminase level in this
serum was 10.6.   There was no subsequent antibody response detectable by hemagglutination, as would be expected if a primary infection had occurred [291].   We therefore interpret this finding
as possibly representing a technical error, e.g., mislabeling of
specimen.

In summary, the results obtained do not support the conclusion
that this lot of HBIG was infectious.   In the light of the high
susceptibility of newly-admitted residents to institutions for the
mentally retarded to infection with hepatitis B virus [263] a much

Table 5. Safety of HBIG: Infectivity of lot 71-1. Results of 4-15 month follow-up of 17 recipients.

CASE	# DOSES HBIG-71-1	# OF SPECIMENS	DURATION (MONTHS)	SGPT # >30	SGPT PEAK	ANTI-HBAg # >32	ANTI-HBAg PEAK	HBAg
SS-1	2	4	6	0	9	0	16	0
SS-4	3	10	12	0	27	0	16	0
SS-5	3	11	10	0	15	1	64	0
SS-7	3	10	9	1	40	0	4	0
SS-8	3	11	11	0	16	1	64	0
SS-9	2	7	8	0	30	0	8	0
SS-14	3	8	7	1	35	0	8	0
SS-16	2	6	4	0	9	0	16	0
SS-17	3	10	10	0	14	4*	512	0
WS-1	4	12	15	0	23	0	32	0
WS-4	4	12	12	0	19	0	16	+**
WS-5	4	12	12	0	30	0	16	0
WS-7	4	12	15	0	19	0	16	0
WS-8	3	7	9	0	20	0	32	0
WS-9	2	6	6	0	25	0	32	0
WS-11	1	4	6	0	16	0	32	0
WS-15	2	4	4	0	16	0	8	0
TOTALS: 17		146	--	2	--	3	--	1
AVERAGE	2.8	8.6	9.2	-	--	-	--	-

* HBAg titer 1:4 prior to first injection of HBIG
**HBAg detectable in single blood specimen 4 weeks after second injection; SGPT = 10.6; no subsequent antibody response. ?? mislabeled tube.

higher clinical and/or serologic response rate would be expected if this material were itself infectious. With the exception of the one case showing an antibody rise who had detectable antibody prior to HBIG administration, the remaining antibody levels were within the range expected due to passive transfer of antibody from the injected HBIG.

We conclude that γ-globulin preparations of conventional or elevated anti-HBAg content are most probably not infectious in man. This hypothesis requires further evaluation by continued careful surveillance during the course of clinical trials now underway.

Safety of HBIG. In our initial report [394] certain possible dangers which could result from clinical use of HBIG were considered, e.g., infectivity and/or attenuation of disease with possible increase in frequency of the chronic carrier states with its attendant

medical complications.   An additional danger has recently come to
our attention.   Administration of antibody to a carrier of large
quantities of circulating antigen could theoretically result in
the formation of immune complexes, fixation of complement, and
liberation of mediators of inflamation or anaphylaxis, e.g., ana-
phylotoxin.   This possibility must be considered especially when
intravenous administration of anti-HBAg is contemplated.   It appears
that this danger is not only theoretical.   Figure 5 summarizes administration of anti-HBAg to two chronic HBAg carriers: (1) Chimp

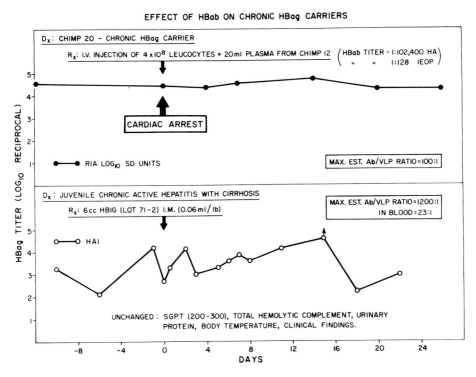

Figure 5.   Possible danger and lack of benefits resulting from
administration of anti-HBAg containing materials to two chronic
HBAg carriers.

20, a chronic HBAg carrier, whom we have followed for three years,
was given 4×10^8 leukocytes from hyperimmunized chimp #12.   The
latter animal had an anti-HBAg titer of 1:128 by IEOP at the time
of plasmapheresis.   The leukocytes were suspended in 20 ml of
plasma from chimp #12 and were injected by slow intravenous injection, (gravity flow from a plastic bag).   After several minutes
blood pressure and pulse became undetectable as a result of ventri-
cular fibrillation and cardiac arrest.   Cardiac massage was immediately instituted.   Atropine and epinephrine were administered;
cardiac function returned to normal over a 30 minute period.   The
above reaction may well have represented passive "systemic" anaphylaxis.   Cardiac arrest has also been observed during administration of anti-HBAg plasma intravenously to two patients with

fulminant hepatitis whose serum contained detectable HBAg (Mosley, J., personal communication; Schaffner, F., personal communication).

These observations suggest that anti-HBAg-containing materials should be administered, whenever possible, only to subjects demonstrably free of HBAg. If it is thought necessary to administer such materials on an emergency basis where HBAg screening cannot be carried out, it would be desirable to carry out a skin test with the anti-HBAg-containing material prior to administration, and then to administrate the anti-HBAg slowly and cautiously under conditions where resuscitative measures are immediately available.

Figure 5 summarizes also administration of HBIG by the IM route to a patient with juvenile chronic active hepatitis and probable cirrhosis. No adverse effects were noted; however, it should also be pointed out that no benefit accrued.

Efficacy - theoretical considerations. We consider it premature to draw conclusions concerning the efficacy of HBIG in prevention, modification, or therapy of hepatitis B infections. The availability of knowledge concerning the number of HBAg particles in carrier plasma (Hall, W.T., personal communication) and estimation of the number of antibody molecules present in HBIG (Table 6) permits theoretical predictions concerning possible dose levels

Table 6. Basis for estimation of number of anti-HBAg molecules.

DATA:	1.	Particle concentration in serum (Cl 98) $\simeq 10^{14}$VLP/ml
	2.	Antibody (Pool 1)
	a)	HA titer = 1:256,000
	b)	Immunological equivalence concentration = 1:4 (Precipitin Curve)

ASSUMPTION: Ab:VLP ratio at equivalence = 50:1

ESTIMATION: $1 \text{ HA unit/ml} = \dfrac{10^{14} \cdot 50 \cdot 4}{2.5 \cdot 10^{14}}$

$\simeq 1 \cdot 10^{11}$ antibody molecules

required in different potential prophylactic applications (Table 7). These estimates are, of course, highly speculative and in particular would be largely invalidated if the antibody to the a specificity is not neutralizing.

The estimates presented in Table 7 suggest that large volumes of HBIG could prevent post-transfusion hepatitis, but that conventional gamma globulin should not be effective in this regard. Furthermore, these estimates suggest that HBIG may be effective in prevention of low dose type infections, (e.g., self-inoculation, oral ingestions) in extremely low doses. Indeed, an intermediate level HBIG, e.g. a preparation having an anti-HBAg titer by hemagglutination of 1:1,000 might be adequate to confer protection for this type of exposure. Clinical trials are currently being initiated to evaluate this hypothesis since such materials could be readily prepared by 1:1000 dilution of hyper-immune HBIG with conventional γ-globulin. Such an approach would make it practical to prepare only one type of "hepatitis immune γ-globulin".

Table 7. A theoretical basis for analysis of potential usefulness of HBIG given prior to exposure in prevention of hepatitis B infection.

Type of Exposure	Estimated # Particles in Challenge Dose*	Estimated # Ab. Molecules Required to Neutralize**	Minimum Volume γ-Globulin Required	
			Conventional (HA titer 1:4)	HBIG (HA titer 1:512,000)
Transf. (200 ml)	2×10^{16}	1×10^{18}	2×10^6 ml	20 ml
Contaminated Inoculation (0.01ml)	1×10^{12}	5×10^{13}	100 ml	0.001 ml
Oral Ingestion	? $<10^{12}$	? $<5 \times 10^{13}$	? <100 ml	? <0.001 ml

*Assuming 10^{14} particles/ml plasma
**Assuming required Ab:Ag ratio = 50:1

Acknowledgements. These studies were aided by Grant #HE-09011 and AI-09516 from the National Institutes of Health, Contract #70-2236 from the National Heart and Lung Institute, and Grants in Aid from the Kresge Foundation and from the Strasburger Foundation. Dr. Prince is a Career Scientist of the Health Research Council of the City of New York under Contract #I-533.

We are grateful for the technical assistance of B. Clinkscale, E. Echenroth, A. M. Moffatt, D. Joss, and J. Friedman and to Drs. J. Soulier, J. Desmyter, G. F. Grady, M. Roumantseff, M. Conrad and B. Holmstrom for kindly supplying samples of their γ-globulin preparations for testing.

49. Discussion
HEPATITIS B IMMUNE GLOBULIN

Saul Krugman

New York University School of Medicine, Department of

Pediatrics, New York, New York

Doctors Prince, Holland, and Alter have emphasized the importance of being aware of the potential hazards of immunoprophylaxis with hepatitis B immune serum globulin (HB-ISG) preparations for the prevention or modification of viral hepatitis, type B. Two important questions have been posed: 1) is it possible that HB-ISG may contain active hepatitis B virus?, and 2) is it possible that the use of HB-ISG may increase the incidence of anicteric infections which are more prone to be associated with a chronic carrier state?

It is clear that the use of standard ISG is not associated with an increased incidence of viral hepatitis, type B. Extensive epidemiological surveys have confirmed the safety of this preparation. The results of a preliminary study by our group [263] indicated that an experimental lot of HB-ISG was not infectious for susceptible recipients. On the other hand, it had a protective and modifying effect. These initial findings are encouraging.

The association of a chronic carrier state following anicteric hepatitis as compared with icteric hepatitis has been well documented. Doctors Holland and Alter have referred to the report of Dr. Barker and his colleagues in this regard. We have had a similar experience during the course of our studies which are summarized in Table 1, Figure 1, and Figure 2. Persistence of HBAg was observed in 56% of 27 cases of anicteric hepatitis as compared with 7% of 14 cases of icteric hepatitis.

During the course of our studies we have had an opportunity to evaluate the effect of immune serum globulin (ISG) for the protection or modification of hepatitis B infection.

Table 1. Correlation of persistence of hepatitis B antigen with presence or absence of jaundice.

Icteric Viral Hepatitis, Type B

Total number of cases	14
Number with transient antigen	13 (93%)
Number with persistent antigen	1 (7%)

Anicteric Viral Hepatitis, Type B

Total number of cases	27
Number with transient antigen	12
Number with persistent antigen	15

Transient = <120 days
Persistent = >120 days

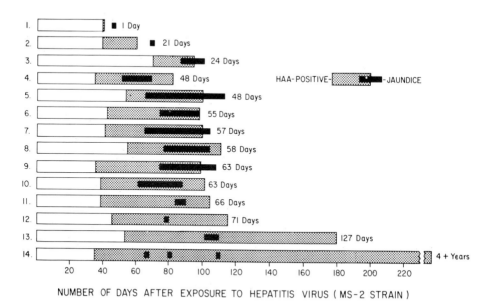

Figure 1. Persistence of hepatitis B antigen (HBAg) in 14 patients with icteric viral hepatitis, type B [260].

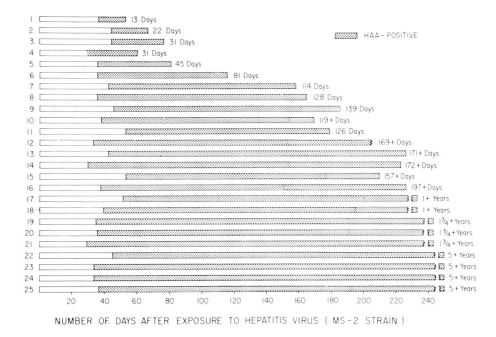

Figure 2. Persistence of hepatitis B antigen (HBAg) in 25 patients with anicteric hepatitis, type B [260].

The ISG was given in one of three ways: 1) it was added to MS-2 serum before inoculation, 2) it was given as a parenteral inoculation of 0.02 ml/lb of body weight, and 3) it was given as HB-ISG in a dose of 0.02 ml/lb of body weight. The use of standard ISG preparations was not associated with a significant decrease in the incidence of hepatitis infection; in contrast, HB-ISG was 70% effective. It was interesting to note, however, that anicteric hepatitis B infection which occurred following ISG prophylaxis was more prone to have a shorter duration of antigen in the serum and a shorter period of abnormal transaminase activity than anicteric infection which occurred without ISG prophylaxis. If these observations are confirmed, it will indicate that the course of anicteric hepatitis associated with gamma globulin prophylaxis is different from the course of unmodified anicteric hepatitis. Consequently, it is possible that ISG may prove to have a beneficial effect, and it is premature to assume that its use is hazardous.

50. HEPATITIS ASSOCIATED WITH THE TRANSFUSION OF HBAg-NEGATIVE BLOOD

Martin Goldfield, Joanne Bill, Henry Black, Wayne
Pizzuti, Sunthorn Srihongse

New Jersey State Department of Health
Trenton, New Jersey

A group at the New Jersey Department of Health has been involved in a large-scale investigation of the blood-service complex,
transfusion practices, risks of transfusion-associated hepatitis,
some attributes of 2,000 cases of transfusion-associated hepatitis
accumulated in the period 1961-1971, and the association of HBAg
with transfusion-associated hepatitis in New Jersey. Approximately
400,000 blood units collected or processed in New Jersey between
July, 1969, and December, 1971, were tested for HBAg in the Department's laboratories by a combination of two or three techniques,
namely: complement fixation, immunoelectrophoresis and agar gel
diffusion. Approximately 15,000 units also have been tested by a
sensitive radioimmunoassay technique. Between July of 1969 and
July of 1970, no attempt was made to perform these tests on a current basis and no reports of results were issued. Beginning in
August of 1970, all known HBAg-positive blood donors were inter-
dicted from donating again, virtually all pints in the State were
pretested and virtually all positive pints were eliminated. As
requested by the conveners of this conference, this presentation
will be limited to information accumulated regarding the occurrence
of hepatitis in recipients of HBAg-negative blood. We shall address
ourselves to two aspects of this subject, namely: 1) what percentage of infectious donors transmitting overt, recognized hepatitis are picked up by conventional HBAg testing, and 2) what percentage of undetected, presumably infectious donors remain undetected because of limitations in the sensitivity of our tests, as
opposed to those donors presumed to be transmitting a variety of
hepatitis unrelated to HBAg.

These studies will be described more fully elsewhere. Hence, a full description of methods employed will, in the interest of brevity, be omitted from this presentation.

Early during the course of these studies, we became aware of the occurrence of transfusion-associated hepatitis following the administration of HBAg-negative blood.

Table 1. Disposition of HBAg-positive and control negative pints

	HBAg-positive		HBAg-negative	
	Number	Percent	Number	Percent
Units as yet untraced	117	-	102	-
All traced units:	760	100	765	100
a) Discarded by bank drawing unit	57	8	20	3
b) Outdated[3]	116	15	129	17
c) Recipients dying in <120 days	200	26	184	24
d) Recipients checked for hepatitis 6 mos. later	387[1]	51	433[2]	57
Number & percent of d) observed to have developed overt hepatitis	56	14.9	14	3.3

[1]One recipient of an HBAg-positive pint had hepatitis when transfused. Nine recipients received two positive pints. Thus the number of recipients at risk of developing hepatitis was 377.
[2]Two recipients of a control negative pint had underlying hepatic disease and another, who developed overt hepatitis, also had received an HBAg-positive pint. Ten recipients each received two control negative pints and one recipient received three control negative pints. Thus the number of recipients at risk of developing hepatitis was 418.
[3]Outdate rate was 10% among units shipped to New Jersey hospitals and 25% among those shipped to hospitals in New York City.

Table 1 summarizes the results of determining the outcome in 387 surviving recipients of pints of HBAg-positive blood as compared to matched controls. It can be seen that 15% of the recipients of a positive unit, as well as 3% of control recipients, developed overt, recognized hepatitis in the ensuing six months. During this period of time, the HBAg rate among units used for transfusion in New Jersey was 6.4/thousand and the average recipient was administered 3.1 units in a six month period. These data permit the following computation. Of 323 recipients per 1,000 pints, 6.4 would be expected to have received a positive pint and 316.1 all negative units. Applying the risk frequencies of 15% and 3%, it becomes simple to compute an estimate that cases of transfusion-associated hepatitis in New Jersey following administration of a negative control pint should be 9.9 fold greater in number than those following administration of a positive unit, i.e. slightly less than

90% of all cases of transfusion-associated hepatitis would be expected to have resulted from the use of HBAg-negative pints. This
result, based as it is on extrapolation of low rates from a very
small sampling of recipients of HBAg-negative pints, and for other
reasons that need not be dwelt on here, was believed to represent
only a vague and inaccurate measure. Nevertheless, it indicated
clearly that only a minority of recipients developing transfusion-
associated hepatitis could be expected to have received a pint
testing positive for HBAg and that exclusion of positive pints would
not prevent a majority of cases of transfusion-associated hepatitis.

Careful prospective studies on recipients of HBAg-positive
and HBAg-negative control units tended to confirm these findings by
revealing the occurrence of overt hepatitis in 19% of recipients
of a positive unit and in 3% of negative recipients. HBAg antigenemia was detected, at some time in their course, in 3% of recipients administered negative control units, most of whom had received no untested pints. It became obvious that at least some
of the donors capable of transmitting HBAg-associated hepatitis
could themselves be found to test negative.

A more direct measure of the sensitivity of HBAg tests of
blood donors is obtainable as follows. All known transfusion-associated cases of hepatitis occurring within New Jersey are investigated, whether uncovered by studies, whether reported by physicians,
or found during the course of a statewide hospital records room
search conducted annually. In view of the tracing of every HBAg-
positive pint to recipients, it should be obvious that recording
of hepatitis among recipients of positive pints is likely to be
more complete than it is among recipients of negative pints. Thus,
this type of analysis will tend to be biased in the direction of
attributing excessive sensitivity to HBAg tests.

Information has been accumulated on 289 New Jersey cases of
transfusion-associated hepatitis where one or more of the units
received had been checked for HBAg in our laboratories and where
all of the bloods used were among the first 132,000 tested. Cases
receiving units of blood beyond the time when disclosure and exclusion of HBAg-positive donors was instituted are omitted from
this analysis (Table 2). Of these, all of the 436 bloods administered to 130 recipients had been checked. In only 25 (19%) of
the 130 cases had there been an HBAg-positive pint administered.
Five hundred and seventy-two (54%) of the 1,056 units administered
to the remaining 159 cases had also been checked. If all 159
cases had received at least one HBAg-positive pint, we would expect that a random selection of 54% of 159 cases, i.e. 86, would
have been revealed to receive a positive pint. Actually, only 16
positive units were found, again amounting to 19% of the expected
number.

Table 2. January 1972. The sensitivity of HBAg testing: an analysis of HBAg test results on units administered to recipients incurring hepatitis.

	No. of cases	No. of units adminis-tered	Units tested No.	Units tested Percent	HBAg-positive units detected Ex-pected* No.	HBAg-positive units detected Ob-served No.	Percent of recipients given an HBAg-positive unit
All tested	130	436	436	100	130	25	19
Some tested	159	1,056	572	54	86	16	19
Total	289	1,492	1,008	-	216	41	19

*Assuming that each recipient received one pint testing positive for HBAg.

Since institution of pre-testing, only about 75 HBAg-positive units have actually been administered to recipients. As indicated in Table 3, only 7 of 154 recipients administered fully tested units and only 4 of 82 recipients given 650 units, 68% of which had been tested, have been found thus far to have received an HBAg-positive pint.

Table 3. HBAg results on units administered to recipients developing hepatitis after institution of prescreening

	No. of cases	No. of units given	Units tested No.	Units tested %	No. of HBAg-positive units observed
All tested	154	547	547	100	7
Some tested	82	650	445	68	4
Total	236	1,197	992	83	11

These results provide ample confirmation of the hypothesis that transfusion-associated hepatitis frequently follows the administration of units of blood and packed cells testing negative for HBAg by relatively sensitive immunoelectrophoretic and complement-fixation techniques. They indicate that only 19% of cases of transfusion-associated hepatitis in New Jersey can be prevented by the application of these techniques for the detection of HBAg. These results, however, do not permit us to estimate the relative frequency of undetected, presumably infectious donors who remain undetected because of limitations in the sensitivity of HBAg tests, as opposed to those donors presumed to be transmitting a variety of hepatitis unrelated to HBAg. Let us address ourselves now to this problem.

Table 4. Distribution of incubation periods in tested recipients
following transfusion with HBAg-positive blood

Incubation period (days)	Recipients with HBAg+ hepatitis		Recipients with HBAg- hepatitis	
	Number	Percent	Number	percent
10-19	-	-	-	-
20-29	-	-	1^1	8
30-39	1	6	2^1	15
40-49	-	-	1	8
50-59	3	17	1	8
60-69	3	17	1	8
70-79	2	11	2^1	15
80+	9	50	5^2	38
Total	18	100	13^5	100

* Recipients who were tested for HB antigen 1-21 days after onset
  of first symptoms of hepatitis

[1]&[2]Indicate number of recipients who tested negative for antigen
  after onset of disease, but had tested positive for antigen during incubation period

During the course of these studies, blood specimens have been
submitted to the laboratories of the New Jersey State Department
of Health on 141 cases of transfusion-associated hepatitis where
a) the specimens had been collected during the first 21 days after
onset, and b) all units of blood administered to them had been
tested here for HBAg. Table 4 outlines the results of testing 31
recipients of an HBAg-positive pint who later developed overt hepatitis and indicates that only 58% of the 31 were themselves found
to test HBAg-positive after onset of disease. Interestingly, five
of the 13 recipients who were negative for HBAg after onset of
symptoms had been monitored by bi-weekly bleedings and been found
to be demonstrably HBAg antigenemic before onset, including two of
the three experiencing incubation periods of less than 40 days.
Thus 23 of these 31 cases of hepatitis presented definite evidence
of HBAg-associated disease, and the presumption is strong that
virtually all were HBAg associated. Nevertheless, only 58% of
these recipients of a positive unit tested positive for HBAg during
the first three weeks after onset of first symptoms.

Table 5 presents information accumulated on 110 recipients of
HBAg-negative pints who developed hepatitis and who themselves
were tested for HBAg during the first three weeks after onset.
Thirty-two percent of the 110 cases were, nevertheless, found to
test positive for HBAg. From the results outlined in the previous
table, it appears safe to assume that only about 58% of the HBAg-

associated cases were actually detected. Consequently, we can
estimate that about 55% of cases of transfusion-associated hepatitis
resulting from the administration of HBAg-negative blood were,
nevertheless, related to viral hepatitis type B. During the period
prior to institution of pretesting all pints for HBAg in New
Jersey, we can now estimate that at least 55% of the 81% of cases
of transfusion-associated hepatitis that followed the administration of HBAg-negative blood were, nevertheless, HBAg-associated,
and that at least 45% plus 19%, or 64% of all cases of transfusion-
associated hepatitis were related to hepatitis B virus infection.

Table 5. Distribution of incubation periods in tested recipients
developing hepatitis following transfusion with HBAg-negative
blood*

Incubation period (days)	Recipients with HBAg- hepatitis		Recipients with HBAg+ hepatitis	
	Number	Percent	Number	Percent
10-19	5	7	1	3
20-29	11	15	-	-
30-39	14	19	-	-
40-49	9	12	1	3
50-59	12	16	4	11
60-69	5	7	4	11
70-79	4	5	1	3
80+	9	12	21	60
Unclassifiable	6	8	3	9
	75	100	35	100

*All units administered to all recipients were tested for antigen
and all recipients were tested for antigen 1-21 days after onset
of first symptoms of illness.

Figure 1 represents a flow diagram which may serve to clarify
the calculations that have been performed. Recipients who were administered an HBAg-positive unit made up 19% of all of the cases.
Recipients who were administered HBAg-negative units may be divided
into three categories: 1) those who had detectable HBAg during
the first three weeks of illness and are considered to have suffered
viral hepatitis type B, 2) those who tested negative for HBAg
but, nevertheless, are estimated to have had viral hepatitis type
B, and 3) those who tested negative for HBAg and are considered
to have incurred hepatitis of unknown etiology, possibly viral hepatitis type A. If this analysis is valid, we can also estimate
that the techniques for HBAg detection used in these studies uncovered less than 30% of the pints resulting in transmission of
overt hepatitis type B or, to put it in other words, for every
HBAg-positive pint detected in New Jersey there were, in all probability, at least 2 1/2 times as many that remained undetected.

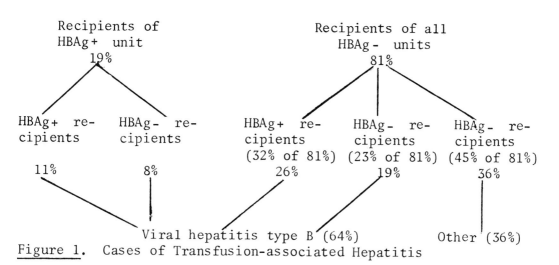

Figure 1. Cases of Transfusion-associated Hepatitis

These results, graphically indicating the need for more sensitive methods for the detection of HBAg, led us to studies of radioimmunoassay techniques. The one presently performed in our laboratory involves the coating of 6 mm glass beads with human anti-HBAg serum, their use in absorbing HBAg from an unknown sample of serum and detection of absorbed HBAg by application of a preparation of highly purified human anti-HBAg antibody tagged with ^{125}I. The technique is relatively simple, easily applied to mass testing, and is between 500 and 1,000 times more sensitive than complement fixation for detection of both ad and ay variants of HBAg antigen. An assessment of the technique's sensitivity with respect to detection of blood units transmitting overt, recognized hepatitis has been completed.

Table 6. The sensitivity of RIA HBAg testing: an analysis of HBAg test results on units administered to recipients incurring hepatitis (March 1972)

	No. of cases	No. of units administered	Units tested No.	Units tested Percent	HBAg-positive units detected Expected* No.	HBAg-positive units detected Observed No.	Percent of recipients given an HBAg-positive unit
All tested	96	266	266	100	96	25	26
Some tested	178	1,144	590	52	93	30	32
Total	274	1,410	856	-	189	55	29

*Assuming that each recipient received one pint testing positive for HBAg.

Table 6 outlines the results of retesting units which had been administered to 274 cases of transfusion-associated hepatitis. Once again, as previously illustrated in Table 2, the analysis is limited to cases that received all of their transfusions in the period prior to exclusion of HBAg-positive donors and prior to institution of pretesting all units for HBAg by conventional techniques. It can be seen that application of this sensitive RIA technique served to detect at least one HBAg-positive unit in only 29% of the cases of transfusion-associated hepatitis studied.

If this result is valid, simple arithmetic permits us to calculate that application of the RIA technique would reveal HBAg-positive pints in 12% of cases of transfusion-associated hepatitis who received units of blood testing HBAg-negative by conventional complement-fixation and immunoelectrophoretic techniques. Table 7 presents results of retesting units which had been administered to 211 recipients in New Jersey after institution of prescreening who, nevertheless, developed hepatitis. It can be seen that a positive unit was detected by the RIA technique in 11% of these cases, substantially as predicted. Thus, studies of cases of transfusion-associated hepatitis indicate that the application of an RIA technique 500-1,000 times as sensitive as complement-fixation, and probably more than 1,000-2,000 times as sensitive as immunoelectrophoresis, would prevent no more than 29% of all cases of transfusion-associated hepatitis in New Jersey and no more than 45% of the cases associated with hepatitis B virus infection.

Table 7. The sensitivity of RIA HBAg testing, recipients developing hepatitis after institution of prescreening**

	No. of cases	No. of units administered	Units tested No.	Units tested Percent	HBAg-positive units detected Expected* No.	HBAg-positive units detected Observed No.	Percent of recipients given an HBAg-positive unit
All tested	112	398	398	100	112	7	6.3
Some tested	99	707	449	64	63	13	
Total	211	1,105	847	-	175	20	21
							11

 *Assuming that each recipient received one pint testing positive for HBAg.
**Cases receiving CF or IE HBAg-positive bloods are omitted from this tabulation.

Up to now, the sole technique employed for estimating the relative frequency of disease related to hepatitis A virus and B virus infection among recipients of blood has been by analysis of incubation periods. The evidence presented in Tables 4 and 5 indicates probable overlap in incubation periods of cases associated with HBAg (assumed to be due to hepatitis B virus) and with others which are presumed to be related to hepatitis A virus infection. Analyses based on distribution of incubation periods, though useful, must be considered to be of relatively limited validity. This paper presents a new approach in estimating the relative frequency of hepatitis B virus infection among cases related to blood transfusion, based on other varieties of epidemiologic information, including studies of HBAg among donors and recipients of blood.

In conclusion, our studies have revealed that about 19% of blood donors transmitting overt, recognized hepatitis in New Jersey can be found to test positive for HBAg by conventional complement-fixation and immunoelectrophoretic techniques, that at least 64% of cases of transfusion-associated hepatitis in the State have been HBAg-associated and that conventional HBAg techniques have revealed less than 30% of the donors involved in hepatitis B virus transmission. Following exclusion of all blood donations by persons testing positive for HBAg by complement-fixation and immunoelectrophoretic techniques in New Jersey, at least 55% of the recipients developing hepatitis can, nevertheless, be expected to do so as a result of hepatitis B virus infection. Application of a sensitive RIA technique for the screening of blood donors would serve to prevent 29% of the cases of transfusion-associated hepatitis or 45% of those related to hepatitis B virus. If all blood donations testing positive by the RIA technique were to be excluded in New Jersey, approximately 49% of the recipients developing hepatitis can be expected, nevertheless, to do so as a result of hepatitis B virus infection.

Clearly, HBAg testing is not yet a panacea and should not detract from our efforts to decrease the excessive usage of blood and the deplorable reliance on commercial donors.

Acknowledgements. These studies were supported, in part, by contract no. NIH-DBS-70-2026 from the Division of Biologics Standards of the National Institutes of Health.

51. Discussion

HEPATITIS ASSOCIATED WITH THE TRANSFUSION OF HBAg-NEGATIVE BLOOD

Herbert F. Polesky

Minneapolis War Memorial Blood Bank

Minneapolis, Minnesota

Dr. Goldfield's interesting and extensive studies on trans-fusion-associated hepatitis in New Jersey point out several impor-tant facts that must be considered in evaluating screening programs for HBAg-positive donors. His data suggests that only 15% of re-cipients given a unit of HBAg (Au, HAA)-positive blood will develop overt hepatitis. Dr. Gocke has recently reported [166] that 33% (28/84) of recipients of HBAg-positive blood in his prospective study done in New York developed overt hepatitis (defined by a bili-rubin in excess of 4 mg/100 ml). Taken together these studies sup-port what many of you suspect, i.e., not all or even most HBAg-posi-tive transfusions result in overt hepatitis.

Dr. Goldfield further documents that 3.3% of recipients of HBAg-negative blood developed overt hepatitis which is similar to the 2.1% (2/94) observed by Gocke.

From these figures Dr. Goldfield suggests that 90% of trans-fusion-associated hepatitis in New Jersey would still occur if units HBAg-positive by CEP or CF were detected. He fails to point out that a recipient is five times more likely to get hepatitis from such units and that there are two donor populations in New Jersey; one of which (Commercial donors - 35% of total bloods) has six times the risk as the other [173].

In asking the question as to the risk of hepatitis from HBAg-negative units we have compared the incidence of overt transfusion-associated hepatitis in Minneapolis before and since HBAg screening has been instituted [380] (Table 1). From our data it appears that more hepatitis has occurred in spite of our testing program.

Table 1. Transfusion associated hepatitis

	HBAg Pos. CEP	RIA	Number Tested
Recipients	9	10	19
Donors	3*	9	191/228
% Total Cases With a pos. donor	16	44	
% Cases given Single donor components	23	62	

* Before routine testing initiated

Table 2. Transfusion associated hepatitis

	1964 - 69	1970 - 71
Units issued	221,891	75,436
Pts. transfused (3 units/pt.)	73,963	25,145
Cases observed	* 30 - 50	* 12 - 18
per 1000 units	0.135 - 0.225	0.159 - 0.239
per 1000 pts.	0.405 - 0.675	0.477 - 0.716

* Single donor components only

I think this partially confirms Dr. Goldfield's observation on the risks of negative units but also can be explained by better reporting of cases since there has been so much publicity about HBAg. Note the first number refers to those recipients getting components from single donors while the larger number includes those getting high risk derivatives such as fibrinogen and Konyne™ [380].

The other very important point illustrated by these data is the lack of sensitivity of the current test methods (Table 2). When radioimmunoassay [295] (RIA) is used to screen implicated donors a positive donor was found in 8/19 (44%) of the cases and if only recipients of a single donor components are considered, a positive donor was found in 8/13 (62%) cases. This suggests that more sensitive screening tests will lessen the risk to the recipient of HBAg-negative blood.

Acknowledgements. The technical assistance of Miss Carol Olson, M.T. (ASCP) and Mrs. Margaret Hanson, M.T. (ASCP) BB, for HBAg testing and Miss Margaret Helgeson, M.T. (ASCP) BB, and Mr. Tom Hoff for art work is greatefully acknowledged.

52. IMMUNOPROPHYLAXIS: VACCINATION

Saul Krugman

Department of Pediatrics, New York University School of

Medicine, New York, New York

Last year Dr. Joan P. Giles, Dr. Jack Hammond and I reported the results of studies on active immunization against viral hepatitis, type B [262]. A heat inactivated preparation was non-infectious, immunogenic, and protective when given to a small group of children. Of 14 children who received one or two inoculations of the experimental vaccine, nine were protected and antibodies have persisted until the present time. The unprotected children had a modified type of viral hepatitis, type B.

This study which has been repeated in a larger group is currently in progress. The final data will not be available for another month or two. In the meantime, the preliminary results are very encouraging. If the present trend continues, the studies on active immunization will be confirmed.

The immunogenic effect of the inactivated vaccine was observed after it was given to an immune individual who had no detectable complement fixation (CF) antibody to HBAg but did have a titer of 1:128 when a passive hemagglutination assay was used. Seven days later there was a 16-fold increase in passive hemagglutination assay was used. Seven days later there was a 16-fold increase in passive hemagglutination titer, rising to a level of 1:16 [384]; the CF titer rose to 1:16. This study confirmed the immunogenic capacity of the inactivated vaccine.

53. OPEN DISCUSSION : POST-TRANSFUSION HEPATITIS

Marcel E. Conrad

Walter Reed Army Institute of Pathology, Washington D.C.

The older literature contains several articles that suggest that gamma globulin administration provides protection against serum (transfusion-associated) hepatitis [184,241,322] while others state that gamma globulin injections have no protective effect [105,213]. An obvious possibility to explain the apparent disparity in results of these studies is that there is some difference in the lots of gamma globulin used. Presently, it seems logical to attribute this difference to the anti-HBAg titer of the gamma globulin.

There are two clinical studies that suggest that the anti-HBAg titer of the gamma globulin may be an important factor in protecting subjects against HBAg hepatitis. One is a study performed from our institution in which we observed that a lot of gamma globulin with an elevated anti-HBAg titer (as compared to several other lots of available gamma globulin) significantly diminished the incidence of HBAg hepatitis [106,164]. The other study was performed at Willowbrook [263] and showed that a specially prepared lot of gamma globulin with a high anti-HBAg titer protected children against HBAg (MS-2) hepatitis. In both of these studies the protection afforded in the gamma globulin-treated groups is convincing, but the relationship between the anti-HBAg titers in the gamma globulin and the salutory effect is conjectural. In our studies, the protective gamma globulin had a reciprocal dilution titer of 1280 by radioimmunoassay, whereas several commercial lots of gamma globulin had titers varying from 20 to 180. However, passive hemagglutination assay of our protective gamma globulin showed only a titer of 4. Further, in the published study from Willowbrook there is no convincing evidence that the gamma globulin preparation with a passive hemagglutination titer for anti-HBAg of 1:260,000 was significantly more protective than a lot of gamma globulin with a

titer of 1:16.

During recent months we have collected aliquots of the gamma globulin that was used in the varius transfusion studies referenced in paragraph 2 above, and made comparisons with our gamma globulin preparations. Aliquots were sent in a coded manner both to Dr. Purcell of NIH and Dr. Overby of Abbott Laboratories. Dr. Purcell has verbally reported that he found no significant titers of anti-HBAg in any of the preparations. Dr. Overby has provided a comprehensive analysis using both a sandwich type radioimmunoassay and a precipitation method of radioimmunoassay for both subtypes ad and ay. Selected findings are shown in Table 1 and reported as standard deviations from a negative control.

Table 1.

	Sandwich Method		Precipitating Method	
	ad	ay	ad	ay
Korean Study [106]				
Lot 3	113	21	52	30
Lot 4	11	20	46	35
Mirich et al. [322]				
California Lot	37	15	22	17
Katz et al. [241]				
Swiss Lot	--	--	23	42
Armour Lot	--	--	0	3
Holland et al. [213]				
Squibb 357	48	22	30	16
Squibb 337	22	12	25	12
Armour	23	15	31	19
Cooperative Study [105]				
Squibb RC-5	46	36	46	27
Squibb 337-3	20	14	27	21
Squibb RC-7	65	33	43	35
Merch C7270	12	10	26	21

Gamma globulin from screened AGD negative plasma 9-26
Gamma globulin from AGD positive plasma >500
*Swiss type gamma globulin

It is evident from the above data that it would be difficult to predict that protection against HBAg hepatitis would be observed in the first three studies but not in the last two. Aside from the consideration that the protection observed in the first three studies was due to chance, four possibilities must be considered to explain these findings:
  1. Australia antibody (anti-HBAg) is not the protective factor in gamma globulin (perhaps we should be screening for antibodies against Dane particles rather than for anti-HBAg);

2. methods for testing anti-HBAg are crude and of insufficient sensitivity;
3. different methods of preparing gamma globulin may produce changes in the antibody protective effect disproportionate to "in vitro" observations; and
4. different periods of storage (3-10 years) and variable storage temperatures (4°C., -15°C.) may sufficiently alter antibody titers so that the recent anti-HBAg testing does not reflect the anti-HBAg titers in the gamma globulin at the time the human studies were performed.

For the reasons stated above, I believe that studies of the effect of gamma globulin containing various amounts of anti-HBAg must contain a control group receiving a non-gamma-globulin placebo solution for comparison with groups receiving gamma globulin that contains either a low titer of anti-HBAg or a high titer of anti-HBAg. Otherwise, the results of experiments may be uninterpretable. We safely used an albumin potassium glutamate solution as a placebo with no difficulty in more than 40,000 soldiers in Korea. Since the value, the lack of value, and perhaps even the unsalutory effects of gamma-globulin in certain types of studies remain to be determined, this approach would seem to be ethically defensible and essential from a scientific viewpoint.

PROPAGATION OF VIRAL CANDIDATES

Chairman: F. Deinhardt

54. RECENT HEPATITIS TYPE A VIRUS (HAV) CANDIDATES

Joseph L. Melnick

Department of Virology and Epidemiology, Baylor

College of Medicine, Houston, Texas

Recovery of an etiological agent from type A hepatitis patients has generally been unsuccessful, as previously reviewed by Mosley and others [329,342]. However, several recent attempts to propagate the virus in tissue culture or in subhuman primates and to detect an interfering factor deserve comment.

Studies in marmosets. Deinhardt and co-workers [127,129,215] have produced biochemical and histological evidence of hepatitis without clinical manifestations in marmosets, particularly white-lipped, following inoculation of certain human acute phase hepatitis type A sera. With one particular sample, Barker (serum obtained from the marmosets during the acute phase of their infection, i.e. when transaminase elevations and liver changes occurred) was capable of transmitting the infection to other marmosets in series. Despite these encouraging reports, (a) standard commercial human gamma globulin preparations capable of neutralizing hepatitis type A virus (HAV) in man, (b) convalescent human serum from HAV patients, and (c) convalescent marmoset serum failed to neutralize the infectivity of the Barker hepatitis agent in marmosets [127,374]. However, marmosets were resistant to a second inoculation of the Barker strain. Animals which developed "subclinical" hepatitis after inoculation with other HAV material, particularly with the MS-1 strain, remained fully susceptible to the Barker strain [127]. A virus indistinguishable from the Barker strain in its properties and its antigenicity has been isolated from sham-inoculated and biopsied cotton-topped marmosets [373]. Cotton-topped marmosets have proven fully susceptible to the Barker isolate [127,129,374], but have responded less well [215] or not at all [373] when inoculated with acute human sera obtained from viral hepatitis type A patients, including those proven to contain infectious HAV. However,

Holmes et al. [215] present further evidence of the marmoset response to plasma of hepatitis type A patients. In this study, 14
specimens (acute phase hepatitis type A or normal control sera)
were inoculated under code into groups of marmosets and were correctly identified. Marmosets developed biochemical and histological
evidence of hepatitis, but the agent has not yet been passed serially and, as indicated above, the responding marmosets fail to
develop immunity to the Barker hepatitis virus.

     Studies in Detroit-6 cells. Boggs et al. studied volunteers
who received an oral dose of MS-1 serum (HAV) or acute phase plasma (K-30) from a patient who developed hepatitis following exposure to MS-1 in a previous study [65,312]. As shown in Table 1,

Table 1. Infectious hepatitis: Transmission to volunteers [312]

Exposed and Control groups studied	Oral Administration			Subcutaneous Administration	
	Phase 1 MS-1 serum 0.05 ml	Phase 2 F-29 plasma 0.1 ml	Phase 3 K-30 plasma 0.1 ml	Phase 4 K-30 0.1 ml	
				infected (MS-1 or K-30 given orally)	resistant (MS-1 or K-30 given orally)
Infected exposed	3/10	0/10	5/10	0/3	2/4
Infected controls*	0/5	0/5	0/5		

* Received bovine plasma or pre-exposure volunteer serum.

three men who developed hepatitis following the oral administration
of HAV showed immunity to the disease when serially rechallenged
subcutaneously 1.5 to 3 years later. However, 2 of 4 other volunteers who had not been infected, clinically or subclinically, after
oral administration of HAV developed clinical hepatitis following
the parenteral inoculation of K-30 plasma. The other two continued
to resist infection. The results suggest that immunity acquired
following natural exposure to HAV may not be solid, but may be
dependent upon the dose or route by which subsequent exposures
occur.

     At the time these studies were being conducted, a Detroit-6
(D6) clone was found to be sensitive to a number of acute phase
sera from the above volunteers [313], as well as to acute phase
sera from type A hepatitis patients in the Houston area. Electron
micrographs of infected D6 cells sometimes showed tremendous accu-
mulations of particles in the 20 nm range (see Figures 1, 2 and 3).

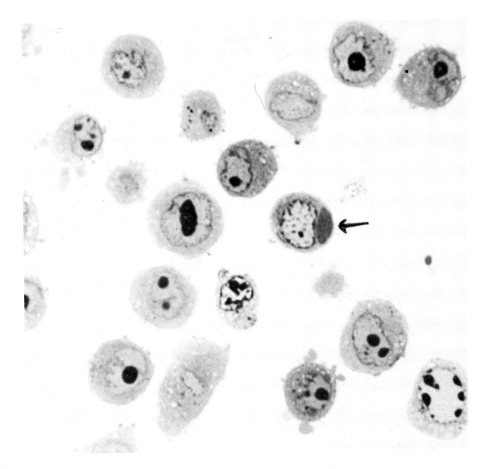

Figure 1. A thin section of D6 cells fixed for electron microscopy. The arrow points to an inclusion body, that is shown at high magnification in Figure 2.

Tissue culture fluids also yielded such particles. On passage this clone was lost. Passage of the virus into other D6 clones led to ready establishment of the Kirk virus, but the new lines were no longer susceptible to the original human materials. The virus being passed in the later D6 cells was identified as a DNA-containing parvovirus (picodnavirus) which is heat-stable and resistant to low pH and overnight ether treatment [323]. Antigenically, it cross-reacts with Kilham's rat virus and with Toolan's H3 virus [130,323] and also with Maynard's HS-3 virus recovered from passage material of human embryonic lung cell cultures originally inoculated with acute phase fecal material from a child with hepatitis type A [306]. Hemagglutination-inhibition antibody to the Kirk agent has been observed in normal rat sera, but not in convalescent sera from patients with hepatitis type A. It is unlikely that an etiological relationship exists between this virus and hepatitis type A. However, acute phase hepatitis specimens, which may contain a factor that interferes with the growth of echovirus [313], may act in the

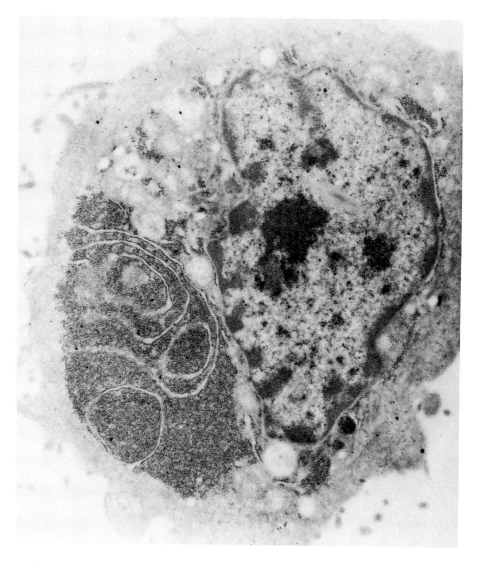

Figure 2. Electron microscopy of a D6 cell infected with Ga virus. Note that the inclusion body shown in the cytoplasm is made of large numbers of 20 nm particles. (x 28,000)

role of a "helper virus", activating a parvovirus latently infecting the D6 cells. The virus ultimately propagated in D6 cells grew poorly unless adenovirus type 7a was added as a helper when the parvovirus yields were increased 100-fold [323].

Interference Tests. The results of the safety tests on samples of plasma from three of the volunteers listed in Table 1 are shown in Table 2. No cytopathic effect (CPE) was detected in any of the GMK or HEK tube cultures inoculated with these samples, or in cultures in which passages were made. No hemadsorbing agents

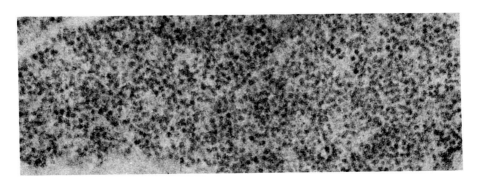

Figure 3. Same cell as shown in Figure 2, but showing the 20 nm particles in the center of the inclusion at a higher magnification.

Table 2. Results of safety tests of plasma from volunteers who received serum containing MS-1 infectious hepatitis virus [313].

Plasma from volunteers*	Cytopathic effect at passage		Hemadsorption at passage		Interference with echovirus at passage**	
	First	Second	First	Second	First	Second
C	none	none	none	none	4	4
F	none	none	none	none	4	4
K	none	none	none	none	0	4
Echovirus 11	---	---	---	---	4	4

* Plasma was obtained 37 days after infection.
**Cultures were challenged with echovirus 10 days after inoculation of plasma. Degree of echovirus cytopathic effect: 0 = no effect; 1 = 25% of cells involved; 2 = 50% of cells involved; 3 = 75% of cells involved; 4 = 100% of cells involved.

were detected in replicate cultures inoculated with either the original plasma or the first-passage material from the original cultures. No agent interfering with echovirus was detected in cell cultures inoculated with plasma obtained from subjects C and F. In these cultures the appearance of the CPE due to echovirus paralleled that in the viral control cultures. In contrast, cultures inoculated with the plasma taken from patient K on day 37 showed complete suppression of CPE due to echovirus 48 hr after challenge, when CPE in the viral controls was 3-4+. This interference effect was lost on passage of harvests of unchallenged replicate cultures in either HEK or GMK cultures.

The possibility existed that the interference was due to the presence of neutralizing antibodies against echovirus 11 in the plasma of K. To exclude this, we tested various samples of plasma from K at a dilution of 1:10 for the presence of neutralizing antibodies. For determination of whether the interference was specific

for the acute-phase sample, additional cell cultures were inoculated
with samples of plasma taken before infection and on days 30, 37,
and 100 after infection. These were challenged with echovirus 10
days after inoculation of the plasma. Results of the tests are
presented in Table 3. None of the samples of plasma neutralized
the echovirus. CPE due to echovirus in cultures inoculated with

Table 3. Assay of samples of plasma from patient K for neutralizing
antibodies to echovirus 11 and for factor that interferes with
replication of this echovirus [313].

Sample	Neutralization	Interference
Serum, before infection	4*	4
Plasma, 30 days after infection	3	0
Plasma, 37 days after infection	3	0
Plasma, 100 days after infection	3	4
Echovirus control	4	4

* Numbers represent degree (on a 0 - 4 scale) of echovirus CPE 36
hr after challenge.

the mixture of virus and plasma developed at the same time as in
the viral controls. When tested for interference, neither the
serum taken before infection nor the plasma taken 100 days after
administration of the virus of infectious hepatitis interfered
with echovirus 11. However, plasmas taken on both day 30 and
day 37 interfered with development of echovirus CPE.

We did experiments to determine if the early agent isolated
in D6 cells from the plasma of K also interfered with the echovirus.
HEK of GMK cells were inoculated, respectively, with 0.1 ml of (a)
K virus after 11 and 15 passages in D6 cells, (b) the virus after
an additional passage in HEK or GMK cells, and (c) harvests of uninoculated, passaged D6 control cells. After adsorption for 1 hr
at 37°C, maintenance medium was added, and cells were incubated
at 37°C for nine days. At this time, 100 $TCID_{50}$ of echovirus was
added to the cultures. The early K virus grown in D6 cells interfered with echovirus, but the ability to interfere was lost after
one passage in HEK or GMK cells. Control material from uninoculated
D6 cells failed to interfere. The titer of the interfering agent
was 10^4 interfering doses/ml, about the same as the $TCID_{50}$ infectivity titer of these passages in D6 cells.

Samples from five volunteers who developed hepatitis after
receiving K-30 [65] were tested for interference (Table 4). The

Table 4. Interference and neutralization tests in African green monkey renal cells with plasma from subjects who ingested plasma taken from patient K 30 days after infection.*

Plasma, patient and day	Interference test	Standard neutralization test
R, 0	No	0
23	Yes	0
25	No	0
27	Yes	0
Mc, 0	No	0
27	Yes	0
30	Yes	0
B, 0	No	0
40	Yes	0
105	No	0
M, 0	No	0
36	No	0
S, 0	NT†	+
49	NT	+

*Taken from reference 313.
†NT indicates no test could be read because of detection of antibody in the tube culture neutralization test.

samples taken from three of the volunteers before infection and the one late sample tested (patient B, day 105) did not interfere with echovirus. In contrast, several samples of acute-phase plasmas interfered with the CPE of echovirus. Samples of plasma taken from R on days 23 and 27 were positive, but the plasma of R on day 25 was negative. Samples of plasma taken from Mc on days 27, 30 and 40 were also positive. It must be emphasized that the interference was usually transitory: CPE of echovirus was delayed for only 24-48 hrs. after the controls had reached a CPE of 4+. However, in cells inoculated with the plasma taken from B on day 40, the CPE due to echovirus did not develop until 72 hrs after the control had reached a CPE of 4+. Samples of plasma from subject S neutralized the echovirus in the tube neutralization test and, therefore, could not be used for testing of interference. Plasma of M taken on day 36 was the only acute-phase sample tested from this patient. It did not interfere with the challenge by echovirus and was also negative in D6 cells.

It should be pointed out that in order to detect the development of an interfering factor at low concentration, sera collected prior to infection and again during infection must be available.

Intrinsic interference test. Carver and Seto [83] have reported other studies on detecting an interfering agent in hepatitis sera from both hepatitis A and hepatitis B patients. As shown in Figure 4, Newcastle disease virus (NDV) is used as the

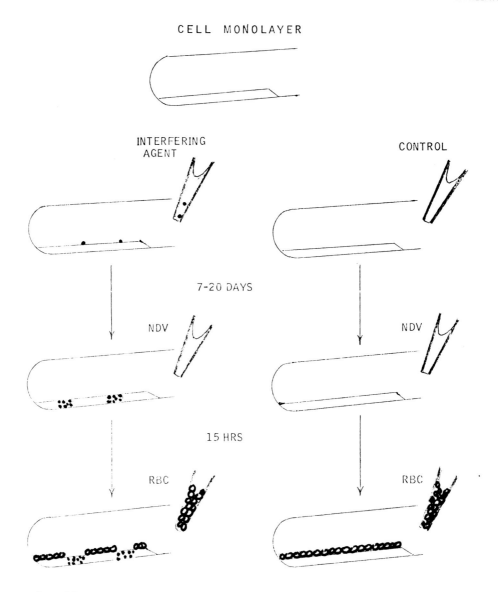

Figure 4. Diagrammatic representation of how bovine red blood cells are adsorbed by cells in which NDV replicates (NDV being the challenge virus). The cells infected with the unknown or test virus are refractory to NDV superinfection and do not adsorb red blood cells.

challenge virus. Bovine red blood cells are adsorbed by cells in which NDV replicates, whereas test virus-infected cells are re-fractory to NDV superinfection and therefore do not adsorb red blood cells (RBC). This type of interference is not mediated through interferon and is termed intrinsic interference. Attempts to confirm this work are being made by Vorndam in our laboratory, who has provided Figures 5, 6, and 7. Figure 5 shows a cell sheet

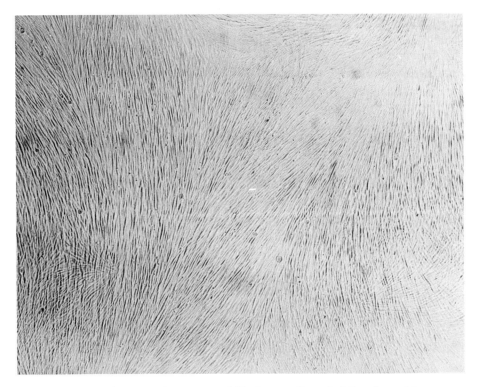

Figure 5. Cell sheet prior to addition of red blood cells.

Figure 6. Control culture treated with NDV and RBC. Complete
hemadsorption is evident, indicating the absence of virus other
than NDV

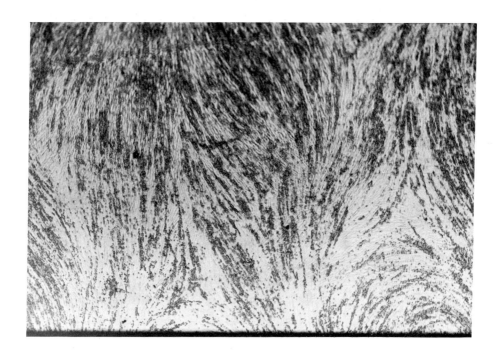

Figure 7. Culture first treated with a positive serum. Note the negative hemadsorption areas which indicate the possible loss of susceptibility to NDV by the cells.

which looks normal, prior to the addition of RBC. Figures 6 and 7 show cell cultures treated with NDV and RBC. Figure 6 shows complete hemadsorption, indicating that no other virus was present. Figure 7 shows a culture that had been treated with hepatitis serum. Negative hemadsorption areas are evident, indicating that the cells had lost their susceptibility to NDV. These results are preliminary and not yet reproducible in our laboratory [473].

Carver and Seto have obtained positive tests for intrinsic interference with HAV samples. The effect has been passed 5 times serially in WI-38 cultures, indicating that an agent is being transferred. Treatment of their HAV with 3 different batches of human gamma globulin prevented the production of interference. Their preliminary results support the most encouraging new candidate hepatitis virus. Unfortunately, the interference is transitory, similar to the transitory interference we noticed with echovirus. This makes the procedure very difficult to control, and several hundred cultures must be used for each test. Nevertheless, if this leads to a test for hepatitis A virus, the effort will be worthwhile.

Acknowledgments. Studies from the Baylor Laboratory were aided by Research Contract DADA 17-67C-7004, from the U.S. Army Medical Research and Development Command.

RECENT HEPATITIS TYPE A VIRUS (HAV) CANDIDATES

Friedrich Deinhardt

Presbyterian-St. Luke's Hospital, Department of
Microbiology
Chicago, Illinois

In this presentation Dr. Melnick raises several questions,
each of which I will consider in some detail.

Studies in marmosets. In discussing studies of hepatitis type
A in marmosets, Dr. Melnick continues to question the origin of the
agents causing hepatitis in marmosets, even though the possibility
that isolation of hepatitis viruses in marmosets represents an activation of latent marmoset agents has been discussed repeatedly
[215, Spl.b-d,i]. There are several points to be made to this issue:

a) in several independent series of experiments, coded specimens of preinoculation sera and acute phase sera from adult, human
volunteers, inoculated with the MS-1 strain of hepatitis type A, have
been correctly identified. No disease was observed in marmosets
inoculated with preinoculation sera, whereas hepatitis was induced
consistently in those marmosets inoculated with acute phase sera.

b) the difficulties encountered in neutralizing the agents
causing hepatitis in marmosets have been discussed previously in
considerable detail [Spl. c,d]. Here, I will just repeat that as
even convalescent sera of marmosets fail to neutralize the agents
in neutralization tests employing an intravenous challenge route,
it is probable that the failure to neutralize agents in marmosets
with human sera or gamma globulin is due to the inadequacy of theee
test system rather than to antigenic differences. In future
experiments we will attempt to enhance neutralization by removing antigen/antibody complexes from neutralization mixture
by use of anti-antibodies, thus preventing antigenic dissociation
after intravenous inoculation of the mixture. In addition, in a

very recent experiment, the induction of hepatitis in marmosets
was prevented or attenuated when the acute phase serum of one of
the MS-1 volunteers was preincubated with the convalescent phase
serum from the same volunteer (Holmes, A. W., Wolfe, L. and Deinhardt, F., unpublished data).

c) several laboratories have isolated agents antigenically
similar to the Barker agent from marmosets inoculated with human
hepatitis materials [299, Spl. a,e]. With the single exception
of Dr. Melnick's own laboratory [373,374] disease was not observed
in control animals, nor were agents indistinguishable in properties
and antigenicity from the Barker agent isolated from sham-inoculated
marmosets.

In this respect it is re-emphasized that before use in such
experiments, marmosets should be fully acclimated to the laboratory
environment and their liver function values must lie within the
normal range. Most wild-caught marmosets have parasitic and other
liver pathology, which is however, easily distinguisable from viral
hepatitis, and elevated serum enzymes can result from many conditions
other than viral hepatitis. However, no hepatitis viruses were
isolated in extensive control experiments with sera selected from
uninoculated, recently imported and not acclimated, marmosets with
indigenous elevated serum enzyme levels, which were inoculated into
other marmosets [f].

d) the lack of cross-protection between MS-1 and Barker does
not support an assumption that hepatitis in marmosets is caused by
activation of latent marmoset agents rather than by the inoculation
of human hepatitis materials, as it is probable that more than one
antigenic type of hepatitis type A viruses exists.

Studies in Detroit-6 cells and interference tests. It is clear
that the "isolation" of K-30 by Boggs, Melnick et al. in D-6 cells
represents laboratory contamination with a strain of the ubiquitous
and highly stable, rodent parvoviruses and is unrelated to human
viral hepatitis [312,323,Spl. d]. The remote possibility that a
human IH virus was carried simultaneously in the D-6 cultures, but
through attenuation had become incapable of producing disease in
marmosets while still capable of infecting and inducing immunity,
was tested by inoculation of the "K-30 agent" into marmosets and
later challenge with original K-30 serum. No animals inoculated
with the "K-30 agent isolated in D-6 cells" developed hepatitis,
and this group of marmosets was as susceptible as control animals
to later inoculation with the original K-30 serum.

The interference observed in Dr. Melnick's laboratory [313],
as well as the "intrinsic interference" reported by Carver and Seto
[83], is interesting but has not yielded a reproducible test system

yet. Results obtained with these tests must be viewed with considerable caution therefore, and at this time I consider that it would be premature to regard them as evidence for the cultivation of hepatitis viruses in cell culture.

56. PRELIMINARY OBSERVATION OF THE TISSUE CULTURE OF THE SERUM HEPATITIS VIRUS

A. J. Zuckerman and Pamela M. Baines

London School of Hygiene and Tropical Medicine,
Hepatitis Unit,
London, Great Britain

The failure to isolate the hepatitis viruses in tissue culture has been a major obstacle to progress in this field. The association between Australia antigen and serum hepatitis or type B viral hepatitis has provided a specific serological marker of infection with, or carriage of, the serum hepatitis virus. There is considerable evidence now that Asutralia antigen represents excess virus-coat material.

Brighton, Taylor and Zuckerman [73] reported the induction of progressive changes in monolayer cultures of human embryo liver cells following inoculation with a known infective hepatitis serum. There was progressive involvement of the normal cellular components of the cultured hepatocytes, as demonstrated by specific fluorescent antibody attachment, first in the cytoplasm, then in the perinuclear membrane and finally marked condensation in the nucleoli. Similar progressive changes were observed in cells of liver cell cultures inoculated with supernatant fluid which has been since passaged in culture twice. Coyne, Millman and Blumberg [131] reported virtually identical fluorescent changes in liver cells cultured from biopsy material obtained from a patient with circulating Australia antigen. After six passages of the cells, the cultured cells were still found to contain Australia antigen in the nuclei and the antigen was also detected by radioimmunoassay in the supernatant fluid.

Baines, Taylor and Zuckerman [28] developed a technique for maintaining successfully human embryo liver organ cultures. These cultures are being used for the inoculation of serum specimens from patients and carriers of type B viral hepatitis and some preliminary results have already been reported [496]. More recently, Zuckerman, Baines and Almeida [498] reported the apparently successful replication of the serum hepatitis virus, as far as it can be based on measurement of Australia antigen, in human embryo liver organ cultures.

A serum specimen, collected from a jaundiced patient, R.B., with viral hepatitis and which was found to contain Australia antigen, was used for inoculation of the cultures. Serum G.C. was obtained from an apparently healthy volunteer blood donor whose blood had caused two deaths from post-transfusion hepatitis in recipients of his blood. Australia antigen has been demonstrated in this serum by serological tests and by electron microscopy.

The inoculated sera were incubated with the organ cultures for 72 hours at 35°C. The organ culture fluid was then replaced with fresh medium and the incubation continued. The culture fluids together with the liver fragments were harvested after 6 and 8 days. This material was rapidly frozen and thawed three times and the resulting fluid used for examination for Australia antigen.

Australia antigen could not be demonstrated in the supernatant fluid by immunodiffusion, complement fixation or by radioimmunoassay after 3 days incubation. Progressive rise in the titre of Australia antigen was obtained, however, with both serum R.B. and G.C., from a complement-fixing titre of 1:4 at 6 days to 1:128 after 8 days in culture. In the two dimensional micro-Ouchterlony technique there was an increase in precipitin titre from 0 at 6 days to a titre of 1:4 with the 8th day's organ culture harvest. The same specimens were also examined by the technique of immune electron microscopy. Examination of the original inocula revealed, in each, small aggregates of particles now associated with Australia antigen. On the 6th day of the original cultures, which were infected with R.B. and G.C., electron microscopy revealed a small number of aggregates built-up with typical Australia antigen particles. These aggregates were small and rather sparse. By day 8 the grids contained numerous large aggregates typical of Australia antigen.

The control preparations and cultures inoculated with a normal serum remained negative by all serological tests for Australia antigen and on electron microscopic examination.

The fluid harvested from the 8 day's cultures, inoculated with both serum R.B. and serum G.C., was passaged into fresh organ cultures. There was no detectable complement-fixing activity in the tissue fluid harvested after 6 days and only a slight rise in the complement-fixing titre to 1:2 with the G.C. passage harvest material at 8 days. The immunodiffusion test on both the 6th and 8th day was negative. No complement-fixing nor precipitin reactions were detected in the 6th day harvest from R.B. passage material. On the other hand, although complement was fixed only to a titre of 1:4 at 8 days with R.B. passage material, a sharply defined precipitin line was obtained in the gel diffusion test, showing a line of immunological identity with known reference Australia antigen.

Immune electron microscopy carried out on the first passage material yielded impressive results. Day 6 of the G.C. passage material showed very scanty small aggregates, and examination of the specimen from day 8 showed only a very small increase in the number of Australia antigen particles. Similar findings were obtained on day 6 of the R.B. first passage material. But, on day 8 the specimen was found to contain considerably more Australia antigen than had been seen in any of the previous specimens, including the original starting serum. Many of the aggregates were too large for high resolution microscopy and only the thinly spread areas at the edge of the aggregates could be photographed.

The passage controls and serum negative controls were entirely negative by complement fixation, immunodiffusion, electron microscopy and radioimmunoassay.

Australia antigen is widely recognized as a specific marker of infection with the serum hepatitis virus. It is concluded therefore, that apparent replication of the serum hepatitis virus, as far as it can be based on measurement of Australia antigen, has taken place in organ cultures of human embryo liver. Further serial passages are in progress and the growth characteristics of the serum hepatitis virus are being studied. It may well be that after a period of adaptation on fetal liver organ cultures the agent of serum hepatitis could be grown on standard continuous cell lines.

Acknowledgments. This work is supported by generous grants from the World Health Organization (Virus Diseases), Pfizer Ltd., Sandwich, Kent and in part by a grant from the Medical Research Council.

It is a pleasure to record our sincere thanks to Dr. H. E. M. Kay and his staff of the Royal Marsden Hospital, London, for the supply of tissue.

57. Discussion

PRELIMINARY OBSERVATION OF THE TISSUE CULTURE OF THE SERUM HEPATITIS VIRUS

Joseph L. Melnick

Baylor College of Medicine, Department of Virology
and Epidemiology,
Houston, Texas

The recent results presented by Dr. Zuckerman augur well for
the future of hepatitis research. Hopefully hepatitis B virus will
be mastered and the conditions will become accurately defined for
its growth in culture. I am somewhat surprised that only 20 nm
particles were found in the culture fluids. Where are the Dane
particles, which, from Almeida's work, may be more representative
of hepatitis virus?

It would appear that we had some modest success in growing
Dane particles in tissue culture. We carried out experiments [234]
in which serum containing hepatitis type B antigen (HBAg) was inoculated onto human lymph node explants and incubated. The inoculum was characterized by an abundance of small 20 nm particles,
some filaments, and a few Dane particles. Ten days post-inoculation,
HBAg could be detected in the tissue culture fluids and Dane-like
particles (30-44 nm in diameter) and filaments were abundant (See
Figure 1). Thin sections also were positive for virus-like particles [234].

Recently, we have observed by electron microscopy some serum
preparations from patients with viral hepatitis type B that were
extremely rich in Dane particles, as demonstrated in Figure 2.
Striking similarities were observed between these particles and
those observed earlier in tissue culture.

In order to more closely compare the two populations, investigations have been undertaken to selectively separate out and
purify the larger particles. However, initial experiments using
the purification procedure of Dreesman et al. [135] have resulted

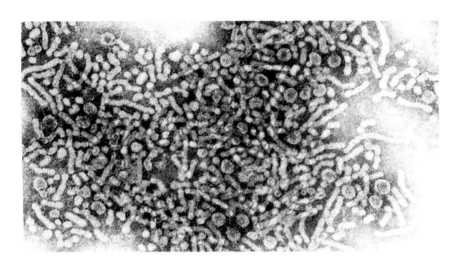

Figure 1. Negative stained preparation of organ culture fluid containing HBAg. 3 distinctive types of particles are shown in this large aggregation: rod-shaped, variable length and diameter; small sperical and ellipsoid-shaped, 18-28 nm diameter; large double-shelled, 30-40 nm diameter (X150,000) [234].

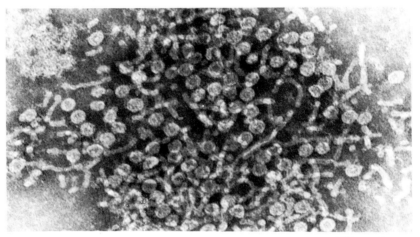

Figure 2. Untreated plasma from a type B hepatitis patient. The sample is extraordinarily rich in Dane particles.

in the disappearance of the Dane particles, leaving only the smaller ones, primarily 22 nm in size. Perhaps the Dane particles become unstable when treated at low pH (2.4), which is a step in the purification method applied. Earlier [234] we called attention to similar variations in morphology of cowpea chlorotic mottle virus that had been studied by Bancroft [29].

        Acknowledgements. Studies from the Baylor laboratory were aided by Research Contract NIH-2231, from the National Heart and Lung Institute, National Institutes of Health.

58. STUDIES OF HEPATITIS CANDIDATE AGENTS IN TISSUE CULTURES AND IN ANIMAL MODELS

J. E. Maynard, K. R. Berquist, and D. H. Krushak

Center for Disease Control, Phoenix Laboratories,

Phoenix, Arizona

Introduction. A viral etiology for both types A and B hepatitis was proposed early in this century by investigators engaged in epidemiologic studies of community outbreaks of disease and of illness following mass inoculation with such human blood-derived products as mumps convalescent plasma and yellow fever vaccine [151, 219, 489]. It was not until the mid 1940's, however, that these etiologies were firmly established in a series of World War II human volunteer experiments [195, 302, 347]. Since that time numerous efforts have been made to propagate the viruses responsible for both forms of hepatitis in cell cultures as well as in animal models.

With the exception of the major breakthrough established with the discovery of the hepatitis B or "Australia" antigen and its subsequent link to the virus of hepatitis B, seldom has so much concentrated research effort yielded so little progress. Part of this sense of frustration is reflected in the changing and imprecise usage of the term "candidate agent" as related to hepatitis. Whereas, in the more rigorous sense this term has been applied to any previously uncharacterized viral agent isolated from appropriate specimen materials, it has also been used to describe already well-characterized agents simply because they were isolated from cases of hepatitis. More recently it has even been applied to classes of physical particles seen in acute illness phase specimens by electronmicroscopy; such particles being often rather optimistically termed "virus like". It is the purpose of this presentation to review briefly some of the recent work related to the study of agents possibly related to hepatitis in tissue culture systems and in animal models.

Tissue Culture. In the late 1940's and early 1950's extensive efforts were made to propagate agents from appropriate specimen materials in embryonated hens' eggs. This work was best represented by that of Henle and associates in 1950 [200]. Lack of
reproducibility of results which looked initially promising led to
a curtailment of efforts in this area. The later reports by Kubelka
of propagation of an agent in eggs initially termed "Motol virus"
and later characterized as a possible paramyxovirus unrelated to
hepatitis resulted in a similar discontinuation of effort with
this cell culture system [269].

With the increase in virologic technical sophistication and
and the successful adaptation and propagation of a wide variety
of cell culture systems in the late 1950's and early 1960's, another
resurgence of effort at the isolation of hepatitis viruses occurred.
To cite a few examples: in 1961 O'Malley reported the isolation
of an agent called A-1 virus in primary rabbit kidney cell cul⁺ure
following inoculation with the NIH icterogenic plasma pool [369].
This agent was later identified as a mycoplasma with no comment as
to its origin [368]. Again in 1961, Chang reported the isolation
of an agent in human liver cell cultures inoculated with acute
illness phase blood from 4 hepatitis patients [90]. The agent was
characterized as a lipovirus and the author later concluded that
its relation to hepatitis was purely fortuitous [91]. In 1962
Hsiung and colleagues reported isolation of a virus on both human
and rhesus-monkey cell cultures inoculated with whole blood from
a fatal case of hepatitis [221]. The agent was found to be immunologically identical to SV5 virus, and although promising results
were found in human serologic testing of hepatitis cases and controls [230], the work was not pursued further. In 1964, Liebhaber
isolated 3 agents in the WI-38 cell line of human diploid fibro-
blasts inoculated with urine and blood from hepatitis patients at
the Willowbrook State School [292]. These agents were later
characterized as myxoviruses related to SV5 virus and probably not
hepatitis causative agents [293].

One of the more interesting series of communications in which
a known group of viruses was associated with type A hepatitis was
initiated by the report of Davis, in 1961, of virus recoveries in
human embryonic lung (HEL) from stools of 14 of 21 children who
became ill during a community outbreak of disease [125]. These
viruses, originally termed "San Carlos" agents were, with one exception, subsequently identified as adenoviruses (types 1 and 3)
[192]. In 1966, Hartwell reported the isolation of adenovirus
type 5 in the same cell culture system from blood clots of 27 of
30 patients ill with hepatitis [190]. The virus was also isolated
from all of 12 family contacts of two of the cases, but from only
one of 70 unrelated individuals without hepatitis. That the association of adenoviruses with hepatitis was not etiologic has been

inferred from the infrequency with which these viruses have been
isolated from hepatitis cases in other laboratories, by the lack
of association of hepatitis with outbreaks of adenoviral illnesses,
and by the failure of human volunteers to develop hepatitis after
infection with adenoviruses.

Perhaps the most protracted and exhaustive studies related to
the isolation of hepatitis viruses in cell culture began with the
initial report of the Parke-Davis group, in 1956, of the recovery
of cytopathic agents in a cloned line of neoplastic human marrow
cells (Detroit-6) inoculated with serum or stool of patients ill
with viral hepatitis [409]. Considerable study of these agents together with extensive efforts to define satisfactorily the sensitivity characteristics of the Detroit-6 (D-6) cell line were followed by a series of human volunteer experiments using several
designated viral prototypes [64]. These experiments produced equivocal results.

Because of the lack of reproducibility of the Parke-Davis
findings in other laboratories and difficulty in working with D-6
cells, further research with these agents and with this tissue
culture cell line was largely discontinued until 1970 when Boggs
and Melnick and associates reported recovery of an agent (Kirk
virus) on D-6 cells inoculated with acute-illness phase plasma of
a volunteer who developed hepatitis 30 days after ingestion of
human serum known to contain the virus of hepatitis A [65, 313].
This agent was subsequently characterized by the Houston group as
a parvovirus immunologically similar to the H-3 group of agents
[323]. It was suggested that the virus might be a latent reacti-
vated tissue culture contaminant not etiologically related to hepatitis A.

We have recently recovered 8 immunologically identical heat-
stable cytopathic agents from HEL cell culture passage material
which had been originally inoculated with acute illness phase stool
filtrates from 8 children with hepatitis A. A strain variant of
adenovirus type 3 was recovered on initial passage in HEL from
each of the 8 specimens. These adenoviruses were destroyed by
heating on subsequent passage. Emergence of the heat-stable agents
occurred on still further passage in HEL. One of these agents
(HS-3) was selected as a prototype, and its ready adaptability to
growth in D-6 cell culture has allowed us to compare it with the
Kirk virus isolated by Boggs and Melnick.

As shown in Table 1, both agents share a similar infectivity
pattern in 6 cell culture systems and common size, ether- and heat-
stability characteristics. Their hemagglutination characteristics
are similar and they are antigenically similar in reciprocal cross
neutralization tests as shown in Table 2. Both are closely related

to the H-3 parvovirus of Toolan as well as to Kilham's rat virus. We have been unable to demonstrate neutralizing or hemagglutination inhibiting (HI) antibody to either Kirk or HS-3 viruses in convalescent sera from children ill with hepatitis A. However, we found HI antibody to these agents in 16 of 22 normal rat sera tested. We have also tested acute-illness phase serum and stool from 12 patients with hepatitis A in D-6 cells for a minimum of 8 passages without recovery of cytopathic agents.

Table 1. Characterization of Kirk-30 and HS-3 Agent

Characteristics	Agent	
	Kirk-30	HS-3
Cytopathic effect in cell culture		
Detroit-6	+	+
HEL	+	+
HEp-2	+	+
PMK	-	-
HAM	-	-
WI-38	-	-
Size	>10 μm <50	>10 μm <50
Ether Sensitivity	-	-
Heat Stability	Stable (60° C for 30 min.)	Stable (60° C for 30 min.)

Table 2. Cross Neutralization Test Results* with K-30 and HS-3 Agents on D-6 Cell Culture

Agent	Rabbit Antiserum		
	K-30	HS-3	PCC**
K-30	256	128	0
HS-3	128	256	0

*Titers expressed as reciprocals of final serum dilution giving complete neutralization.
**Rabbit anti D-6 passed cell control.

These results together with those of the Houston group firmly establish the identity of Kirk and HS-3 agents as parvoviruses probably unrelated to hepatitis. They also indicate that currently available clones of D-6 cells are probably not susceptible to the virus of hepatitis A. The question of source of these viruses as well as the other agents previously discussed must be carefully

considered. Throughout this review the possibility of tissue culture contamination either as reactivation of latent agents carried
for long periods in cell culture or as the result of contemporary
inadvertent introduction of agents exogenous to the inoculated human source materials runs like a recurring thread. In this connection the recent report by Hallauer that 34 out of 41 examined
human permanent cell lines were found to be contaminated with parvoviruses is of great significance [189]. These lines include such
commonly used cells as KB, HeLa, and HEp-2. It now seems clear
that more rigorous efforts to monitor for latent agents in cell
culture will be required and that such a derivation for any agents
isolated in continuous cell strains from hepatitis material be
firmly ruled out before they are seriously advanced to candidacy
as etiologic. Epidemiologic and other supportive evidence such as
the positive effect of pooled gamma globulin for prevention of hepatitis A firmly suggests that human infection with hepatitis
A virus invokes normal immunologic response mechanisms. It would,
therefore, also seem prudent to require that serum antibody rises
between acute and convalescent phase sera in cases of hepatitis,
without such rises in control serum pairs, be demonstrated against
any newly recovered agent before it is posed as a hepatitis A
etiologic candidate.

The most recent report of note concerning the propagation of
hepatitis agents in cell culture has concerned the possible occurrence of intrinsic interference in Wistar 38 cells between Newcastle Disease Virus (NDV) and the virus of hepatitis B [83]. As
described by Carver, this phenomenon can be demonstrated by the
production of hemadsorption negative areas on cell sheets infected
with NDV after prior inoculation with presumed hepatitis B virus-
containing serum, which areas are not observed in comparably
challenged cell sheets not priorly inoculated with this serum.
Confirmation of these observations by other laboratories has been
slow in coming, in no small measure due to the extremely cumbersome
and highly detailed techniques involved. It is to be hoped that
the legacy of failure which must be ascribed to attempts so far
to isolate hepatitis viruses in tissue culture will not be transferred to these most recent efforts...

Animal Models. Another area of intensive research in recent
years has related to attempts to propagate human hepatitis agents
in non-human primates. In 1967 Deinhardt and Holmes reported the
occurrence and serial transmission of biochemically and histologically confirmed hepatitis in marmoset monkeys following inoculation
with acute-illness phase serum from a human case (G.B.) of hepatitis
A [129]. These experiments were later expanded to include an extensive series of successful coded studies in which acute-illness
phase and pre-inoculation plasmas from human volunteers who developed hepatitis after inoculation with the Willowbrook MS-1

strain of hepatitis A virus were inoculated into marmosets [215, 216]. Although Parks and Melnick were able to confirm the original findings of Deinhardt and associates concerning the G.B. strain of hepatitis virus, their attempts to propagate hepatitis agents in animals inoculated with acute-illness phase human hepatitis sera produced equivocal results due to the occurrence of histopathologically and biochemically confirmed hepatitis in animals inoculated with normal human control sera [373]. Their additional findings of hepatitis in uninoculated animals led them to suggest that the marmoset-propagated agents might be indigenous to these animals and not of human origin. However, the positive findings from the heretofore mentioned coded studies together with an independent confirmation by Lorenz and colleagues [299] provides support for the view that marmosets are susceptible to the causative agent of human hepatitis A and that further studies with this animal model system should be encouraged.

The occurrence of viral hepatitis in chimpanzees was documented in 1963 when Hillis reported that biochemical and histopathological abnormalities resembling human viral hepatitis were observed in animals which had been newly imported into this country [206]. This author had earlier suggested that the illness could be transmitted to chimpanzee handlers [205]. Since that time further confirmation of the similarity between human and chimpanzee hepatitis has been published and continued transmission of illness from these animals to man has been documented [268].

Prior to the establishment of the hepatitis B antigen (HBAg) and its antibody (anti-HBAg) as immunologic markers for hepatitis B, the use of chimpanzees as experimental animals for the study of human viral hepatitis did not meet with unqualified success. Early attempts by Atchley [24] and Deinhardt and associates [128] to induce hepatitis in these animals with human specimen material produced equivocal results. Much of the difficulty was undoubtedly related to the unknown susceptibility status of the animals, with resultant unpredictable occurrence of hepatitis in control as well as inoculated chimpanzees.

In 1969 Hirschman and colleagues detected HBAg in two of 128 chimpanzees by agar gel diffusion techniques [207]. Prince similarly found both HBAg and anti-HBAg in 10% of a separate set of 138 animals by the same technique [385]. Also in 1969, Lichter reported the successful immunization of 2 chimpanzees with partially purified HBAg derived from a third animal [291]. This induced serum antibody formed precipitins in agar gel which identified HBAg in the sera of 5 separate chimpanzees.

In our laboratory we studied the identity patterns between naturally occurring chimpanzee and human HBAg and anti-HBAg using a sensitive matrix gel diffusion (MGD) technique [191]. We were able to establish the identity of human and chimpanzee reagent materials by this method. In a later experiment we induced both complement fixing (CF) and MGD serum antibody rises in two animals following immunization with partially purified chimpanzee-derived HBAg. These results for one animal are shown in Figure 1.* The antibody so formed was sensitive and specific for detection of human HBAg and anti-HBAg by both CF and gel diffusion techniques and established the usefulness of chimpanzee reagents for human diagnostics.

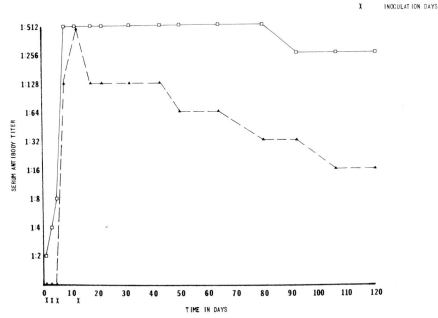

Figure 1. Anti-HBAg complement fixation and matrix gel diffusion titers in serum from chimpanzee MA-196 following inoculation with partially purified HBAg.

We were also able to study the relationship of serum HBAg and anti-HBAg to the occurrence of viral hepatitis in 97 newly imported chimpanzees which had been housed at our laboratories between 1964 and 1970 for periods varying from 2 to 24 months [308]. As shown in Table 3,* 30% of the animals experienced viral hepatitis. Such illness invariably occurred within 30 days of arrival of the animal at our laboratory. Illness-occurrence in relationship to the presence of serum anti-HBAg is shown in Figure 2* for

*Figures 1 and 2 and Table 3 taken from Maynard, J.E., et al: Viral hepatitis and studies of hepatitis associated antigen in chimpanzees. C.M.A. Journal/February 26, 1972/Vol. 106, Special Issue, p. 474.

2 animals in the series. Chimpanzee Faye experienced disease in
the presence of anti-HBAg, while chimpanzee Ruby was the only animal
which developed anti-HBAg just subsequent to the occurrence of
disease. These findings suggest that most viral hepatitis in newly
imported chimpanzees is not related to the virus of hepatitis B.
This view is further supported by our failure to detect HBAg or
anti-HBAg in acute illness phase sera from 5 handlers who acquired
viral hepatitis in our laboratory after exposure to several of the
chimpanzees in the series. The 30% incidence of naturally occurring
hepatitis in these animals also serves to emphasize their limited
usefulness for studies of hepatitis A until some suitable antigenic
markers for the causative agent are found.

Table 3. Occurrence of viral hepatitis in chimpanzees with and
without HBAg or anti-HBAg in sera from serial bleedings

Category	Number of Animals	Number with Hepatitis	Percent with Hepatitis
HBAg - anti-HBAg -	86	27	31
HBAg + anti-HBAg -	6	0	0
HBAg - anti-HBAg +	5	2	40
TOTAL	97	29	30

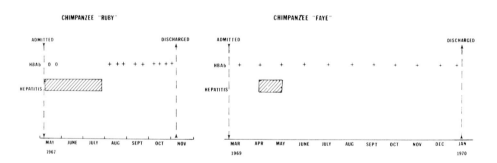

Figure 2. Antibody to HBAg in sera of two chimpanzees in relation
to occurrence of viral hepatitis.

On the other hand, our finding of anti-HBAg sero-conversion
in one animal following the occurrence of disease suggested the
possibility that experimental transmission of hepatitis B in immunologically susceptible chimpanzees might be possible. The
recent availability of extremely sensitive techniques for detection

of anti-HBAg in serum, such as passive hemagglutination (HA) and
radioimmunoassay (RIA), provided a tool for the determination of
susceptibility status.

In an attempt to induce natural infection with hepatitis B
virus, two animals (Xat and Yon), whose susceptibility was inferred
from lack of demonstrable serum anti-HBAg by both HA and RIA
techniques and who had both been held under conditions of isolation
for one year prior to study, were inoculated intravenously with
1.0 ml of a 1:10 dilution of human plasma containing HBAg and
known to cause hepatitis B in human volunteers. As shown in
Figure 3, Xat developed a transient antigenemia 70 days after inoculation with development of HA antibody 36 days later. Antibody
detectable by RIA did not develop until 7 days following appearance
of HA antibody and MGD antibody did not appear until 151 days
after inoculation. When the animal was given an identical reinoc-
ulation after 51 weeks, an immediate boost in HA and MGD antibody
titers occurred and CF antibody appeared for the first time.

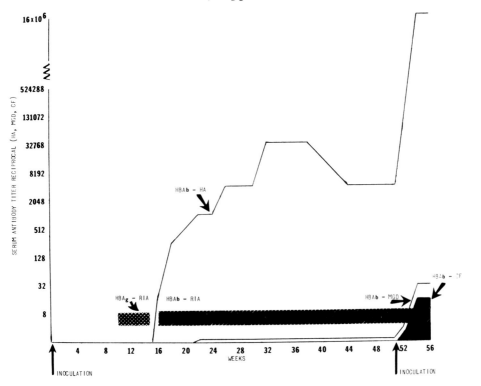

Figure 3. Immunologic response in chimpanzee Xat following inoculation with hepatitis B virus.

Chimpanzee Yon did not demonstrate antigenemia following inoculation, but developed HA antibody after 27 days, RIA antibody
after 32, and MGD antibody after 151 days. As with Xat, no CF
antibody was produced after initial challenge. However, a similar

pattern of boost in HA and MGD antibodies and an initial appearance
of CF antibody occurred when the animal was identically rechallenged
after 51 weeks.

Neither chimpanzee developed clinical, biochemical, or histologic evidence of hepatitis. Barker and colleagues have recently
produced similar immunologic responses as well as chemically and
histologically proven hepatitis in chimpanzees inoculated with the
NIH icterogenic plasma pool and have successfully subpassaged the
effect in a second chimpanzee series [33]. These combined observations leave little doubt that primary infection with the hepatitis
B virus may be induced in susceptible chimpanzees. Our findings
in relation to CF antibody production in chimpanzees suggest that
this antibody is not formed in response to primary infection with
the hepatitis B virus but may appear only as an anamnestic
response to antigenic restimulus.

Concern for the high cost and relative scarcity of chimpanzees
has resulted in a search for other non-human primates as possible
experimental models in hepatitis B research. Deinhardt and colleagues have been unsuccessful in infecting marmosets with hepatitis
B materials. However, Blumberg reported the presence of HBAg in
vervet and squirrel monkeys [59] and it has also been found in
gibbons and orangutans [385]. Using the RIA technique Purcell has
demonstrated anti-HBAg in baboons [397] and we are currently engaged in an attempt to transmit the hepatitis B virus in these
animals. Most recently, London and associates have reported success in the serial transmission of an agent associated with HBAg
in rhesus monkeys [297]. Their inoculum was derived from a human
HBAg carrier with chronic hepatitis. All infections produced were
inapparent and not associated with enzyme elevations or liver
pathology.

It would seem that the chimpanzee and, perhaps, certain other
non-human primates can provide important models for the study of
immune response to hepatitis B virus infection, and as such, may
serve as adjunct systems for the testing of anticipated hepatitis
B vaccines.

59. INFECTION OF CHIMPANZEES WITH HEPATITIS B VIRUS

Alfred M. Prince

The New York Blood Center,

New York, New York

Dr. Maynard has reviewed the frustrating history of attempts to isolate hepatitis viruses, in vitro and in vivo. I should like to present some recent data which appear to indicate conclusively that the chimpanzee represents a useful experimental animal model for human hepatitis B infections. As in the case of the results reported by Dr. Maynard and his co-workers, our results did not become conclusive until the direct radioimmunoassay technique of Ling and Overby was applied.

On August 13, 1970, six young adult chimpanzees, ranging in age from one to four years, were challenged with 70-100 ml of plasma obtained from chimpanzee No. 20, a chronic HBAg carrier whom we have studied since 1969. As ultrasensitive assay techniques for anti-HBAg were not available at the time, we chose to use a "high dose" challenge, i.e., an exposure analogous to transfusion of an HBAg-containing unit of blood to a human recipient.

Materials and Methods. Serum samples were obtained at weekly intervals prior to challenge, on the day of challenge prior to plasma inoculation, and at weekly intervals thereafter for nine months. Follow-up specimens were again obtained from these animals during the 18th month after exposure. Serum was separated from blood with minimal delay and immediately frozen at -70°C prior to assay.

All serum specimens were tested for SGPT by the kinetic spectrophotometric method routinely employed in our laboratory [384]. Our method involves the routine use of frozen serum controls to insure accuracy and reproducibility. The upper limit of normal in our laboratory (95% of volunteer blood donors) is 30 Karmen units. Our experience with serial blood sample collection from approximately 35 chimpanzees during the past three years indicates that chimpanzees do not differ significantly from man in normal mean SGPT levels.

Sera were also tested for HBAg and anti-HBAg by agar gel diffusion (AGD) [384], IEOP [388], passive hemagglutination (HA) and hemagglutination inhibition (HAI) [477] and more recently by the direct radioimmunoassay (RIA) of Ling and Overby utilizing the Ausria$^{(TM)}$ kits supplied by Abbott Laboratories.

Results. The results of this experiment are summarized in Table 1. When the (HA) assay became available, it became feasible to examine the pre-inoculation sera with a sensitive assay for anti-HBAg. This revealed that all except two animals had preexisting levels of this antibody, and had therefore, in all probability, been previously exposed to infection.

Table 1. Results of challenge of 6 chimpanzees with 70-100 ml CH 20 (ad) plasma.

NO.	PREINOCULATION HA TITER (RECIPROCAL)	DURATION OF ANTIGENEMIA (WEEKS) HAI ASSAY	SGPT RISE INCUBATION PERIOD (WEEKS)	PEAK (WEEKS)	ANTIBODY RESPONSE INCUBATION PERIOD (WEEKS)	PEAK TITER
23	32	5	14	150 (16)	-	64
25	<2	4	6	84 (11)	5	2048
27	8	2	8	51 (9)	4	1024
29	64	<1 / 2 WKS BY IEOP	16	141 (17)	2	1024
31	<2	9	18	89 (21)	9	128
38	4	1	14	76 (15)	8	64

Residual inoculated HBAg was detectable by HAI for periods varying between one and nine weeks after challenge. There was no clear-cut correlation between preexisting antibody titers and rate of disappearance of injected antigen.

All animals developed clear-cut transaminase elevations between six and eighteen weeks after challenge. The elevations were mild to moderate (peak SGPT varied between 51 and 150) but were in most cases quite distinct, as illustrated in Figure 1.

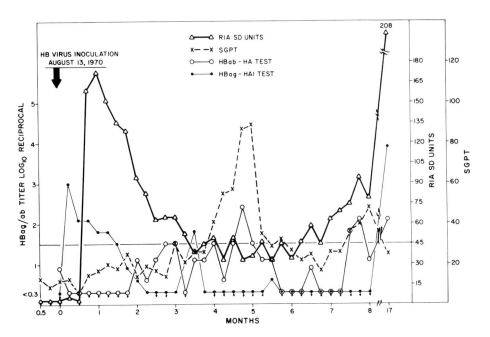

<u>Figure 1.</u> Infection of Chimpanzees with hepatitis B virus.

Distinct seroconversion (four fold or greater rise in anti-
HBAg titer detected by passive hemagglutination) was seen in all
except one animal. The initially sero-negative animals No. 25
and No. 31, and chimpanzee number 38, who had a pre-inoculation
titer of 1:4, showed antibody rises occurring between five and
nine weeks after exposure i.e., typical primary antibody responses.
Chimpanzee 29, who had the highest pre-inoculation HA titer, showed
an anamnestic type response two weeks after exposure. The above
results were strongly suggestive but did not prove infection.

Through the kindness of Drs. King and Overby of Abbott Laboratories, we have been able to examine the sera from this experiment
by their direct RIA technique. The most convincing results were
those found when the sera of chimpanzee No. 31 were examined (Figure 1). It will be seen that by RIA technique, antigen never became nondetectable: indeed, beginning three to four months after
exposure a chronic antigen carrier state became apparent. Initially
(during the period between three and nine months) antigen remained
at relatively low levels detectable only by RIA. The RIA was, however, very strongly positive throughout this period (greater than
30 standard deviations from the mean of control sera). The quantity of circulating antigen began to rise at about six months,
reaching levels corresponding to about 90 standard deviation units.
A follow-up specimen taken 17 months after exposure revealed antigen to be detectable by RIA, HA inhibition, and now even by AGD
and IEOP.

The above experiments unequivocally demonstrate that chimpanzees are susceptible to infection with hepatitis B virus of chimpanzee origin. As indicated by Dr. Maynard and others, the antigens of this virus are immunologically indistinguishable from those present on human hepatitis B associated particles. The disease induced is clinically entirely analogous to anicteric post-transfusion hepatitis. Replication of hepatitis B antigen has been clearly demonstrated. It has been shown, as might be expected on the basis of post-transfusion follow-up studies in man, that past immunity does not protect against reinfection; or against the development of at least mild forms of hepatitis.

These experiments establish the existence of an animal model for this important human disease. Future studies of immuno-prophylaxis and immunotherapy of hepatitis B infections should be based on prior exploration of possible risks and benefits in this or other available animal models.

Acknowledgements. These studies were aided by Grant #HE-09011 and AI-09516 from the National Institutes of Health, Contract #70-2236, from the National Heart and Lung Institute, and Grants in Aid from the Kresge Foundation and from the Strasburger Foundation. Dr. Prince is a Career Scientist of the Health Research Council of the City of New York under Contract #1-533.

We are grateful for the technical assistance of B. Clinkscale, Edwina Echenroth, Annie May Moffatt, Dan Joss and Judy Friedman, and especially Mr. Wayne Johnson, Mr. Bill Tyrell, and ten co-workers at the Laboratory for Experimental Medicine and Surgery in Primates, Sterling Forest, New York.

EPILOGUE

H. A. Perkins

Irwin Memorial Blood Bank

San Francisco, California

The proceedings make amply clear the areas in which full
agreement has been achieved as well as those in which further
information is urgently needed. These have been fully discussed,
and there is no need for me to dwell on them further.

I shall limit my remarks to the prospects of early improvement in procedures in routine blood banking to minimize transfusion-associated hepatitis.

The data presented at this conference indicate even more
strongly than we had previously suspected that we are not only
failing to detect blood donors who are carriers of hepatitis A
virus but, with current routine technics, are missing a considerable proportion of the hepatitis B carriers.

We are all in agreement that blood donors must be tested
for HBAg. With current routine technics--most commonly counterelectrophoresis (CEP)--a group of high risk donors is excluded.
More sensitive technics, such as hemagglutination inhibition (HAI)
and radioimmunoassay (RIA) are under investigation. HAI, despite
its sensitivity, misses many HBAg carriers in most laboratories,
presumably because of failure of the reagents employed to detect
all subtypes. RIA has not been reported to exhibit the same
difficulty for reasons unclear to me; but many variations of the
RIA test are under investigation, and reproducibility within and
between laboratories is often poor. Although one commercially
developed RIA kit appears to have been successfully employed,
the test takes 20 hours. In many areas, such a large proportion
of blood components will have been transfused before the test has

been completed that its increased sensitivity might result in no
added protection for the recipients.

We have heard, also, that blood donors with such low levels
of HBAg that they are detected only by RIA are less likely to
transmit hepatitis than donors with HBAg detected by CEP. Conversely, we have heard that when HBAg-positive hepatitis followed
transfusion of CEP-negative blood, the original donor samples
did not, in most instances, reveal HBAg by RIA. It is obvious that
more data are needed before the conclusion can be drawn that routine
testing of donors by RIA, or some other similarly sensitive test,
should be a requirement.

It seems likely, therefore, that transfusion-associated
hepatitis will not be eliminated by the employment of more sensitive tests for HBAg. It seems possible that, with increasingly
sensitive tests, we will be approaching the point of diminishing
returns because with very low levels of virus, many recipients
may have sufficient immunity to prevent signs of infection by the
hepatitis B virus. Moreover, although hepatitis A virus seems to
result in a less serious form of the disease, evidence was presented that it may account for a considerable proportion of cases
of transfusion-associated hepatitis with jaundice and associated
symptoms.

Further suggestions to minimize transmission of hepatitis by
blood transfusion included the old suggestion to eliminate donors
with a high level of transaminase, and the suggestion to request
a reply from all transfused patients at the end of six months to
ensure complete reporting of all transfusion-associated hepatitis.

The cost of blood transfusions will be considerably increased
if all these suggestions are followed and if more sensitive and
complicated tests are employed. Blood banks can be counted on to
follow any recommendations on which there is general agreement,
but we must avoid recommendations which will (1) seriously decrease the already limited supply of blood for transfusion and
(2) eliminate so few cases of hepatitis that the added cost to
the bill of all patients is not justifiable.

The conference now ending makes evident numerous areas in
which there is general agreement regarding hepatitis and its
relation to the Australia antigen. It also points out the topics
on which data are inadequate and provides an indication of the
areas in which vigorous research is being pursued in many laboratories. The next year or two can be expected to provide a
wealth of new data with implications of both fundamental and
practical importance.

BIBLIOGRAPHY

1. Aach R.D., Grisham J., Parker C., Proc. Nat. Acad. Sci., US/, 68:1056, 1971.
2. Aach R.D., Hacker E.J., Parker C.W., in Viral Hepatitis and Blood Transfusion, Ed. G.N. Vyas et al., Grune & Stratton, New York, 1972.
3. Ahmed M.N., Huang S.N., Spence L., Arch. Path., 92:66, 1971.
4. Akdamar K.A., Maumus L., Cherrie-Epps A., et al., Lancet, i:909, 1971.
5. Allen J.G., Dawson D., Sayman W.A., et al., Ann. Surg., 150: 455, 1959.
6. Allison A.C., Blumberg B.S., Lancet, i:634, 1961.
7. Almeida J.D., Le Bouvier G.L., (Unpublished Data).
8. Almeida J.D., Rubenstein D., Stott E.J., Lancet, ii:1225, 1971.
9. Almeida J.D., Waterson H.P., Lancet, ii:983, 1969.
10. Almeida J.D., Waterson A.P., Trowell J.M., et al., Microbios, 6:145, 1970.
11. Almeida J.D., Zuckerman A.J., Taylor P.E., et al., Microbios, 2:117, 1969.
12. Alpert E., Issalbacher K., Schur P., N. Eng. J. Med., 285: 185, 1971.
13. Alter H.J., Blumberg B.S., Blood, 27:297, 1966.
14. Alter H.J., Holland P.V., Lander J.L., et al., Amer. Soc. Micro. Symposium on Australia Antigen, Philadelphia, Pa., Nov. 9., 1971.
15. Alter H.J., Holland P.V., Purcell R.H., J. Lab. Clin. Med., 77:1000, 1971.
16. Alter H.J., Holland P.V., Purcell R.H., et al., Residual hepatitis after exclusion of the commercial and HBAg positive blood donor, (In Preparation).
17. Alter H.J., Holland P.V., Schmidt P.J., Lancet, ii:142, 1970.
18. Alter H.J., Polesky H.F., Holland P.V., J. Immun., 108:358, 1972.
19. Anderson N., Nunley C., Rankin C., Anal. Biochem., 31:255, 1969.
20. Andrassy E., Ritz R., Deutsch. Med. Wschr., 95:2467, 1970.
21. Annotation, Nature, 235:364, 1972.
22. Apostolov K., Bauer D.J., Selway J.W.T., et al., Lancet, i:1274, 1971.

23. Ashcavai M., Peters R.L., Amer. J. Clin. Path., 55:262, 1971.
24. Atchley F.O., Kimbrough R.D., Lab. Invest., 15:1520, 1966.
25. Aynaud M., Compt. Rend. Soc. Biol., 70:54, 1911.
26. Baggenstoss A.H., Soloway R.D., Summerskill W.H.J., et al., Gastroenterology (Abstract in Press).
27. Bagshawe A.F., Parker A.M., Jindani A., Brit. Med. J., 2:88, 1971.
28. Baines P.M., Taylor P.E., Zuckerman A. J., Arch. ges. virusfors., 1972, (In Press).
29. Bancroft J.B., Bracker C.E., Wagner G.W., Virology, 38:324, 1969.
30. Bancroft W.H., Mundon F.K., Russell P.K., (Submitted for Publication).
31. Banke O., Dybkjaer E., Nordenfelt E., Lancet, i:860, 1971.
32. Barandun S., Kistler P., Jeunet F., et al., Vox Sang., 7:157, 1962.
33. Barker L.F., (Personal Communication).
34. Barker L.F., Murray R., J. Am. Med. Ass., 216:1970, 1971.
35. Barker L.F., Peterson M.R., Murray R., Vox Sang., 19:211, 1970.
36. Barker L.F., Shulman N.R., Murray R., et al., J. Am. Med. Ass., 211:1509, 1970.
37. Barker L.F., Smith K.O., Gehle W.D., et al., J. Immun., 102:1529, 1969.
38. Bar-Shany S., Naggan L., Wolpiansky N., Israel J. Med. Sci., 8:1, 1972.
39. Bayer M.E., Blumberg B.S., Werner B., Nature, 218:1057, 1968.
40. Berg H.C., Diamond J.M., Marfey P.S., Science, 146:64, 1965.
41. Berg R., Björling H., Berntsen K., et al., Vox Sang., 1972, (In Press).
42. Bjomebre M., Prytz H., Orskow F., Lancet, i:58, 1972.
43. Blainey J.D., Earle A., Flewett T.H., et al., Lancet, i:797, 1971.
44. Blumberg B.S., Bull. N.Y. Acad. Med., 40:377, 1964.
45. Blumberg B.S., J. Clin. Invest., 45:988, 1966 (Abstract).
46. Blumberg B.S., Tokyo J. Med. Sci., 76:324, 1968.
47. Blumberg B.S., Bull. Acad. Med. Toronto, 45:45, 1972.
48. Blumberg B.S., Allison A.C., Proc. II Int. Congr. Hum. Genet., Rome, 1961, p. 733, 1963.
49. Blumberg B.S., Alter H.J., Visnich S., J. Am. Med. Ass., 191:541, 1965.
50. Blumberg B.S., Dray S., Robinson J.C., Nature, 194:656, 1962.
51. Blumberg B.S., Friedlaender J.S., Woodside A., et al., Proc. Nat. Acad. Sci., 62:1108, 1969.
52. Blumberg B.S., Gerstley B.J.S., Hungerford D.A., et al., Ann. Int. Med., 66:924, 1967.
53. Blumberg B.S., Gerstley B.J.S., Sutnick A.I., et al., Ann. N.Y. Acad. Sci., 171:486, 1970.
54. Blumberg B.S., London W.T., Sutnick A.I., Amer. J. Med., 48:1, 1970.

55. Blumberg B.S., London W.T., Sutnick A.I., Postgrad. Med., 50:70, 1971.
56. Blumberg B.S., Melartin L., Guinto R.A., et al., Am. J. Hum. Genet., 18:594, 1966.
57. Blumberg B.S., Melartin L., Guinto R.A., et al., J. Chronic Dis., 23:507, 1970.
58. Blumberg B.S., Millman I., Sutnick A.I., et al., J. Exp. Med., 134:320, 1971.
59. Blumberg B.S., Sutnick A.I., London W.T., Bull. N.Y. Acad. Med., 44:1566, 1968.
60. Blumberg B.S., Sutnick A.I., London W.T., Amer. J. Med., 48: 1, 1970.
61. Blumberg B.S., Sutnick A.I., London W.T., et al., CRC Critical Reviews Clin. Lab. Sci., 2:473, 1971.
62. Blumberg B.S., Sutnick A.I., London W.T., et al., in Perspectives in Virology VII, Ed. by M. Pollard, p. 223, Academic Press, New York and London, 1971.
63. Blumberg B.S., Sutnick A.I., London W.T., et al., in Viruses Affecting Man and Animals, Ed. by M. Sanders and M. Schaeffer, p. 250, Warren H. Green, Inc., St. Louis, Mo., 1971.
64. Boggs J.D., Capps R.B., Weiss C.F., et al., J. Am. Med. Ass., 177:114, 1961.
65. Boggs J.D., Melnick J.L., Conrad M.E., et al., J. Am. Med. Ass., 214:1041, 1970.
66. Boklan B.F., Ann. Int. Med., 74:298, 1971.
67. Bond H.E., Hall W.T., J. Infect. Dis., 125:263, 1972.
68. Bone J.M., Tonkin R.W., Marmion B.P., et al., Proc. Eur. Dial. Trans. Assoc., 8:189, 1971.
69. Bothwell P.W., Martin D., Macara A.W., et al., Brit. Med. J., 2:1613, 1963.
70. Boyden S.V., J. Exp. Med., 93:107, 1951.
71. Boyer J., in Viral Hepatitis and Blood Transfusion, Ed. by G.N. Vyas, et al., Grune & Stratton, New York, 1972.
72. Boyer J.L., Klatskin G., N. Eng. J. Med., 283:1063, 1970.
73. Brighton W.D., Taylor P.E., Zuckerman A.J., Nature New Biol., 232:57, 1971.
74. Brussin A.M., Kalajev A.W., Z. Immunitatsforsch, 70:497, 1931.
75. Bulkley B.H., Heizer W.D., Goldfinger S.E., et al., Lancet, ii:1323, 1970.
76. Bull. Wld. Hlth. Org., 39:935, 1968.
77. Bunnel I.L., Furcolow M.L., Pub. Health Rep., 63:299, 1948.
78. Byrne E.B., J. Am. Med. Ass., 195:362, 1966.
79. Cameron J.D.S., Quart. J. Med., 12:139, 1943.
80. Candeias J.A.N., Rev. Microbiol., 2:129, 1971.
81. Capps R.B., Bennett A.M., Stokes J. Jr., J. Clin. Invest., 29:802, 1950.
82. Carbonara A.O., Trinchieri G., Bedarida G., et al., Vox Sang., 19:288, 1970.
83. Carver D.H., Seto D.S.Y., Science, 172:1265, 1971.

84. Carver D., Seto D., Gerin J., et al., Perspectives in Virology VIII, 1972, (In Press).

85. Catt K., Tregear G.W., Science, 158:1570, 1967.

86. Cawley L.P., in A Seminar on Basic Immunology, p. 111, Am. Assoc. Blood Banks, Chicago, 1971.

87. Ceppellini R., Bedarida G., Carbonara A.O., et al., Minerva Medica Torino, p. 53, 1970.

88. Chalmers T.C., Forrest J.N., Grady G.F., Trans. Am. Clin. Climatol. Assoc., 80:15, 1968.

89. Chalmers T.C., Koff R.S., Grady G.F., Gastroenterology, 49: 22, 1965.

90. Chang R.S., Proc. Soc. Expt. Biol. Med., 107:135, 1961.

91. Chang R.S., Pan I.H., Rosenau B.J., J. Exp. Med., 124:1153, 1966.

92. Cherry W.T., Goldman M., Corski T.R., Public Health Ser. Pub. No. 729, U.S. Government Printing Office, Washington, D.C., 1960.

93. Cherubin C.E., Lancet, i:627, 1971.

94. Cherubin C.E., Hargrove R.L., Prince A.M., Am. J. Epid., 91: 510, 1970.

95. Cherubin C.E., Prince A.M., Transfusion, 11:25, 1971.

96. Chilgren R.A., Quie P.G., Meuwissen H.J., et al., Lancet, ii: 688, 1967.

97. Chung W.K., Moon S.K., Gershon R.K., et al., Arch. Int. Med., 113:535, 1964.

98. Cohen S.N., Daugherty W.J., J. Am. Med. Ass., 203:427, 1968.

99. Cohn E.J., Strong L.E., Hughes W.L., et al., J. Am. Chem. Soc., 68:459, 1946.

100. Coller J.A., Millman I., Halbherr T.C., et al., Proc. Soc. Expt. Biol. Med., 138:249, 1971.

101. Combes B., Shorey J., Barrera A., et al., Lancet, i:234, 1971.

102. Combes B., Stastny P., Shorey J., et al., Lancet, ii:234, 1971.

103. Cook G.C., Mulligan R., Sherlock S., Quart. J. Med., 40:159, 1971.

104. Coons A.H., in General Cytochemical Methods, VI, Ed. by J.F. Danielle, Academic Press, Inc., New York, 1958.

105. Cooperative Study, J. Am. Med. Ass., 214:140, 1970.

106. Cooperative Study conducted by Walter Reed Army Institute of Research, Arch. Int. Med., 128:723, 1971.

107. Cossart Y.E., (Personal Communication).

108. Cossart Y.E., Vox Sang., 19:404, 1970.

109. Cossart Y.E., Field A.M., Lancet, i:848, 1970.

110. Cossart Y.E., Le Bouvier G.L., (Unpublished Data).

111. Cossart Y.E., Vahrman J., Brit. Med. J., 1:403, 1970.

112. Coyne V.E., Blumberg B.S., Millman I., Proc. Soc. Expt. Biol. Med., 138:1051, 1971.

113. Coyne V.E., Millman I., Blumberg B.S., Bact. Proc. (Abstr.), p. 175, 1971.

114. Coyne V.E., Millman I., Cerda J., et al., J. Exp. Med., 131: 307, 1970.
115. Creutzfeldt W., Severidt H.-J., Brachmann H., et al., Deutsch. Med. Wschr., 91:1905, 1966.
116. Cross G.F., Waugh M., Ferris A.A., Aus. J. Exp. Biol. Med. Sci., 49:1, 1971.
117. Crowder J.G., Gilkey G.H., White A.C., Arch. Int. Med., 128: 247, 1971.
118. Crowder J.G., White A., J. Lab. Clin. Med., 75:128, 1970.
119. Csapo J., et al., Acta Ped., 4:195, 1963.
120. Culliford B.J., Nature, 201:1092, 1964.
121. Curtain C.C., J. Histochem. Cytochem., 9:484, 1961.
122. Daguet G.L., Brit. J. Ven. Dis., 32:96, 1956.
123. Dane D.S., Cameron C.H., Briggs M., Lancet, i:695, 1970.
124. David J.R., Al-askari S., Lawrence H.S., et al., J. Immun., 93:264, 1964.
125. Davis E.V., Science, 133:2059, 1961.
126. De Groote J., Desmet V., Gedigh P., et al., Lancet, ii:626, 1968.
127. Deinhardt F., in Infections and Immunosuppression in Subhuman Primates, p. 55, Balner & Beveridge, Copenhagen, Denmark, 1970.
128. Deinhardt F., Courtois G., Dherte P., et al., Amer. J. Hyg., 75:311, 1962.
129. Deinhardt F., Holmes A. W., Capps R.B., et al., J. Exp. Med., 125:673, 1967.
130. Deinhardt F., Holmes A. W., Wolfe L., et al., in International Virology II, Ed. J. L. Melnick, S. Karger, Basel, Switzerland, 1972, (In Press).
131. Dejanov I.I., Trajkovski B., Sotirovska Lj., et al., Lancet, ii:164, 1971.
132. Del Prete S., Costantino D., Doglia M., et al., Lancet, ii: 579, 1970.
133. Delrez L., Govaerts P., Compt. Rend. Soc. Biol., 81:53, 1918.
134. Dodd R.Y., Levin J.J., Ni L., et al., in Viral Hepatitis and Blood Transfusion, Ed. G.N. Vyas, et al., Grune & Stratton, New York, 1972.
135. Dreesman G.R., Hollinger F.B., McCombs R.M., et al., Inf. & Immun., 5:213, 1972.
136. Dubin I.N., Sullivan B.H., Legolvan P.C., et al., Amer. J. Med., 29:55, 1960.
137. Duke H.L., Wallace J.M., Parasitology, 22:414, 1930.
138. Duncan G.C., Christian H.A., Stokes J. Jr., et al., Am. J. Med. Sci., 213:53, 1947.
139. Dunn E., Peters R., Schweitzer I., et al., Hepatitis Scientific Memoranda, January 1972, (Personal Communication).
140. Edgington T., Ritt D., J. Exp. Med., 134:871, 1971.
141. Editorial, Lancet, i:80, 1972.
142. Editorial, Transfusion, 10:1, 1970.
143. Ekbloom L., Olsson P., Aberg T., Acta Chir. Scand., 133:351, 1967.

144. Espmark A., (Personal Communication).
145. Federal Register, 35:14229, 1970.
146. Federal Register, 36:1470, 1971.
147. Ferguson A., Carswell F., Brit. Med. J., 1:75, 1972.
148. Ferraresi R.W., Dedrick C.T., Raffel S., J. Immun., 102:852, 1969.
149. Ferris A.A., Kaldor J., Gust I.D., et al., Lancet, ii:243, 1970.
150. Fields A., Cossart Y., Lancet, ii:91, 1971.
151. Findlay G.M., MacCallum F.O., Trans. Roy. Soc. Trop. Med. Hyg., 31:297, 1937.
152. Findlay G.M., Martin N.H., Lancet, i:678, 1943.
153. Findlay G.M., Wilcox R.R., Lancet, i:212, 1945.
154. Fritz R.B., Rivers S.L., J. Immun., 108:108, 1972.
155. Fudenberg H.H., in A Seminar on Basic Immunology, Am. Assoc. of Blood Banks, Chicago, 1971.
156. Fudenberg H.H., Faulk W.P., Vyas G.N., et al., in Immunologic Methods, Ed. H. Friedman and C.C. Thomas, 1972, (In Press).
157. Gellis S.S., Stokes J. Jr., Brother G.M., et al., J. Am. Med. Ass., 128:1062, 1945.
158. Gerin J., Holland P., Purcell R., J. Virol., 7:569, 1971.
159. Gerin J., Purcell R., Hoggan M., et al., J. Virol., 4:763, 1969.
160. Giblett E.R., in Genetic Markers of Human Blood, I Edition, Ed. F.A. Davis, Philadelphia, Penn., 1969.
161. Giles J.P., Leibhaber H., Krugman S., et al., Virology, 24: 107, 1964.
162. Giles J.P., McCollum R.W., Berndtson L.W. Jr., et al., N. Eng. J. Med., 281:119, 1969.
163. Ginsberg A.L., Bancroft W.H., Conrad M.E., J. Lab. Clin. Med., 1972, (Submitted for Publication).
164. Ginsberg A.L., Conrad M.E., Bancroft W.H., et al., N. Eng. J. Med., 286:562, 1972.
165. Giorgini G.L., Hollinger F.B., Leduc L., et al., 1972, (Submitted for Publication).
166. Gocke D.J., J. Am. Med. Ass., 219:1165, 1972.
167. Gocke D.J., Greenberg H.B., Kavey N.B., J. Am. Med. Ass., 212:877, 1970.
168. Gocke D.J., Howe C., J. Immun., 104:1031, 1970.
169. Gocke D.J., Kavey N.B., Lancet, i:1055, 1969.
170. Gocke D.J., Morgan C., Lockshin M., et al., Lancet, ii: 7684, 1970.
171. Goeser E., London T., Sutnick A., et al., Clin. Res., 18: 380, 1970.
172. Goldfield M., (Personal Communication).
173. Goldfield M., A Progress Report on Hepatitis Studies in New Jersey Presented at Soc. for Epidemiologic Research, Minneapolis, Minn., June 1970.
174. Goldfield M., Black H.C., (Personal Communication).

175. Goodman M., Wainright R.L., Weir H.F., et al., Pediatrics,
      48:907, 1971.
176. Gordon I., Berberian M., Stevenson D., et al., J. Infect.
      Dis., 1972, (In Press).
177. Grady G.F., Bennett A.J., Chalmers T.C., et al., J. Am.
      Med. Ass., 214:140, 1970.
178. Grady G.F., Bennett A.J.E., Chalmers T.C., et al., J. Am.
      Med. Ass., 1972, (In Press).
179. Grady G.F., Bennett A.J.E., Culhane P.O., et al., J. Infect.
      Dis., 1972, (In Press).
180. Grady G.F., Chalmers T.C., N. Eng. J. Med., 271:337, 1964.
181. Greenberg H.B., Gocke D.J., J. Infect. Dis., 123:356, 1971.
182. Greenwood F.C., Hunter W.M., Glover J.S., Biochem. J., 39:
      114, 1963.
183. Grob P.J., Jemelka H., Lancet, i:206, 1971.
184. Grossman E.B., Stewart S.G., Stokes J. Jr., J. Am. Med. Ass.,
      129:991, 1945.
185. Guardia J., Bacardi R., Hernandea J.M., et al., Lancet, ii:
      465, 1970.
186. Gust I.D., Aus. J. Exp. Biol. Med. Sci., 1972, (In Press).
187. Gust I.D., Kaldor J., Nastasi M., Lancet, i:797, 1971.
188. Hadziynnis S., Ciba Foundation Symposium, London, 1970.
189. Hallauer C., Kronauer G., Siegl G., Arch. ges. virusfors.,
      35:80, 1971.
190. Hartwell W.V., Love G.J., Eidenbock M.P., Science, 152:1390,
      1966.
191. Hartwell W.V., Maynard J.E., Berquist K.R., Appl. Microbiol.,
      21:623, 1971.
192. Hatch M.H., Siem R.A., Am. J. Epid., 84:495, 1966.
193. Havens W.P. Jr., J. Exp. Med., 83:251, 1946.
194. Havens W.P. Jr., J. Exp. Med., 84:403, 1946.
195. Havens W.P. Jr., Paul J. R., J. Am. Med. Ass., 129:270, 1945.
196. Havens W.P. Jr., Ward R., Drill V.A., et al., Proc. Soc. Expt.
      Biol. Med., 57:206, 1944.
197. Hawkes R.A., Med. J. Australia, p. 519, September 19, 1970.
198. Heisto H., Julsrud A.C., Acta Med. Scand., 164:349, 1959.
199. Hellerstein L.J., Deykin D., N. Eng. J. Med., 284:1039, 1971.
200. Henle W., Harris S., Henle G., et al., J. Exp. Med., 92:271,
      1950.
201. Hepatitis Surveillance Report No. 31, Jan. 1, 1970, p. 15,
      Center for Disease Control, US Dept. of Health, Education
      and Welfare, Atlanta, Georgia.
202. Herbert W.J., in Handbook of Experimental Immunology, Ed.
      D.M. Weir, Blackwell Scientific Publications, Oxford, 1967.
203. Hersh T., Goyal R.K., Grubb M.N., et al., Lancet, i:908, 1971.
204. Hershgold E.J., Pool J.G., Pappenhagen A.R., J. Lab. Clin.
      Med., 67:23, 1966.
205. Hillis W.D., Amer. J. Hyg., 73:316, 1961.
206. Hillis W.D., Transfusion, 3:445, 1963.

207. Hirschman R.J., Shulman R., Barker L.F., et al., J. Am. Med.
      Ass., 208:1667, 1969.
208. Hirschman S., Vernace S., Schaffner F., Lancet, i:1099, 1971.
209. Hoag M.S., Johnson F.F., Robinson J.A., et al., N. Eng. J.
      Med., 280:581, 1969.
210. Holland P., Alter H., Purcell R., et al., Vox Sang., 20:464,
      1971.
211. Holland P.V., Alter H.J., Purcell R.H., et al., The Infectiv-
      ity of Blood Containing the Australia Antigen, Presented
      at the Symposium on Australia Antigen of the American
      Society for Microbiology, Philadelphia, November 9, 1971,
      (Proceedings in Press).
212. Holland P.V., Purcell R.H., Smith H., et al., J. Immun.,
      1972., (Submitted for Publication).
213. Holland P.V., Rubinson R.M., Morrow A.G., et al., J. Am. Med.
      Ass., 196:471, 1966.
214. Hollinger F.B., Vorndam V., Dreesman G.R., J. Immun., 107:
      1099, 1971.
215. Holmes A.W., Wolfe L., Deinhardt F., et al., J. Infect. Dis.,
      124:520, 1971.
216. Holmes A.W., Wolfe L., Rosenblate H., et al., Science, 165:
      816, 1969.
217. Holper J.C., Proc. Soc. Expt. Biol. Med., June 1972, (In
      Press).
218. Holper J.C., Jambazian A., Transfusion, 11:157, 1971.
219. Homologous Serum Jaundice: Memorandum prepared by Medical
      Officers of the Ministry of Health, Lancet, i:83, 1943.
220. Hsia D.Y.Y., Kennell J.H., Gellis S.S., Am. J. Med. Sci.,
      226:261, 1953.
221. Hsiung G.D., Isacson P., McCollum R.W., J. Immun., 88:284,
      1962.
222. Hsu K.C., in Methods in Immunology and Immunochemistry, I,
      Ed. C.A. Williams and N.M. Chase, Academic Press, Inc.,
      New York, p. 397, 1967.
223. Huang S.N., Amer. J. Path., 64:483, 1971.
224. Huang S.N., Millman I., O'Connell A., et al., Amer. J. Path.,
      1972, (In Press).
225. Hunter W.M., Greenwood F.C., Nature, 194:495, 1962.
226. Huntsman R.G., Hurn B.A., Ikin E.W., et al., Brit. Med. J.,
      1508, 1962.
227. Ibrahim A.B., Ph.D. Dissertation, University of California,
      Berkeley, California, 1971.
228. International Group, "Morphological criteria in viral
      hepatitis," Lancet, i:333, 1971.
229. Irwin G.R. Jr., Hierholzer W.J. Jr., McCollum R.W., J.
      Infect Dis., 125:73, 1972.
230. Isacson P., McCollum R.W., Hsiung G.D., J. Immun., 88:300,
      1962.
231. Israel H.L., Sones M., N. Eng. J. Med., 273:1003, 1965.

232. Ivey K.J., Clifton J.A., Gastroenterology, 59:630, 1970.
233. Jandl J.H., Simmons R.L., Brit. J. Hemat., 3:19, 1957.
234. Jenson A.B., McCombs R.M., Sakurada N., et al., Exp. Mol.
      Path., 13:217, 1970.
235. Jindani A., Bagshawe A., Forrester A.T.T., East Afric. Med.
      J., 47:138, 1970.
236. Jokelainen P., Krohn K., Prince A., et al., J. Virol.,
      6:685, 1970.
237. Joswiak W., Koscielak J., Madalinski K., et al., Nature
      New Biol., 229:92, 1971.
238. Juji T., Yokochi T., Japan J. Exp. Med., 39:615, 1969.
239. Kafuko G.W., Baingana N., Knight E.M., et al., East Afric.
      Med. J., 46:414, 1969.
240. Kaszewska-Jablonska L., Pol. Arch. Med. Wewn., 47:231, 1971.
241. Katz R., Rodriguez J., Ward R., N. Eng. J. Med., 285:925,
      1971.
242. Kim C.Y., Bissell D., J. Infect. Dis., 123:470, 1971.
243. Kim C.Y., Tilles J.G., J. Infect. Dis., 123:618, 1971.
244. Kim C.Y., Tilles J.G., J. Infect. Dis., 124:512, 1971.
245. Kingdon H.S., Ann. Int. Med., 73:656, 1970.
246. Kissling R.E., (Personal Communication).
247. Kistler P., Nitschmann H., Vox Sang., 7:414, 1962.
248. Klatskin G., Amer. J. Med., 25:333, 1958.
249. Klatskin G., Presented at A.S.M. Symposium on Australia
      Antigen, Philadelphia, 1971.
250. Kliman A., N. Eng. J. Med., 284:109, 1971.
251. Kliman A., Reid N.R., Lilly C., et al., N. Eng. J. Med.,
      285:783, 1971.
252. Knepp C.S., Coleman C.N., Shulman N.R., Clin. Res., 18:442,
      1970.
253. Koff R.S., Grady G.F., Chalmers T.C., the Boston Inter-
      Hospital Liver Group, Under-reporting of viral hepatitis,
      (Unpublished Observations).
254. Kohn J., Morgan J.R., J. Clin. Path., 24:673, 1971.
255. Kritschewski I.L., Tscherikower R.S., Z. Immunitatsforsch,
      42:131, 1925.
256. Kritschewski I.L., Tscherikower R.S., Z. Immunitatsforsch,
      57:234, 1928.
257. Krugman S., N. Eng. J. Med., 269:195, 1963.
258. Krugman S., et al., J. Am. Med. Ass., 218:1665, 1972.
259. Krugman S., Giles J.P., J. Am. Med. Ass., 212:1019, 1970.
260. Krugman S., Giles J.P., Canad. Med. Ass. J., 106:442, 1972.
261. Krugman S., Giles J.P., Hammond J., J. Am. Med. Ass., 200:
      365, 1967.
262. Krugman S., Giles J.P., Hammond J., J. Am. Med. Ass., 217:
      41, 1971.
263. Krugman S., Giles J.P., Hammond J., J. Am. Med. Ass., 218:
      1655, 1971.
264. Krugman S., Ward R., Giles J.P., et al., N.Eng. J. Med.,
      261:729, 1959.

265. Krugman S., Ward R., Giles J.P., et al., J. Am. Med. Ass.,
      174:823, 1960.
266. Krugman S., Ward R., Giles J.P., Amer. J. Med., 32:717,
      1962.
267. Krugman S., Ward R.W., Giles J.P., in Perspectives in
      Virology III, Ed. Morris Pollard, p. 159, Harper and Row
      Publisher Inc., New York, 1963.
268. Krushak D.H., Lab. Anim. Care., 20:52, 1970.
269. Kubelka V., Sousek O., Srajez E., Trans. Gastroent., 7:230,
      1964.
270. Kukowski Sister Kay, London W.T., Sutnick A.I., et al.,
      Human Biol., 1972, (In Press).
271. Kunin C.M., Am. J. Med. Sci., 237:293, 1959.
272. Kunkel H.G., in Methods of Biochemical Analysis I, Ed. D.
      Glick, Interscience Press, Inc., New York, 1954.
273. Lamanna C., Bacteriol. Rev., 21:30, 1957.
274. Lamanna C., Hollander D.H., Science, 123:889, 1956.
275. Lander J.J., Alter H.J., Purcell R.H., J. Immun., 106:1166,
      1971.
276. Lander J.J., Giles J.P., Purcell R.H., et al., N. Eng. J.
      Med., 285:303, 1971.
277. Lander J.J., Holland P.V., Alter H.J., et al., J. Am. Med.
      Ass., 1972, (In Press).
278. Landsteiner K., in The Specificity of Serological Reactions,
      Revised Ed., Harvard University Press, Cambridge, Mass., 1945.
279. Larson D.L., Blondin J., Seshul M.B., et al., J. La. State
      Med. Soc., 122:69, 1970.
280. Laveran A., Mesnil F., Ann. Inst. Pasteur, 15:673, 1901.
281. Lawrence J.S., Lancet, i:41, 1946.
282. Leach J.M., Ruck B.J., Brit. Med. J., 4:597, 1971.
283. Le Bouvier G.L., J. Infect. Dis., 123:671, 1971.
284. Le Bouvier G.L., Amer. J. Dis. Child., 123:420, 1972.
285. Le Bouvier G.L., Barker L.F., Prince A.M., et al.,
      (Unpublished Data).
286. Le Bouvier G.L., Marmion B.P., Tonkin R.W., et al., (In
      Preparation).
287. Lennette E.H., in Diagnostic Procedures for Viral and
      Rickettsial Diseases, Ed. L.H. Lennette and N.J. Schmidt,
      III Edition, p. 1, American Public Health Association,
      New York, 1964.
288. Leupold F., Z. Hyg. Infektionskrankh, 109:144, 1929.
289. Levaditi C., Ann. Inst. Pasteur, 15:894, 1901.
290. Levene C., Blumberg B.S., Nature, 221:195, 1969.
291. Lichter E.A., Nature, 224:810, 1969.
292. Liebhaber H., Krugman S., Giles J.P., et al., Virology,
      24:107, 1964.
293. Liebhaber H., Krugman S., McGregor D., et al., J. Exp. Med.,
      122:1135, 1965.
294. Liman A., N. Eng. J. Med., 284:109, 1971.

295. Ling C.M., Overby L.R., Austria test system, (Personal
      Communication).
296. London W.T., Proc. Nat. Acad. Sci., 66:235, 1970, (Abstract).
297. London W.T., Alter H.J., Lander J., et al., J. Infect. Dis.,
      1972, (In Press).
298. London W.T., Di Figlia M., Sutnick A.I., et al., N. Eng. J.
      Med., 281:571, 1969.
299. Lorenz D., Barker L., Stevens D., et al., Proc. Soc. Expt.
      Biol. Med., 135:348, 1970.
300. Lous P., Skinhoj P., Olesen H., Vox Sang., 19:379, 1970.
301. Lurman A., Berlin Klin. Wschr., 22:20, 1885.
302. MacCallum F.O., Bradley W.H., Lancet, ii:228, 1944.
303. Madalinski K., Krawczynski K., Sztachelska A., et al., J.
      Infect. Dis., 124:517, 1971.
304. Magnius L.O., Espark A., Acta Path. Microbiol. Scand.
      (Section B)., 1972, (In Press).
305. Malin S.F., Edwards J.R., Nature New Biology, 235:182, 1972.
306. Maynard J.E., Berquist K.R., (Personal Communication).
307. Maynard J.E., Hartwell W.V., Berquist K.R., et al., Bact.
      Proc., p. 175, 1971.
308. Maynard J.E., Hartwell W.V., Berquist K.R., J. Infect. Dis.,
      126:660, 1971.
309. McCollum R.W., Proc. Soc. Exp. Biol. Med., 81:157, 1952.
310. McKenna P.J., et al., Lancet, ii:214, 1971.
311. Melartin L., Blumberg B.S., Nature, 210:1340, 1966.
312. Melnick J.L., Boggs J.D., Canad. Med. Ass. J., 106:461, 1972.
313. Melnick J.L., Boucher D.W., Craske J., et al., J. Infect.
      Dis., 124:76, 1971.
314. Midgley A.R., Endocrinology, 79:10, 1966.
315. Miller W.V., Watson L.E., Holland P.V., et al., Vox Sang.,
      21:1, 1971.
316. Millman I., Huhtanen H., Merino F., et al., Bact. Proc.,
      p. 176, 1971, (Abstract).
317. Millman I., Loeb L.A., Bayer M.E., et al., J. Exp. Med.,
      131:1190, 1970.
318. Millman I., Zavatone V., Gerstley B.J.S., et al., Nature,
      222:181, 1969.
319. Millman I., Ziegenfuss J.F. Jr., Raunio V., et al., Proc.
      Soc. Expt. Biol. Med., 133:1426, 1970.
320. Milne G.R., Barr A., Wallace J., Lancet, i:77, 1971.
321. Mirick G.S., Shank R.E., Trans. Am. Clin. Climatol. Assoc.,
      71:176, 1959.
322. Mirick G.S., Ward R., McCollum R.W., N. Eng. J. Med., 273:
      59, 1965.
323. Mirkovic R.R., Adamova V., Boucher D.W., et al., Proc. Soc.
      Expt. Biol. Med., 138:626, 1971.
324. Mistilis S.P., Blackburn C.R.B., Amer. J. Med., 48:484, 1970.
325. Mollison C.L., in Blood Transfusion in Clinical Medicine,
      Second Ed., Ed. F.A. Davis, Philadelphia, Penn., 1967.

326. Morbidity and Mortality Weekly Report, Center for Disease Control, Atlanta, Georgia, 20:123, 1971.

327. Morgan W.T.J., Watkins W.M., Brit. Med. Bull., 25:30, 1969.

328. Morrison M., Bayse G.S., Webster R.G., Immunochem., 8:289, 1971.

329. Mosley J.W., in Progress in Liver Disease, Ed. H. Popper and F. Schaffner, p. 252, Grune & Stratton, New York, 1970.

330. Mosley J.W., Canad. Med. Ass. J., 106:427, 1972.

331. Mosley J.W., in Viral Hepatitis and Blood Transfusion, Ed. G. N. Vyas et al., Grune & Stratton, New York, 1972.

332. Mosley J.W., Ann. Int. Med., 1972, (In Press).

333. Mosley J.W., Barker L.F., Shulman N.R., et al., Nature, 225:953, 1970.

334. Mosley J.W., Dull H.B., Anesthesiol., 27:409, 1966.

335. Mosley J.W., Edwards V.M., Meihaus J.E., et al., Am. J. Epid., 1972, (In Press).

336. Mosley J.W., Galambos J.T., in Diseases of the Liver, Ed. L. Schiff, 3rd Ed., p. 428, Lippencott, Philadelphia, 1969.

337. Muniz F.J., Malyska H., Levin W.C., N. Eng. J. Med., 284: 501, 1971.

338. Murray R., Bull. N.Y. Acad. Med., 31:341, 1955.

339. Murray R., Oliphant J.W., Tripp J.T., et al., J. Am. Med. Ass., 157:8, 1955.

340. Myrvik Q.N., Leake E.S., Fariss B., J. Immun., 86:128, 1961.

341. Natali P.G., Tan E.M., J. Immun., 108:318, 1972.

342. National Academy of Sciences, Symposium on Laboratory Propagation and Detection of the Agent of Hepatitis, National Academy of Sciences, National Research Council Publication No. 322, Washington, D.C., 1954.

343. National Academy of Science - National Research Council, Panel of the Committee on Plasma and Plasma Substitute, Transfusion, 103:1, 1970.

344. Neefe J.R., Gambescia J.M., Kurtz C.H., et al., Ann. Int. Med., 43:1, 1955.

345. Neefe J.R., Gellis S.S., Stokes J., Amer. J. Med., 1:3, 1946.

346. Neefe J.R., Stokes J. Jr., J. Am. Med. Ass., 128:1063, 1945.

347. Neefe J.R., Stokes J. Jr., Gellis S.S., Am. J. Med. Sci., 210:561, 1945.

348. Neefe J.R., Stokes J. Jr., Reinhold J.G., Am. J. Med. Sci., 210:29, 1945.

349. Nefzger M.D., Chalmers T.C., Amer. J. Med., 35:299, 1963.

350. Nelson D.S., Nelson R.A., Yale J. Biol. Med., 31:185, 1959.

351. Nelson J.M., Barker L.F., Danovitch S.H., Lancet, i:773, 1970.

352. Nelson M., Cooke B., Med. J. Australia, 2:950, 1971.

353. Nelson R.A., Brit. J. Ven. Dis., 28:160, 1952.

354. Nelson R.A., Science, 118:733, 1953.

355. Nelson R.A., Proc. Roy. Soc. Med., 49:55, 1956.

356. Nelson R.A., II Int. Symp. on Immunopath., p. 245, 1962.

357. Nelson R.A., Nelson D.S., Yale J. Biol. Med., 31:201, 1959.

358. Newman S.J., Madden D.L., Gitnick G.L., et al., Amer. J. Dis. Child., 122:129, 1971.
359. Nielsen J.O., Dietrichson O., Elling P., et al., N. Eng. J. Med., 285:1157, 1971.
360. Nishioka K., J. Immun., 90:86, 1963.
361. Nishioka K., Linscott W.D., J. Exp. Med., 118:767, 1963.
362. Nordenfelt E., Kaij K., Ursing B., Vox Sang., 19:371, 1970.
363. Notkins A.L., Mahar S., Scheele C., et al., J. Exp. Med., 124:81, 1966.
364. Nowoslawski A., Brzosko W.J., Madalinski K., et al., Lancet, i:494, 1970.
365. Ohbayashi A., Mayumi M., Okochi K., Lancet, i:244, 1971.
366. Okochi K., Mayumi M., Haguino Y., et al., Vox Sang., 19:332, 1970.
367. Okochi K., Murakami S., Vox Sang., 15:374, 1968.
368. O'Malley J.P., McGee Z.A., Barile M.F., et al., Proc. Nat. Acad. Sci., 56:895, 1966.
369. O'Malley J.P., Meyer H.M. Jr., Smadel J.E., Proc. Soc. Expt. Biol. Med., 108:200, 1961.
370. Oncley J.L., Melin M., Pichart D.A., et al., J. Am. Chem. Soc., 71:541, 1949.
371. Ouchterlony Ö., Progr. Allergy, 5:1, 1958.
372. Parker C.W., Prog. Clin. Path., 1972, (In Press).
373. Parks W.P., Melnick J.L., J. Infect. Dis., 120:539, 1969.
374. Parks W.P., Melnick J.L., Voss W.R., et al., J. Infect. Dis., 120:548, 1969.
375. Paul J.R., Havens W.P. Jr., Sabin A.B., et al., J. Am. Med. Ass., 128:911, 1945.
376. Pennell R.B., in Hepatitis Frontiers, Ed. F.W. Hartman, G. A. LoGrippo, J.G. Matew and J. Barron, p. 297, Little Brown, Boston, 1957.
377. Peters R.L., Ashcavai H., Gastroenterology, 58:284, 1970.
378. Peterson E.A., Sober H.A., J. Am. Chem. Soc., 78:751, 1956.
379. Phillips L.L., Surg. Gyn. Obst., 121:551, 1965.
380. Polesky H.F., Human Path., 2:441, 1971.
381. Porter J.E., Shapiro M., Maltby G.L., et al., J. Am. Med. Ass., 153:17, 1953.
382. Prevention of post-transfusion hepatitis by γ-globulin: preliminary report: a cooperative study, J. Am. Med. Ass., 214:140, 1970.
383. Prince A.M., Amer. J. Trop. Med. Hyg., 19:872, 1970.
384. Prince A.M., Proc. Nat. Acad. Sci., 60:814, 1968.
385. Prince A.M., in Proc. 2nd Conf. Exptl. Med. Surg. in Primates, N.Y., 1969, S. Karger, 1972, (In Press).
386. Prince A.M., Vox Sang., 1972, (In Press).
387. Prince A.M., Brotman B., Cherubin C.E., Amer. J. Dis. Child., 1972, (In Press).
388. Prince A.M., Burke K., Science, 169:593, 1970.
389. Prince A.M., Gershon R.K., Transfusion, 5:120, 1965.

390. Prince A.M., Hargrove R.L., Szmuness W., et al., N. Eng. J. Med., 282:987, 1970.

391. Prince A.M., Ikram H., Brotman B., Abstracts 24th Ann. Meeting Amer. Ass. Blood Banks, Chicago, Sept. 1971.

392. Prince A.M., Szmuness W., Brotman B., et al., in Viral Hepatitis and Blood Transfusion, Ed. G.N. Vyas et al., Grune & Stratton, New York, 1972.

393. Prince A.M., Szmuness W., Hargrove R.L., et al. Virol., 7:241, 1971.

394. Prince A.M., Szmuness W., Woods K.R., et al., N. Eng. J. Med., 285:933, 1971.

395. Propert S.A., Brit. Med. J., 1:677, 1938.

396. Prophylactic gamma globulin for prevention of endemic hepatitis. Effects of U.S. gamma globulin upon the incidence of viral hepatitis and other infectious diseases in U.S. soldiers abroad, A cooperative study, Arch. Int. Med., 128:723, 1971.

397. Purcell R.H., (Personal Communication).

398. Purcell R.H., Gerin.J.L., Holland P.V., et al., J. Infect. Dis., 121:222, 1970.

399. Purcell R.H., Holland P.V., Walsh J.H., et al., J. Infect. Dis., 120:383, 1969.

400. Purcell R.H., Holland P.V., Walsh J.H., et al., J. Infect. Dis., 121:550, 1970.

401. Raffel S., Amer. J. Hyg., 19-20:416, 1934.

402. Raunio V., London W.T., Sutnick A.I., et al., Proc. Soc. Expt. Biol. Med., 134:548, 1970.

403. Redeker A., in Viral Hepatitis and Blood Transfusion, Ed. G.N. Vyas et al., Grune & Stratton, New York, 1972.

404. Redeker A.G., Hopkins C.E., Jackson B., et al., Transfusion, 8:60, 1968.

405. Redeker A.G., Peters R.L., Yamahiro H.S., Presented to the Western Association of Physicians, Carmel, California, January 31, 1968.

406. Remington J.S., Gaines J.D., Gilmer M.A., Lancet, i:413, 1972.

407. Rhodes K., Markham R.L., Maxwell P.M., et al., Brit. Med. J., 2:439, 1969.

408. Rieckenberg H., Z. Immunitatsforsch, 26:53, 1917.

409. Rightsel W.A., Keltsch R.A., Tekushan F.M., et al., Science, 124:226, 1956.

410. Rittner C., Schwinger E., Stockhausen F.G., et al., Vox Sang., 19:280, 1970.

411. Rodbard D., Ruder H.J., Vaitukaitis J., et al., J. Clin. Endocrin. Metab., 33:343, 1971.

412. Ross C.A.C., Pringle R.C., Lancet, ii:434, 1971.

413. Rowe A.W., Eyster E., Kellner A., Cryobiology, 5:119, 1968.

414. Saint E.G., King W.E., Joshe N.A., Austral. Ann. Med., 2:113, 1953.

415. Salaman M.H., Wedderburn N., Bruce-Chwatt L.J., J. Gen. Microbiol., 59:383, 1969.

416. Schaffer F., Editorial, N. Eng. J. Med., 283:1108, 1970.
417. Schmidt N.J., Gee P.S., Lennette E.H., Appl. Microbiol.,
     22:165, 1971.
418. Schmidt N.J., Lennette E.H., J. Immun., 105:604, 1970.
419. Schmidt N.J., Lennette E.H., Health Lab. Sci., 8:238, 1971.
420. Schmidt N.J., Lennette E.H., Amer. J. Clin. Path., (In Press).
421. Schroeder D.D., Mozen M.M., Science, 168:1462, 1970.
422. Schroeder D.D., Mozen M.M., (Unpublished Data).
423. Schweitzer I., Wing A., McPeak C., et al., J. Am. Med. Ass.,
     1972, (In Press).
424. Sela M., Givol D., Mozes E., Biochim. Biophys. Acta., 78:
     649, 1963.
425. Senior J.R., Goeser E., Dahlke M., et al., Gastroenterology,
     60:752, 1971.
426. Serpeau D., Mannoni P., Dhumeaur D., et al., Lancet, ii:1266,
     1971.
427. Shaffer W.E., Vyas G.N., Shahed A., et al., Vox Sang., 22:
     366, 1972.
428. Sherlock J., Fox R.A., Niazi S.P., et al., Lancet, i:1243,
     1970.
429. Shorey J., (Personal Communication).
430. Shulman N.R., Amer. J. Med., 49:669, 1970.
431. Shulman N.R., Ann. Int. Med., 72:257, 1970.
432. Shulman N.R., Barker L.F., Science, 165:304, 1969.
433. Simon J.B., Canad. Med. Ass. J., 105:618, 1971.
434. Simons M.J., Yap E.H., Yu M., et al., Lancet, i:1149, 1971.
435. Singleton J.W., Fitch R.A., Merrill D.A., et al., Lancet, ii:
     785, 1971.
436. Skinhøj P., Thulstrup H., Scand. J. Clin. Lab. Invest., 27:
     61, 1971.
437. Smith C.E., Whiting E.G., Baker E.E., et al., Amer. Rev.
     Tuberc., 57:330, 1948.
438. Smithwick E.M., Go S.C., Lancet, ii:1080, 1970.
439. Solaas M.H., Scand. J. Haemat., 7:506, 1970.
440. Soulier J.P., Thromb. Diath. Haemorrh. Supplement, XLV:449,
     1971.
441. Soulier J.P., Blatrix Ch., Courouce A.M., et al., Amer. J.
     Dis. Child, 1972, (In Press).
442. Soulier J. P., Courouce-Pauty A.M., Benamon-Djiane D., Rev.
     Fr. Transfus., 12:361, 1969.
443. Soulier J.P., Courouce-Pauty A.M., Benamon-Djiane D., Vox
     Sang., 19:345, 1970.
444. Spector S., J. Pharmacol. Exp. Ther., 178:253, 1971.
445. Stokes J.Jr., Blanchard M., Neefe J.R., J. Am. Med. Ass.,
     138:336, 1948.
446. Stokes J. Jr., Farquhar J.A., Drake M.E., et al., J. Am.
     Med. Ass., 147:714, 1951.
447. Stokes J. Jr., Neefe J.R., J. Am. Med. Ass., 127:144, 1945.
448. Sukeno N., Shirachi R., Yamaguchi J., et al., J. Virol.,
     9:182, 1972.

449. Sutnick A.I., Levine P.H., London W.T., et al., Lancet, i:1200, 1971.
450. Sutnick A.I., London W.T., Blumberg B.S., et al., J. Nat. Can. Inst., 44:1241, 1970.
451. Sutnick A.I., London W.T., Gerstley B.J.S., et al., J. Am. Med. Ass., 205:670, 1968.
452. Sutnick A.I., London W.T., Millman I., et al., Med. Clin. N.A., 54:805, 1970.
453. Sutnick A.I., Millman I., London W.T., et al., Ann. Rev. Med., 1972, (In Press).
454. Szmuness W., Pick R., Prince A.M., Am. J. Epid., 92:51, 1970.
455. Szmuness W., Prince A.M., Am. J. Epid., 94:585, 1971.
456. Szmuness W., Prince A.M., Lancet, ii:433, 1971.
457. Szmuness W., Prince A.M., Cherubin Ch. E., Brit. Med. J., 2:198, 1971.
458. Szmuness W., Prince A.M., Zirnis M., et al., (In Press).
459. Taswell H.F., (Unpublished Data).
460. Taswell H.F., Shorter R., Maxwell N.G., Mayo Clin. Proc., 47:98, 1972.
461. Taswell H.F., Shorter R., Poncelet T.K., et al., J. Am. Med. Ass., 214:142, 1970.
462. Thiry L., Clinet G., Cremer M., et al., Lancet, ii:547, 1971.
463. Tong M., Shih-Chien S., Schaeffer B., et al., Ann. Int. Med., 75:687, 1971.
464. Torii A., Nakano S., Miyazato Y., in Proc. 10th Congr. Int. Soc. Blood Transf., Stockholm 1964, S. Karger, p. 1055, 1965.
465. Triger D.R., Alp M.H., Wright R., Lancet, i:60, 1972.
466. Turner G.C., Brit. J. Hosp. Med., 5:296, 1971.
467. Turner G.C., Field A.M., Lasheen R.M., et al., Arch. Dis. Child., 46:616, 1971.
468. van Kooten Kok-Doorschodt H.J., van den Akker R., Gispen R., J. Infect. Dis., 1972, (In Press).
469. Velasco M., Sorenson R., Daiber A., et al., Lancet, i:1183, 1971.
470. Vischer T.L., Brit. Med. J., 2:695, 1970.
471. Voegt H., Munchen. med. Wschr., 89:76, 1942.
472. Vogel C.L., Anthony P.P., Mody M., et al., Lancet, ii:621, 1970.
473. Vorndam V., 1972, (Unpublished Observations).
474. Vyas G.N., (Personal Communication).
475. Vyas G.N., in Viral Hepatitis and Blood Transfusion, Ed. G.N. Vyas et al., Grune & Stratton, New York, 1972.
476. Vyas G.N., Fudenberg H.H., Pretty H.M., et al., J. Immun., 100:274, 1968.
477. Vyas G.N., Shulman N.R., Science, 170:332, 1970.
478. Vyas G.N., Williams E.W., Klaus G.G.B., et al., J. Immun., 108:1114, 1972.
479. Waldorf D.S., Sheagren J.N., Trautman J.A., Lancet, ii:773, 1966.
480. Wallace J.M., Wormall A., Parasitology, 23:346, 1931.

481. Wallis C., Melnick J.L., Appl. Microbiol., 21:867, 1971.
482. Walsh J.H., Purcell R.H., Morrow A.G., et al., J. Am. Med. Ass., 211:261, 1970.
483. Walsh J.H., Yalow R., Berson S.A., J. Infect. Dis., 121:550, 1970.
484. Ward R., Krugman S., Giles J.P., et al., N. Eng. J. Med., 258:407, 1958.
485. Ward R., Krugman S., Giles J.P., Postgrad. Med., 28:12, 1960.
486. Washburn T.C., Medearis D.N. Jr., Childs B., Pediatrics, 35: 57, 1965.
487. Wedderburn N., Lancet, ii:1114, 1970.
488. Wenzel R.P., Le Bouvier G.L., Beam W.E., J. Am. Med. Ass., 220:707, 1972.
489. Williams H., J. Am. Med. Ass., 80:532, 1923.
490. Winslow C.-E.A., Tech. Quart., 14:110, 1901.
491. Wright R., Vox Sang., 19:320, 1970.
492. Wroblewski F., LaDue J.S., Proc. Soc. Expt. Biol. Med., 91:571, 1956.
493. Ziegenfuss J.R. Jr., Miller J., Rossman D., N. Eng. J. Med., 284:1104, 1971.
494. Zieve L., Hill E., Nesbitt S., et al., Gastroenterology, 25:495, 1953.
495. Zuckerman A.J., Nature, 223:569, 1969.
496. Zuckerman A.J., Vox Sang., 19:304, 1970.
497. Zuckerman A.J., Brit. Med. J., 1:49, 1972.
498. Zuckerman A.J., Baines P.M., Almeida J.D., Nature New Biol., 1972, (In Press).
499. Zuckerman A.J., Taylor P.E., Amer. J. Dis. Child., 1972, (In Press).
500. Zuckerman A.J., Taylor P.E., Almeida J.D., Brit. Med. J., 1:262, 1970.
501. Zuckerman A.J., Taylor P.E., Bird R.G., Clin. Exp. Immun., 7:439, 1970.
502. Zuckerman A.J., Taylor P.E., Bird R.G., et al., J. Clin. Path., 24:2, 1971.

SUPPLEMENTARY BIBLIOGRAPHY

a. Casey, H.L., Pub. Health Monograph No. 74, 1965.
b. Deinhardt, F., Canad. Med. Assoc. J., 106:479, 1972.
c. Deinhardt, F., Holmes, A.W., and Wolfe, L.G., J. Infect. Dis., 121:353, 1970.
d. Deinhardt, F., Wolfe, L., Junge, U. and Holmes, A.W., Canad. Med. Assoc. J., 106:468, 1972.
e. Kent, J.F. and Fife, E.H., Amer. J. Trop. Med. and Hyg., 12:103, 1963.
f. Kohler, H., Apodaca, J. and Lang, W., personal communication, 1970.
g. Krugman, S. and Giles, J.P., Tr. Assoc. Amer. Phys., 83:133, 1970.
h. Liu, C., Voth, D.W. and Cho, C.T., personal communication, 1972.
i. Melnick, J.L., Parks, W.P., J. Infect. Dis., 121:353, 1970.
j. Sever, J.L., J. Immunol., 88:320, 1962.
k. Wright, R., McCollum, R.W., Klatskin, G., Lancet 2:117, 1969.
l. Maynard, J. E., Berquist, K. R., Hartwell, W.V. and Krushak, D.H., Canad. Med. Assoc. J., 106: 475, 1972

AUTHOR INDEX

Aach, R. D., 155
Adelberg, S., 251
Alter, H. J., 61
Aronoff, A., 235
Baines, P. M., 387
Barker, L. F., 197
Berquist, K. R., 393
Bill, J., 353
Black, H., 353
Blumberg, B. S., 63,235
Bond, H. E., 221
Boyer, J. L., 43
Brotman, B., 147,299,335
Cabasso, V. J., 289
Caggiano, V., 323
Chalmers, T. C., 277
Chen, E., 181
Coleman, C. R., 257
Conrad, M. E., 367
Coyne, V., 235
Deinhardt, F., 383
Dodd, R. Y., 175
Ehrich, C., 335
Finlaysen, N. C. D. C., 335
Gault, H., 235
Gerin, J. L., 205
Giles, J. P., 9
Gocke, D. J., 115, 319
Goldfield, M., 353
Gordon, I., 111
Grady, G. F., 309
Greenwalt, T. J., 175
Hacker, E. J., Jr., 155
Hall, W. T., 227
Hirsch, R. L., 299
Holland, P. V., 275,331
Hollinger, F. B., 167
Huang, S. N., 235
Ibrahim, A. B., 251
Ikram, H., 147,335

Jamieson, G. A., 175
Katz, R., 325
Knepp, C. S., 257
Krugman, S., 9,269,349,365
Krushak, D. H., 393
Lange, R. F., 257
Le Bouvier, G., 97
Lederberg, J., 89
Lennette, E. H., 125
Levin, J. J., 175
Lippin, A., 335
Marston, R. Q., 3
Mason, M. A., 137
Maynard, J. E., 393
Melnick, J. L., 373,391
Millman, I., 235
Mosley, J. W., 23
Mozen, M. M., 289
Ni, L., 175
Ockner, R. K., 53
O'Connell, A., 235
Panick, J. M., 319
Parker, C. W., 155
Perkins, H. A., 181,407
Perkins, S. L., 181
Petrakis, N., 85
Pizzuti, W., 353
Polesky, H. F., 121,363
Prince, A. M., 147,299,335,403
Purcell, R. H., 311
Redeker, A. G., 55
Roberto, R. R., 37
Rodriguez, J., 325
Schmidt, N. J., 125
Schroeder, D. D., 289
Shulman, N. R., 133,257
Srihongse, S., 353
Stryker, M., 335
Szmuness, W., 299,335
Taswell, H. F., 271